Royal College of Radiologists' Clinical Oncology symposia previously published:

Thyroid Cancer
Edited by William Duncan

Prostate Cancer
Edited by William Duncan

Colorectal Cancer
Edited by William Duncan

Paediatric Oncology
Edited by William Duncan

Lung Cancer
Edited by William Duncan

Ovarian Cancer
Edited by Norman M. Bleehen

Tumours of the Brain

Edited by

Norman M. Bleehen

With 90 Figures and 32 Tables

Springer-Verlag
Berlin Heidelberg New York Tokyo

Professor Norman M. Bleehen
University Department of Clinical Oncology and Radiotherapeutics,
Addenbrooke's Hospital, Hill's Road, Cambridge CB2 2QQ, UK.

ISBN 978-1-4471-3439-8 ISBN 978-1-4471-3437-4 (eBook)
DOI 10.1007/978-1-4471-3437-4

Library of Congress Cataloging-in-Publication Data. Main entry under title: Tumours of the brain. Edited papers from a symposium held in London in Feb. 1985, sponsored by the Royal College of Radiologists. Includes bibliographies and index. 1. Brain-Tumors-Congresses. I. Bleehen, Norman M., 1930– . II. Royal College of Radiologists (Great Britain) III. Tltle: Tumors of the brain. [DNLM: 1. Brain Neoplasms-congresses. WL 358 T9247 1985] RC280.B7T854 1986 616.99'281 85-17375 ISBN 978-1-4471-3439-8

Softcover reprint of the hardcover 1st edition 1986

Typeset by Wenden Typesetting Services Limited, Saffron Walden, Essex

2128/3916-543210

Preface

The seventh annual multidisciplinary symposium on clinical oncology organised by the Royal College of Radiologists discussed the subject of malignant brain tumours. It was held in London in February 1985 and this volume collects together the edited texts of the papers which were presented at the meeting.

Primary tumours of the central nervous system account for about 9% of all malignant diseases but as much as 20% of all paediatric neoplasms. The prognosis ranges from excellent for some of the less aggressive tumours, through good for children's tumours such as medulloblastoma, to appalling for the high-grade adult astrocytomas. Improvements in pathological diagnosis and surgical and radiotherapeutic techniques have led to considerable sequential improvements in outcome over those obtained in the past. In contrast the response to chemotherapy over the whole range of tumours remains disappointing, and clearly awaits new drugs and methods of delivery.

The relative rarity of individual types of tumours, apart from the commoner high-grade adult astrocytomas, has made progress in terms of clinical trials difficult to organise. In spite of this much investigative work is in progress. The symposium, and the present volume, were designed to provide a comprehensive overview of the subject by experts, with an emphasis on the possible routes to future progress. The topics included aspects of pathology, imaging, diagnosis and treatment of both the common and uncommon primary tumours. It is hoped the papers will stimulate further interest and activity in this difficult area of clinical therapy and investigation.

I wish to express my thanks to all the speakers for making the symposium a success and for agreeing to provide manuscripts for publication. Mr Michael Jackson of Springer-Verlag has continued to give advice and support in the production of this volume. I should also like to thank my secretaries Miss Lesley Sargeant and Mrs Fiona Brown for help with the organisation of the meeting and editing of the manuscripts. Finally my thanks are due to Mr A.J. Cowles, General Secretary of the Royal College of Radiologists, and to his staff who contributed to the organisation and management of the symposium.

Royal College of Radiologists, Norman M. Bleehen
38 Portland Place, London W1N 3DG

April 1985

Contents

List of Senior Authors

R.O. Barnard
Department of Neuropathology, National Hospital for Nervous Diseases, Maida Vale, London W9 1TL, UK

R.P. Beaney
MRC Cyclotron Unit, Hammersmith Hospital, Du Cane Road, London W12 0HS, UK

H.J.G. Bloom
Department of Radiotherapy and Oncology, Royal Marsden Hospital, Fulham Road, London SW3 6JJ, UK

G.M. Bydder
Department of Diagnostic Radiology, Royal Postgraduate Medical School, Hammersmith Hospital, Du Cane Road, London W12 0HS, UK

H.B. Coakham
Department of Neurosurgery, Frenchay Hospital, Bristol BS16 1LE, UK

J.R.W. Gleave
Department of Neurological Surgery and Neurology, Addenbrooke's Hospital, Hills Road, Cambridge CB2 2QQ, UK

J.L. Hildebrand
Department of Neurology, Université Libre de Bruxelles, Hôpital Erasme, Route de Lennik 808, B-1070 Brussels, Belgium

A.E. Jones
Department of Radiotherapy, St Bartholomew's Hospital, London EC1A 7BE, UK

I.F. Moseley
Lysholm Department of Radiology, National Hospital for Nervous Diseases, Queen Square, London WC1N 3BG, UK

G.E. Sheline
Department of Radiation Oncology, University of California, San Francisco, San Francisco, California 94143, USA

D.G.T. Thomas
Gough Cooper Department of Neurological Surgery, Institute of Neurology, National Hospitals for Nervous Diseases, Queen Square, London WC1N 3BG, UK

R.O. Weller
University Department of Neuropathology, Southampton General Hospital Tremona Road, Southampton SO9 4XY, UK

P. Workman
MRC Clinical Oncology and Radiotherapeutics Unit, Hills Road, Cambridge CB2 2QH, UK

1 The Pathology of Brain Tumours

R. O. Barnard

Introduction

The pathological diagnosis of brain tumour may be reached in several ways. Cytological examination of the cerebrospinal fluid (CSF) may provide very useful information in many cases, especially where current methods such as cytocentrifugation are employed in experienced hands. Good results are often obtained with those tumours, such as metastatic carcinoma, that tend to shed cells into the CSF, but are much less constant in neuroectodermal tumours with the exception of medulloblastoma cerebelli.

In most cases the diagnosis is reached by examination of material removed at operation, either by craniotomy, burr hole biopsy or more recently, by multiple biopsy guided by computerised tomography. Often, material is used for rapid preparations (smears and frozen sections) which can give helpful information during the course of the operation. The diagnostic accuracy of the immediate smear method is high in experienced hands. (Adams et al. (1981) claim 93%) but there are various pitfalls awaiting the inexperienced and unwary. The existence of these problems means that it is essential that material also be examined in the usual way by paraffin wax embedding and sectioning. The smear technique, however, can yield results of outstanding cytological detail (Fig. 1.1).

The clinical requirement of the examination of biopsied tissue is to establish the nature of the lesion, estimate its potential for malignant behaviour and thereby indicate possible therapy. There is also a need to give some guidance towards prognosis. The behaviour of different types of brain tumour is reasonably well established, but disparity between the clinical behaviour and pathological findings is not uncommon.

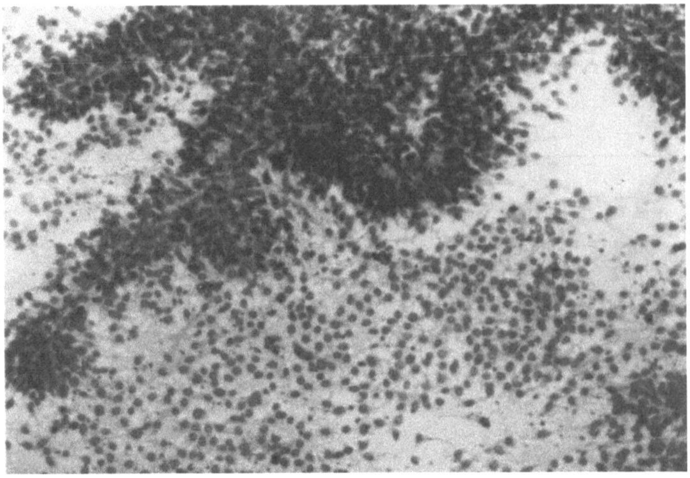

Fig. 1.1. Rapid smear preparation; ependymoma cells clustered around blood vessels and spreading to form a regular film. H & E, × 100.

Classification

Twentieth-century schemes of classification are mainly based upon the pioneer work of Bailey and Cushing (1926) who related the appearance of glioma cells to the cells found in the course of normal development. Subsequent further classifications haved aimed towards simplification. They have laid increasing stress on the importance of anaplasia and other factors influencing the prognosis that may be assessed microscopically. In the 1940s a series of papers from Kernohan and his colleagues at the Mayo Clinic proposed the use of a numerical grading scheme from 1 to 4 to indicate the degree of cellular anaplasia in a glioma. They found that a good correlation could be made with 5-year survival in the case of the astrocytomas, though it was less impressive with oligodendrogliomas (Earnest et al. 1950). The recent classification sponsored by the World Health Organisation (Zülch 1979) is an attempt to present a scheme of nomenclature that can be widely accepted. Even so, proposals to modifiy parts of this scheme are already being discussed.

The description of the pathological features of different tumours that follows is, of necessity, concise and cannot be, in any sense, comprehensive. The reader is referred for more detailed information to standard texts (Rubinstein 1972, Burger and Vogel 1976, Russell and Rubinstein 1977).

Astrocytomas

Glial tumours whose cells resemble astrocytes are common. They form a rather heterogeneous group which includes some slow-growing, highly differentiated tumours as well as the commoner, rapidly progressive and destructive, malignant examples. Subdivision of astrocytomas follows their microscopical pattern and cellular detail. In protoplasmic astrocytoma few fibrils are demonstrable (Fig. 1.2). Fibrillary astrocytoma contains numerous fibrils, which may be thick or fine. Gemistocytic astrocytoma is composed of swollen astrocytes with plentiful eosinophilic cytoplasm and an eccentric nucleus; fibrils can be demonstrated at the periphery of the cell (Fig. 1.3). 'Benign' examples of these gliomas (grade 1) exist but are uncommon; signs of anaplasia may be found, and the gemistocytic type is especially prone to develop malignant features and pursue a rapid course. Pilocytic

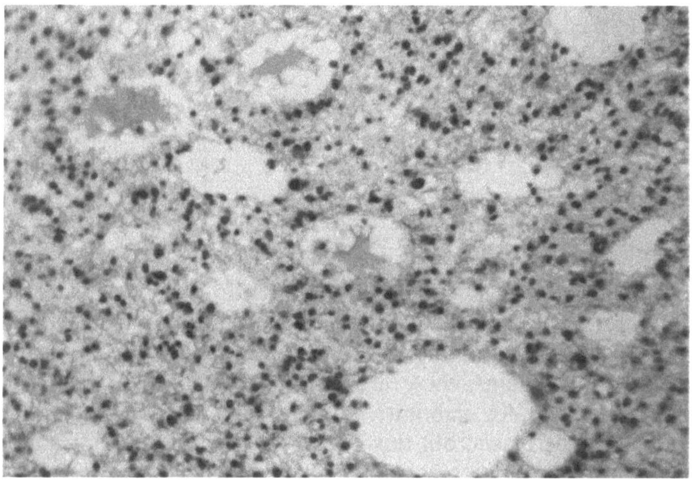

Fig. 1.2. Protoplasmic astrocytoma with microcysts. H&E, ×160.

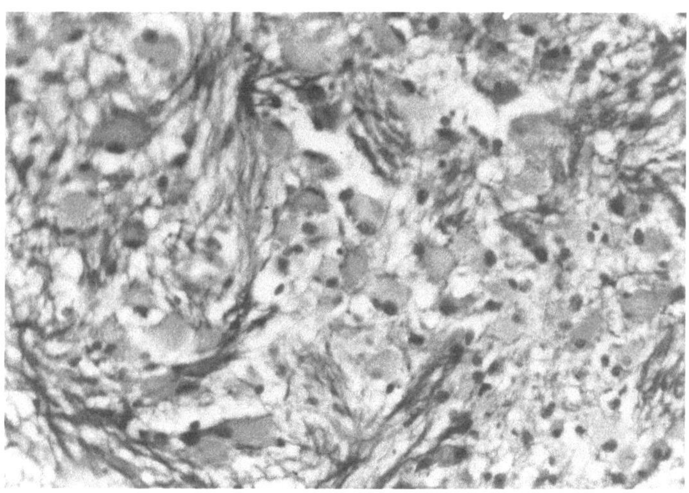

Fig. 1.3. Gemistocytic astrocytoma with plentiful fibrils. PTAH, ×279.

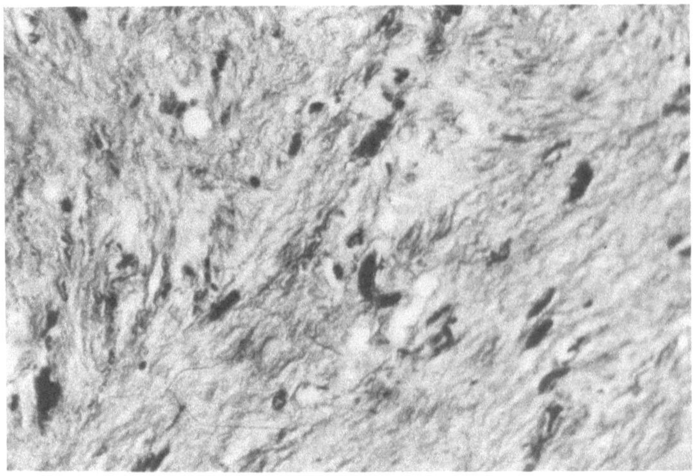

Fig. 1.4. Pilocytic astrocytoma showing very fine hair like processes and solid, dark-staining Rosenthal fibres. PTAH, ×212

astrocytoma is a special type with delicate hair-like processes arising from elongated or fusiform cells; the majority of cerebellar, optic nerve and infundibular gliomas are of this type. Cysts of all sizes are common. Rosenthal fibres (Fig. 1.4) and granular bodies are sometimes found; these are brightly eosinophilic masses of material derived from astrocytes. An elaborate vascular pattern may be present, sometimes with endothelial hyperplasia, but this carries no prognostic implication: the majority of pilocytic astrocytomas are grade 1. The subependymal giant cell astrocytoma, arising in the ventricular wall or floor, is associated with tuberous

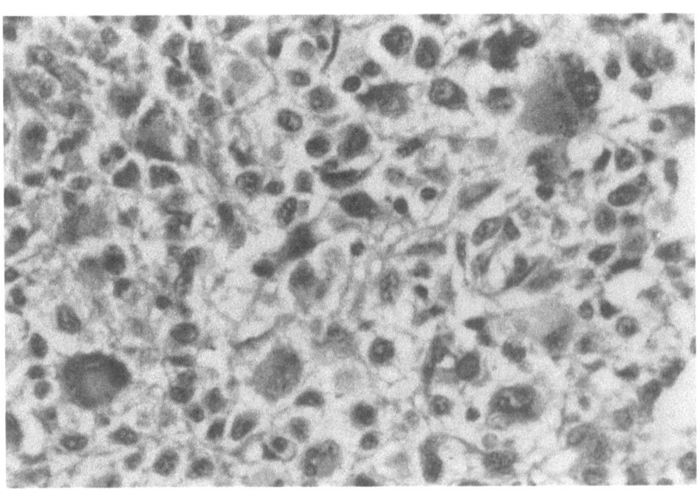

Fig. 1.5. Glioblastoma including giant cells with multiple nuclei. H&E, ×290.

sclerosis. The large size of the component astrocytic cells may suggest malignancy, but in fact this is a benign tumour.

Malignant astrocytoma (anaplastic astrocytoma) is a common hemispheric tumour, and corresponds to grade 3. The features that distinguish it are high cellularity and pleomorphism, mitotic figures, vascular overgrowth with endothelial hyperplasia, and necrosis of tissue. These features are also characteristic of the highest grade of glioma, often called glioblastoma (grade 4), and the lines of distinction between these two are not well defined. In general, the malignant astrocytoma should contain a fair proportion of cells of clearly astrocytic type, as well as anaplastic forms. Necrosis of tissue should not be an overwhelming feature. Prognosis is not good, but in some series it is evidently slightly more favourable than for the grade 4 tumour. It is of interest that perivascular lymphocytic cuffing is commoner in astrocytomas grade 2 and 3 than in grade 4 and is most common in the gemistocytic type.

Glioblastoma

Despite attempts in some quarters to avoid its use, the term glioblastoma is still in current use for tumours of the highest malignancy rating where only a small proportion of cells are differentiated and where vascular changes and necrosis of tissue are widespread. The cellular components vary within wide limits. Some "giant-cell" glioblastomas contain very large cells with single or multiple nuclei (Fig. 1.5), and their atypical appearance has, in the past, led to their interpretation as ganglioneuromas or monstrocellular sarcomas. Many examples justify the traditional term multiforme by their pleomorphism; yet other glioblastomas are almost uniformly small-celled. Angiogenesis is clearly apparent. Thus endothelial proliferation resulting in glomeruloid tangles and solid masses of mesenchymal cells is a common feature. Angioma-like blood channels sometimes occluded by thrombus are also seen. Examination of nearby white matter often reveals extension of the prolific capillaries beyond the edges of the tumour. The atypical vascular proliferation may itself be neoplastic with the formation of a combined glioblastoma-sarcoma. In this case a mottled pattern can be seen with islands of remaining glioma alternating with tracts of vascular connective tissue. Necrosis may be massive, with only small fragments of viable tumour remaining, or may be in the form of elongated serpiginous zones bordered by small fibrillated cells in a pseudo-palisade arrangement. Mitotic figures are sometimes of granular type (Swaen et al. 1964), and more typical mitotic figures are often seen in the vascular endothelium.

The natural history of malignant gliomas is one of progressive expansion, often with destruction of brain tissue. Some gliomas of low histological malignancy, such as the pontine astrocytoma of childhood, can infiltrate extensively without destruction of tissue, producing great enlargement of the affected structure.

In the case of the pons or medulla this results in an impossible situation to treat effectively. More malignant gliomas may spread along pre-existing white matter pathways, including the corpus callosum and internal capsule. Then on reaching the ependyma they will tend to breach the surface producing nodules of growth projecting into the cavity, whence cells may easily be swept away by the CSF to implant and resume growth in other areas. Another important mode of spread is via

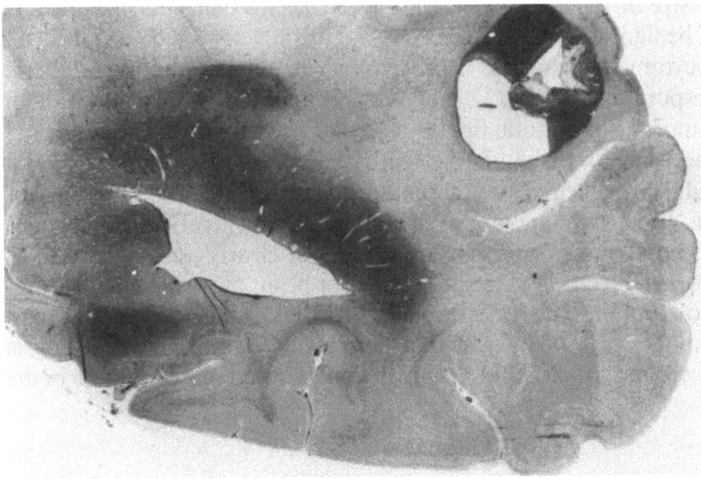

Fig. 1.6. An apparently circumscribed cystic glioblastoma in the posterior parietal white matter which could be seen with the naked eye. Microscopical examination also revealed diffuse neoplastic infiltration around the margins of the horn of the ventricle. Nissl, × 1.6.

the leptomeninges. Penetration here may stimulate a desmoplastic reaction and a florid overgrowth of connective tissue merges with the glioma. This effect is, perhaps, most familiar in medulloblastoma. Subsequent attachment to the dura may occur, with the production of a hard mass whose appearance mimics that of meningioma. Some glioblastomas, however, appear to be well-circumscribed solitary tumours confined to one part of the brain: microscopical study is necessary to demonstrate the extent of the infiltration that is found in such cases (Fig. 1.6).

Oligodendroglioma

Oligodendrogliomas are less common than tumours of the astrocytic type, and probably account for only 8% or less of intracranial gliomas. The typical oligodendroglioma is a slow-growing hemispheric tumour, calcified at its periphery, and with correspondingly long-standing clinical symptoms. The familiar microscopical picture is of cells whose rounded nuclei appear to float in clear cytoplasm within a honeycomb-like network of well-defined cell membranes, with narrow capillaries branching at right angles to subdivide the tissue into compartments (Fig. 1.7). Many oligodendrogliomas, however, have a much more complex cell composition and cells of astrocytic type, especially perivascular astroblasts, may be included, together with cells that appear to be less differentiated but of oligodendrocytic type. Anaplastic cellular features together with necrosis and excessive vascular overgrowth may be found focally, or may be so predominant that a diagnosis of glioblastoma is made.

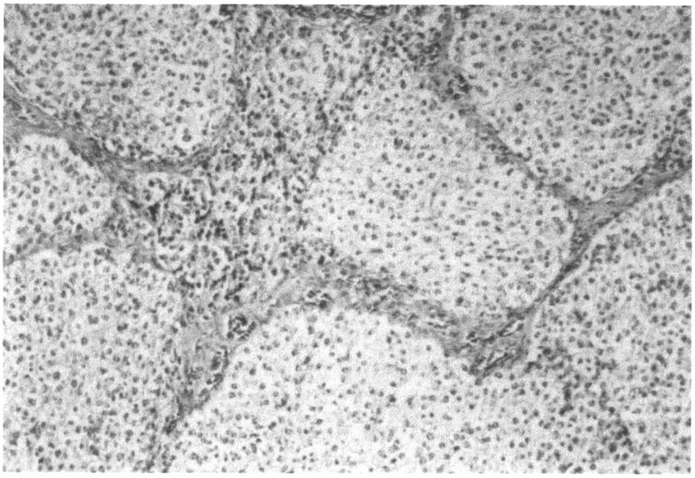

Fig. 1.7. Well-differentiated oligodendroglioma of typical appearance. The tissue is subdivided by fibrovascular trabeculae and the nuclei appear to float in clear cytoplasm. HVG, × 100.

It is always difficult to give an accurate prognosis in any oligodendroglioma. A well-differentiated example usually merits consideration as grade 2. The presence of mitotic figures or of hyperplastic capillary vessels does not seem to carry an unfavourable prognostic significance. Tumours in which poorly differentiated cells or astrocytic cells are numerous, in which the typical architectural pattern is destroyed and in which necrosis of tissue is conspicuous are usually referred to grade 3. Some unusual architectural patterns such as rhythmic palisade-like arrangement (Fig. 1.8; also illustrated by Rubinstein 1972) or a perivascular grouping of cells may be found, without any special significance as regards prognosis.

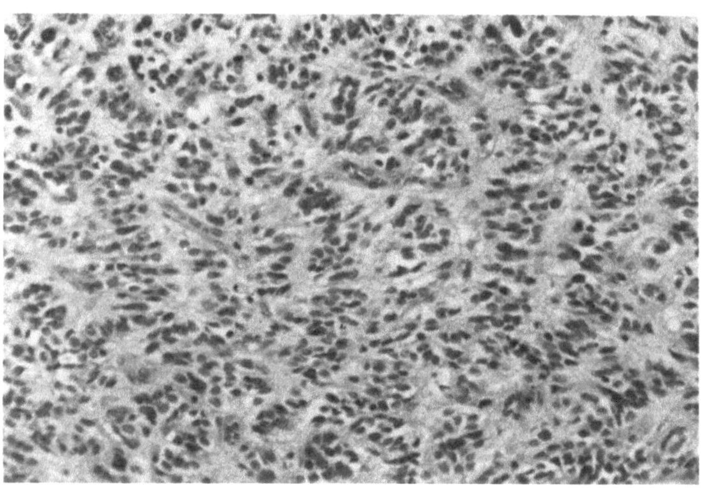

Fig. 1.8. Rhythmic pattern of cells with nuclei arranged in rows in an oligodendroglioma. H & E, × 160.

Highly malignant behaviour may be found, though not commonly, in oligodendrogliomas even of highly differentiated type. Extensive spread via the CSF may result in implantation all over the neuraxis. Histopathological malignancy and 5-year survival do not always correlate, and this is especially true of oligodendroglioma.

Ependymoma

Tumours whose cells resemble ependyma are found associated with all the cerebral ventricles, especially the fourth, and form the commonest type of intramedullary tumour in the spinal cord. It is rare to find microscopical signs of malignancy, apart from in the rare ependymoblastoma (Rubinstein 1970) which is a highly malignant tumour of infancy. Ependymomas tend to form well-demarcated, often papillary masses which grow slowly and fill available space without destruction of tissues. It is characteristic for the fourth ventricle to be filled, producing obstruction to the flow of CSF, and for a tongue of tumour to extend beside the medulla to the cisterna magna.

The microscopical appearances are usually typical. Unlike those in other neuroepithelial tumours the cells often have a clearly epithelial appearance, and taken together with their tendency to form tubules, the appearances may be mistaken for those of metastatic carcinoma. The cells tend to have very regular oval nuclei with delicately stippled chromatin, and to be arranged in a papillary or tubular structure (Fig. 1.9). Alternatively they may be clustered around blood vessels, or form rosettes in which the cells taper towards a central lumen. In smear preparations the perivascular clusters of cells often bear some resemblance to a tree with branches and leaves. Ependymoma cells may or may not be associated with glial fibrils, and

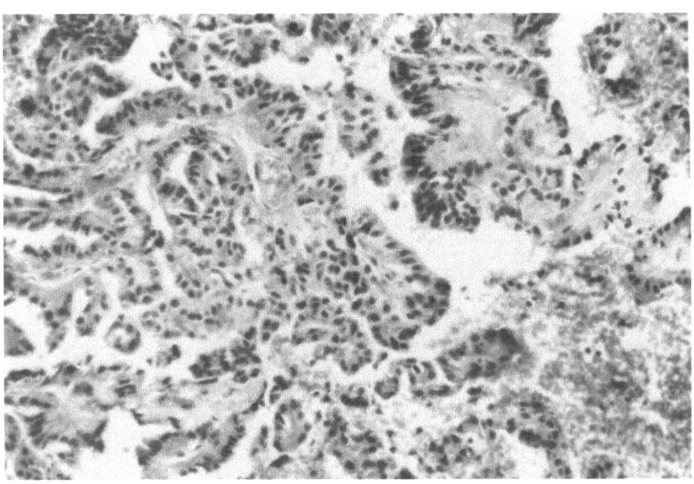

Fig. 1.9. Ependymoma showing tubulopapillary pattern. The distinction from choroid plexus papilloma may be difficult. H&E, × 160.

appropriate staining may demonstrate variation between one part of a tumour and another. Blepharoplasts, which are tiny rod-shaped bodies, may be found clustered near the nucleus. These structures correspond to the basal bodies at the ends of the cilia (Brightman and Palay 1963), and are a positive identification for ependymal cells.

Certain variants of ependymoma merit attention.The myxopapillary ependymoma is a subtype in which there is extensive mucoid material in the stroma: it seems to be restricted to the cauda equina region. The subependymoma is a variant in which groups of cells of ependymal type are found in a matrix very rich in glial fibrils. Such tumours may be asymptomatic and be found only at post-mortem examination, where they present as small hard nodules projecting into the ventricular cavity. Even those examples removed surgically appear very benign. While many ependymomas can be regarded clinically and pathologically as benign, in the sense of being slow-growing and well differentiated, there is no doubt that over the years they can spread and disseminate in the nervous system. They may even be responsible for extraneural metastases.

Choroid Plexus Papilloma

Papillary tumours of the choroid plexuses of the fourth ventricle and lateral ventricles are uncommon in adults, the majority being found in the first decade of life. They form papillary masses of cells resembling normal choroid mounted on a simple vascular stalk. Large specimens present a cauliflower-like appearance and usually cause considerable hydrocephalus. Carcinoma of the choroid (Lewis 1967) is rare; there is then evident anaplastic change, loss of papillary structure and invasion of brain.

Colloid Cyst

The colloid cyst is a developmental curiosity, but a potentially dangerous one. This is because of its location: commonly a pedunculated mass in the third ventricle. Sudden, acute blockage of the foramen of Monro may result from its ball-valve action. The pathological features are of a single layer of cuboidal epithelium covering a homogeneous core.

Medulloblastoma

The medulloblastoma is in several ways quite distinct from the other tumours of neuroepithelial origin. It is believed to arise only at one site, that is in the cerebellum. In contrast to the other tumours there is strong evidence from experimental studies using organ culture systems (Herman and Rubinstein 1984) to suggest that the cell of origin is capable of both neuronal and glial differentiation as proposed originally by Bailey and Cushing (1926).

The peak incidence is in the first two decades of life, and the most common situation is in the vermis. However medulloblastomas may also occur in adult life and in these cases the growth is sometimes laterally placed. Indeed, they may then appear to be extracerebellar by reason of strong meningeal attachments.

Typically, the picture is of high cellularity, with the cells being darkly stained and the oval, round or pointed nucleus dominant with little cytoplasm visible. Often there is no defined pattern and the tumour cells are simply arranged in solid sheets. There may be perivascular pseudo-rosettes, or a tendency for the cells to be arranged in parallel rows. The true rosettes, regarded as a hallmark of neuroblastic differentiation, are not always present: they consist of small groups of cells arranged in a roughly circular manner with processes tapering toward the centre.

Following invasion of the leptomeninges a vigorous overgrowth of connective tissue can be excited and a pattern of trabeculae of tumour cells separated by strands of reticulin may result. On occasion this "desmoplastic" type of appearance has been misinterpreted as sarcoma. In common with other highly cellular malignant tumours the medulloblastoma is characteristically invasive. Thus multiple foci of growth within the cerebellum are often seen, the fourth ventricle is commonly occupied, and the growth readily disseminates over the neuraxis, reaching the spinal cord (Fig. 1.10) as easily as the frontal or temporal region (Fig. 1.11). Extraneural metastases have been recorded.

Neuroblastic or glioblastic differentiation has been observed but is generally unusual. The presence of melanin or of muscle tissue (medullomyoblastoma as recently reviewed by Smith and Davidson 1984) is very rare. Any medulloblastoma must be given grade 4 malignancy.

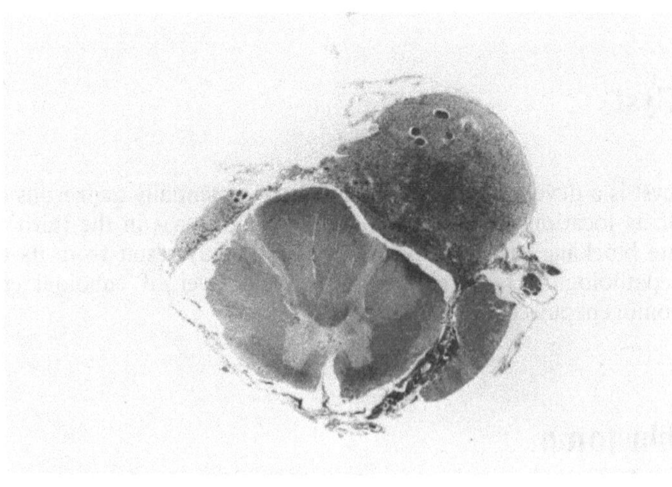

Fig. 1.10. Transverse section of thoracic spinal cord with a huge meningeal nodule resulting from spread of a medulloblastoma. PTAH, ×4.5.

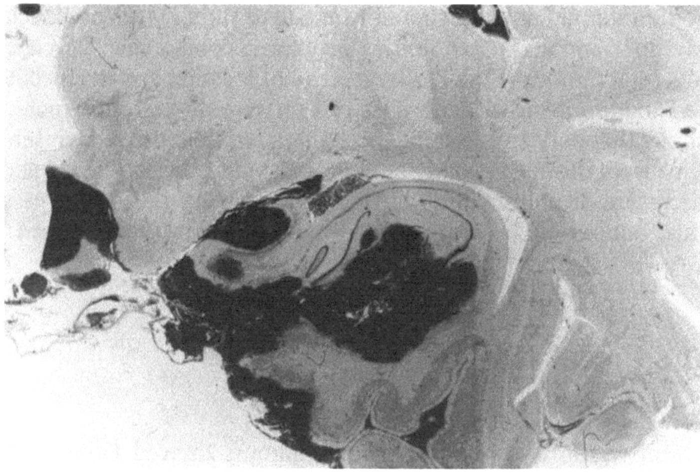

Fig. 1.11. Medulloblastoma infiltrating temporal lobe from the meninges. Nissl, ×0.18.

Neuroblastoma

Primary cerebral neuroblastoma (Horten and Rubinstein 1976) has similarities with the cerebellar medulloblastoma: it occurs most often as a large mass discovered in the first decade of life but is very much less common. The cell composition is usually that of a largely undifferentiated neoplasm but typical rosettes or axonal structures may be found.

Ganglioglioma

The ganglioglioma and ganglioneuroma group are, in essence, extremely uncommon lesions in which ganglion cells form an element of the neoplastic process. To make this diagnosis it is essential to exclude the possibility that the ganglion cells concerned are not merely normal neurons engulfed within an extending glioma. Because of the varied nature of these lesions no overall prognosis can be given, as this depends on the maturity of the different components. Neuroblastic foci in such a tumour would clearly be a sign of ill-omen, but the majority of cases seem to be slow-growing and of maldevelopmental origin.

Primitive Neuroectodermal Tumour

The inherent difficulty of interpreting the appearances of an undifferentiated neuroepithelial tumour, especially if only limited amounts of material are available, has led to the suggestion that an attempt should be made to simplify the nomenclature. All the poorly differentiated, or primitive neoplasms would then be called primitive neuroectodermal tumour (PNET), irrespective of location and irrespective of any line of differentiation being evident. This category would therefore include not only those examples that defy any attempt at classification, but also recognisable medulloblastomas, neuroblastomas, ependymoblastomas and others. This topic is currently under discussion (Rubinstein 1985). It seems unlikely that the present concepts of individual tumour entities in the childhood group will be abandoned.

Tumours of the Pineal Region

Tumours of the pineal region can be divided into tumours derived from pineal parenchymal cells and the group of midline germinomas and teratomas that often are found in the pineal location. The latter are the commoner.

The true pineal tumours should be classified with other neuroepithelial tumours and their features do not overlap at all with those of the germinoma-teratoma group. The pineoblastoma, similar to the cerebellar medulloblastoma in cellular appearance, is also similar in its malignant behaviour and frequency of cerebrospinal metastasis. The pineocytoma shows a greater degree of differentiation which may be towards astrocytes or ganglion cells (Herrick and Rubinstein 1979). The distinction has some practical importance since the only benign tumours in this group are those with ganglionic differentiation.

Germinoma may be found at the pineal site, or in the suprasellar region, or both. There may be extensive involvement of the ventricular system and spinal meninges (Dayan et al. 1966). These malignant tumours have characteristic microscopical

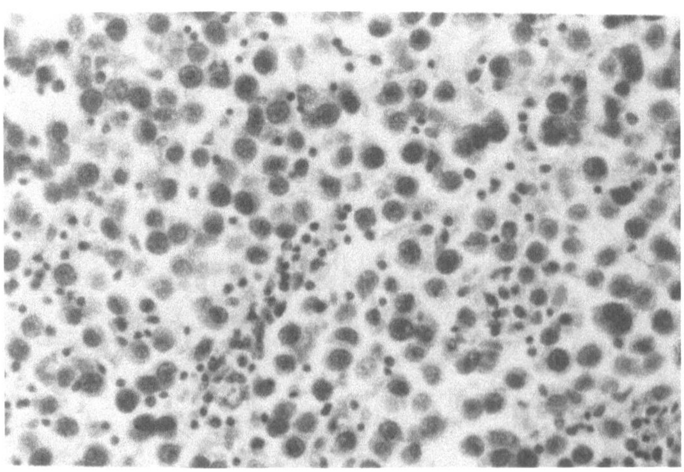

Fig. 1.12. Germinoma composed of large spheroidal cells with prominent nucleoli. Groups of perivascular lymphocytes are also found. H & E, × 250.

appearances. They have large spheroidal cells with large nuclei containing prominent nucleoli, and mitotic figures are a consistent feature (Fig. 1.12). Tracts of small lymphocytes often extend between groups of these cells, but there are no intermediate forms between one cell type and the other. In a proportion of cases other tissue elements are present and indicate clearly the teratomatous nature of the lesion. More typical teratomas, embryonal carcinoma and chorion carcinoma are also found at the pineal site.

Lymphoma

Primary cerebral lymphomas usually show distinctive pathological features and can be separated from instances of systemic lymphoma and leukaemia with secondary neural involvement because in the latter group meningeal and nerve root infiltration are common and intraparenchymal spread rare. One notable association of cerebral lymphoma that has come to assume some importance is with conditions of inherited or acquired immune deficiency. Thus, patients given immunosuppressive therapy for organ transplantation were quickly seen to carry a specially high risk (Hoover and Fraumeni 1973). It is interesting to speculate whether or not the spread of AIDS will generate a disproportionate number of cases.

A variety of synonyms has been used for this type of tumour. One of the most popular has been microglioma (Russell et al. 1948), indicating that the cells are derived from the cerebral histiocyte or microglial cell. While these tumours are accompanied by a remarkable microglial (and astrocytic) proliferation it is now clear from immunocytochemical studies that many cases are truly B cell lymphomas (Henry et al. 1974). But other types of lymphoma such as Burkitt's type may also rarely be found (Kobayashi et al. 1984). The microscopical features in routine sections are quite characteristic and have long been recognised. The infiltration is usually multifocal and more extensive than could be anticipated from the naked-eye appearances, and the subependymal regions and leptomeninges are frequently involved (Fig. 1.13). The perivascular spaces are distended with cells, and their reticulin fragmented with a lamellar appearance (Fig. 1.14). Large cells of immunoblastic type are often present, together with cells closer to plasma cells in appearance, typical microglia and mature lymphocytes (Fig. 1.15). Mitotic figures are often present and the tissues between the affected perivascular spaces may be necrotic. The pattern of infiltration frequently resembles a "malignant" meningoencephalitis. Only a detailed post-mortem study can accurately demonstrate the extent of the lesions.

Meningeal Tumours

The histological classification of meningiomas is complicated by the variety of appearances they can assume and, fortunately, only a few varieties carry an unfavourable prognosis. The majority remain circumscribed, even encapsulated,

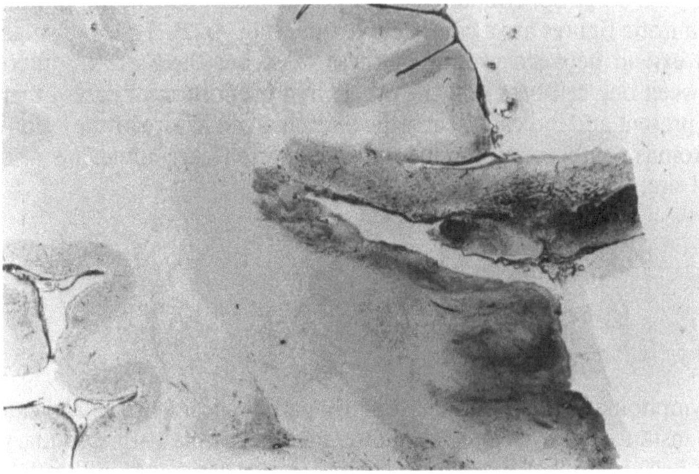

Fig. 1.13. Infiltration of perivascular spaces in corpus callosum and subependymal region and leptomeninges in cerebral lymphoma. Nissl, × 1.8.

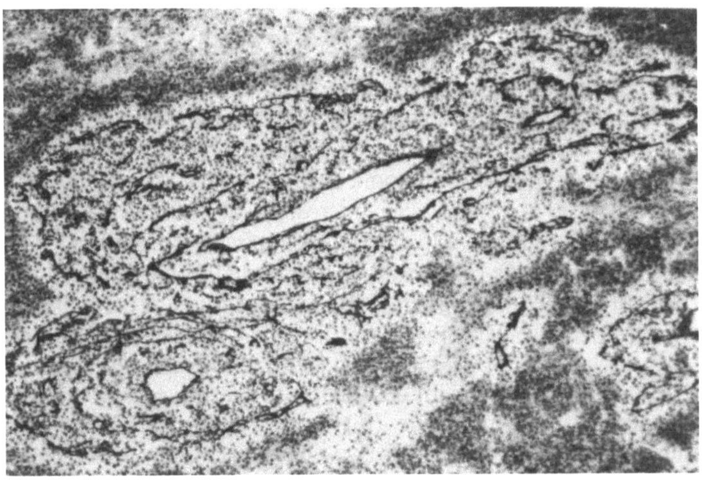

Fig. 1.14. Fragmentation of reticulin in distended perivascular spaces in a cerebral lymphoma. Gordon & Sweet, × 100.

and grow by expansion and not by infiltration. The WHO group histological typing (Zülch 1979) used the terms meningotheliomatous (syncytial) (Fig. 1.16), fibrous (fibroblastic), transitional (mixed), psammomatous, angiomatous, haemangioblastic, haemangiopericytic, papillary and anaplastic (malignant). Only tumours in the last three categories can be expected to behave in an unusually aggressive manner. The haemangiopericytic meningioma resembles the haemangiopericytoma found in other parts of the body. It is highly cellular, with numerous mitotic figures,

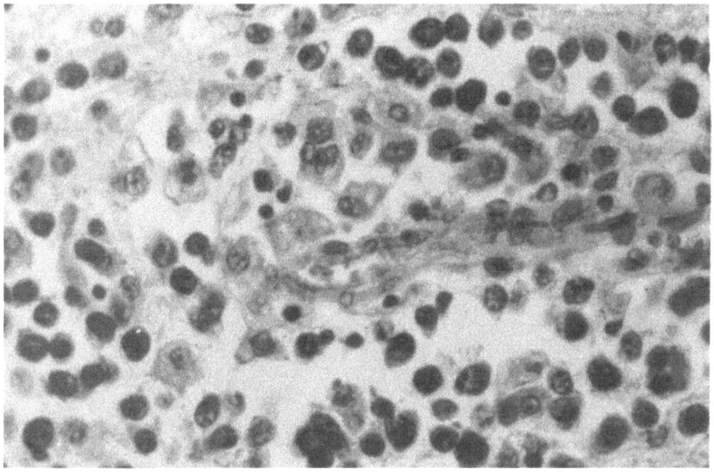

Fig. 1.15. Cerebral lymphoma: variety of cells present in perivascular infiltration. H&E, ×530.

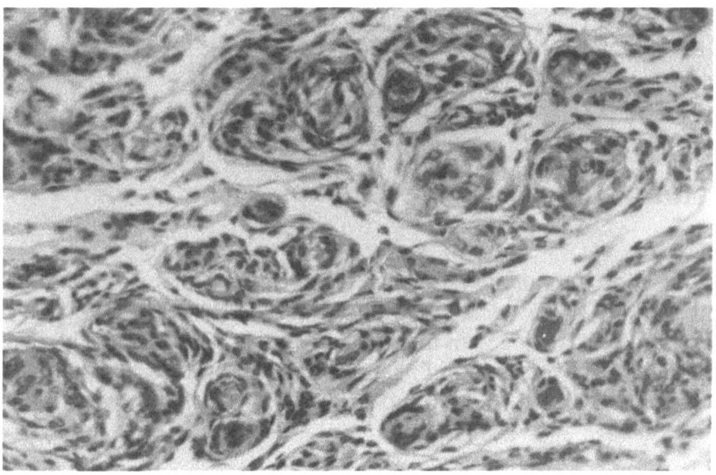

Fig. 1.16. Syncytial meningioma with whorling. H&E, ×200.

and the cells are disposed in relation to slit-like capillaries (Fig. 1.17). Growth, and recurrence, follow a rapid sequence. This variety has been given a grading of 2.

The rare papillary meningioma shows a papillary pattern of growth. It is often associated with malignancy and was graded 2–3 by the WHO group. Anaplastic meningiomas display frankly malignant characteristics, but can be separated from the sarcomas. Within the group of highly malignant meningeal tumours are the primary fibrosarcoma, the polymorphic cell sarcoma and the primary undifferentiated sarcoma of childhood. Primary meningeal melanoma must also be included.

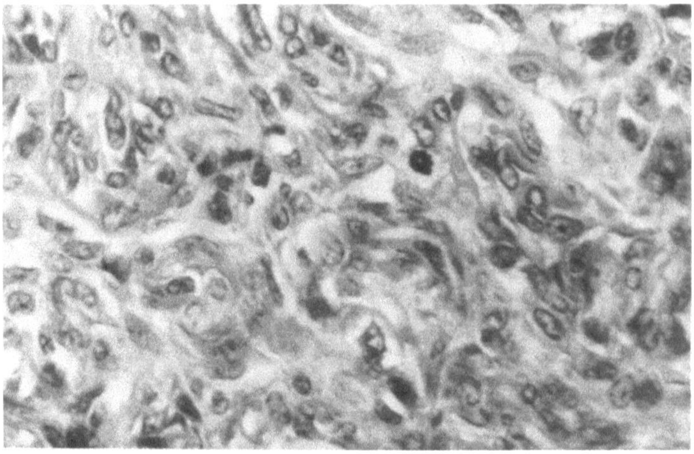

Fig. 1.17. Haemangiopericytic meningioma showing slit-like spaces; among the cells mitotic figures are noted. H&E, ×450.

Nerve Root Tumours

The commonest nerve root tumour is the benign Schwannoma or neurilemmoma more often present on the VIIIth nerve than any other. Its structure is that of a proliferation of Schwann cells arranged in interlacing bundles with nuclei tending to be aligned in parallel. Unlike the situation in neurofibroma (of von Recklinghausen's disease) axons are not involved within the tumour, though they may be adherent at one edge.

Blood Vessel Tumours

Excluding the angiomata, which are considered here as malformations, the only common blood vessel tumour is the capillary haemangioblastoma found in the cerebellum and, less commonly, in the pia covering the brain stem and cord. These growths may be solid or cystic, and are composed of many capillaries with intervening stromal cells, and often a densely gliotic capsule. They have a familial incidence and may be accompanied by lesions in other organs including the retina in von Hippel-Lindau's disease.

Involvement with Other Local Tumours

The brain may be involved by compression from a pituitary adenoma, from a craniopharyngioma or chordoma. More rarely, other bony tumours may infiltrate the brain.

Metastatic Tumours

Probably over 20% of brain tumours are metastatic (Fig. 1.18), the commonest primary source being the respiratory tract. In carcinomatous meningitis extensive infiltration only one or two cells thick may be found and provide a diagnostic problem. This may be resolved by examination of the CSF for malignant cells. One case arising from an unsuspected thyroid primary has been illustrated (Barnard et al. 1976, pp. 142–4). Solitary metastasis is unusual, but in such cases—particularly in renal cell carcinoma and chorion-carcinoma—treatment may be worthwhile.

The author wishes to thank Mr Trevor Scott for the photomicrographs and Mrs C. ard for secretarial help.

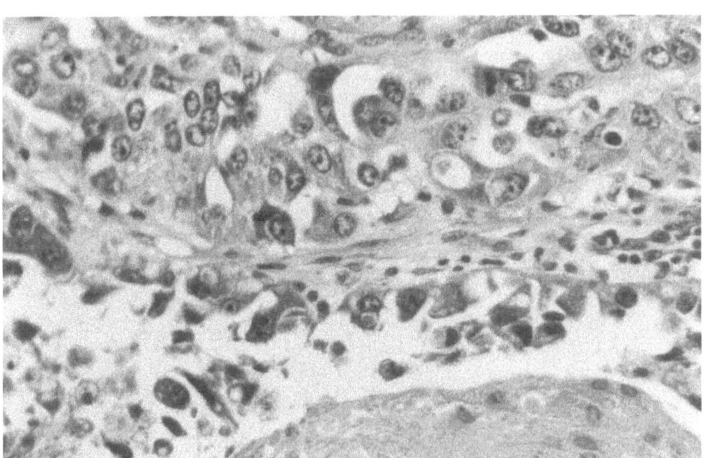

Fig. 1.18. Metastatic carcinoma of poorly differentiated type infiltrating neural tissue. H&E, ×290.

References

Adams JH, Graham DI, Doyle D (1981) Brain biopsy: the smear technique for neurosurgical biopsies. Chapman and Hall, London

Bailey P, Cushing H. (1926) A classification of tumors of glioma group. Lippincott, Philadelphia

Barnard RO, Logue V, Reaves PS (1976) An atlas of tumours involving the central nervous system. Balliere Tindall, London

Brightman MW, Palay SL (1963) The fine stucture of ependyma in the brain of the rat. J Cell Biol 19: 415–439

Burger PC, Vogel FS (1976) Surgical pathology of the nervous system and its coverings. Wiley, New York

Dayan AD, Marshall AHE, Miller AA, Pick FJ, Rankin NE (1966) Atypical teratomas of the pineal and hypothalamus. J Pathol Bact 92: 1–28

Earnest F III, Kernohan JW, Craig WMcK (1950) Oligodendrogliomas (review of 200 cases). Arch Neurol Psychiatr 63: 964–976

Henry JM, Heffner RR Jr, Dillard SH, Earle KM, Davis RL (1974) Primary malignant lymphomas of the central nervous system. Cancer 34: 1293–1302

Herman MM, Rubinstein LJ (1984) Divergent glial and neuronal differentiation in a cerebellar medulloblastoma in an organ culture system: In vitro occurrence of synaptic ribbons. Acta Neuropathol 65: 10–24

Herrick M Kaarsoo, Rubinstein LJ (1979) The cytological differentiating potential of pineal parenchymal neoplasms (true pinealomas): A clinicopathological study of 28 tumours. Brain 102: 289–320

Hoover R, Fraumeni JF Jr (1973) Risk of cancer in renal transplant recipients. Lancet II: 55–57

Horten BC, Rubinstein LJ (1976) Primary cerebral neuroblastoma. A clinicopathological study of 35 cases. Brain 99: 735–756

Kobayashi H, Sano T, Ii K, Hizawa K (1984) Primary Burkitt-type lymphoma of the central nervous system. Acta Neuropathol 64: 12–14

Lewis P (1967) Carcinoma of the choroid plexus. Brain 90: 177–186

Rubinstein LJ (1970) The definition of the ependymoblastoma. Arch Pathol 90: 35–45

Rubinstein LJ (1972) Tumours of the central nervous system. Atlas of tumor pathology, second series, fascicle 6. Armed Forces Institute of Pathology, Washington, DC

Rubinstein LJ (1985) Embryonal central neuroepithelial tumors and their differentiating potential. J Neurosurg 62: 795–805

Russell DS, Rubinstein LJ (1977) Pathology of tumours of the nervous system, 4th edn. Edward Arnold, London

Russell DS, Marshall AHE, Smith FB (1948) Microgliomatosis (a form of reticulosis affecting the brain). Brain 71: 1–15

Smith TW, Davidson RI (1984) Medullomyoblastoma: A histological, immunohistochemical and ultrastructure study. Cancer 54: 323–332

Swaen GJV, Vossenar T, Wyers HJG (1964) Abnormal mitosis in gliomas. J Pathol Bact 87: 75–78

Zülch KJ (1979) Histological typing of tumours of the central nervous system. World Health Organisation, Geneva

2 The Immunopathology of Brain Tumours

Roy O. Weller

Introduction

Immunological techniques and concepts have been applied to the pathology of brain tumours in two major areas: the localisation of specific proteins, marker antigens, by immunocytochemical techniques; and the evaluation of immunological responses to the presence of a brain tumour. Immunocytochemistry, in particular, has been of great value in the study of the biology of brain tumours, in their histological diagnosis, and in the assessment of prognosis.

Marker Antigens in Normal and Tumour Brain Tissue

During the last 100 years a number of tinctorial stains have been developed to study the histology of the normal brain and the tumours arising from the central nervous system. Electron microscopy has also contributed to our understanding of the morphological aspects of tumour cells and their relationships to normal tissue elements. With the introduction of the peroxidase–antiperoxidase (PAP) technique in the 1970s (Sternberger 1979) it became possible to identify proteins either within cells or on the surface of cells with the specificity only attainable by immunological techniques. Monoclonal or polyclonal antibodies are now widely used in biology and in pathology for the immunocytochemical identification of cell and tissue proteins.

Antibodies to a variety of proteins in the brain are now available and can be used to increase the accuracy of diagnosis of brain tumours. Furthermore, the greater

Table 2.1. Marker antigens most commonly used for the immunocytochemical study of intracranial tumours

Marker antigen	Normal cell type
Intermediate filaments	
Glial fibrillary acidic protein (GFAP)	Astrocytes: some ependymal cells
Neurofilament proteins	Neurons and axons
Vimentin	Fetal brain, and other tissues
Cell proteins and enzymes	
Neuron-specific ($\gamma\gamma$) enolase (NSE)	Neurons
S-100 protein	Glia and Schwann cells
Carbonic anhydrase C	Choroid plexus; oligodendrocytes
Myelin basic protein	Myelin; oligodendrocytes in infants
Factor-VIII-related antigen	Endothelial cells
Hormones	
Pituitary hormones	Anterior pituitary
Cell surface antigens	
Monoclonal antibodies	Various brain cell types; lymphocyte subsets; macrophages etc.

understanding obtained through immunocytochemical studies of the activities of brain tumour cells may allow better evaluation of prognosis and treatment. Some of the proteins which can be identified in the normal brain and in brain tumours are listed in Table 2.1. Such marker proteins are not necessarily specific for one cell type but, by the judicious use of controls, they have proved to be very useful for the analysis of histological and cytological features of brain tumours.

Intermediate filaments, 9–11 nm in diameter, provide some of the most useful marker proteins in different tissues of the body. In the brain, glial fibrillary acidic protein (GFAP) is composed of protein subunits with a molecular weight of 47 000 (Eng 1980) and is extensively used as a marker for fibrillary astrocytes; it is also present in some ependymal cells. Neurofilaments are the 9 nm intermediate filaments in neurons and axons. They are composed of protein triplets with subunits of molecular weight 68 000, 145 000 and 200 000 (Schlaepfer et al. 1981), but not all three proteins are present in all neurons or in all parts of the neuron (Bonnin and Rubinstein 1984). Vimentin is the first intermediate filament to appear in the brain in embryological development; in the mouse it is present in fetal and adult astrocytes but not in oligodendrocytes or neurons (Schnitzer et al. 1981).

A number of cytoplasmic proteins and enzymes are very useful marker antigens for cells in the nervous system. Neuron-specific ($\gamma\gamma$) enolase (NSE) is an enzyme in the glycolytic pathway; this isoenzyme is virtually confined to neurons and cells of the peripheral neuroendocrine system (Schmechel et al. 1978). S-100 protein is a cytoplasmic protein of unknown origin with a molecular weight of 21 000 (Eng 1980, Bonnin and Rubinstein 1984); it is present in glial cells but is most useful for the identification of Schwann cells and other cells of neural crest origin. Carbonic anhydrase C has proved to be particularly useful for the identification of normal adult oligodendrocytes and cells of the choroid plexus epithelium (Weller et al. 1985). Myelin basic protein is also present in oligodendroglial cell bodies and processes but only in infants; in adults this protein is confined to myelin (Bonnin and Rubinstein 1984). Factor-VIII-related antigen is confined to endothelial cells in the brain (Weller et al. 1981) and is a useful blood vessel marker for normal and neoplastic tissue.

Antibodies raised against enzymes in the synthetic pathways of neurotransmitters, and antibodies to neuropeptides, have been used extensively in the elucidation of neurological pathways within the brain, but, as yet, these antibodies have not been applied extensively to the study of brain tumours. On the other hand, the immunocytochemical localisation of pituitary hormones has been used widely, not only for the study of the normal pituitary but also for the clarification of hormonal secretion by pituitary adenomas (Martinez et al. 1980).

There is extensive overlap in the use of polyclonal and monoclonal antibodies. For example, either type of antibody may be raised to GFAP or neurofilament proteins. Antibodies to cell surface proteins, however, are usually raised as monoclonal antibodies. Both types of antibody are of great value in the identification of different cell types in the brain and, as will be seen later, they play a role in tumour diagnosis.

The Use of Marker Antigens in the Diagnosis and Assessment of Prognosis of Brain Tumours

Immunocytochemical techniques are used in tumour pathology:

a) to identify a tumour
b) to characterise its cell of origin
c) to establish its degree of differentiation
d) as another parameter by which to judge how the tumour will behave and respond to treatment.

If firm differences between tumour cells and normal cells can be established, more selective therapy for the elimination of brain tumours may be possible.

As a general principle, the histological appearance of brain tumours tends to correlate with their biological behaviour. Anaplasia is associated with rapid growth and invasiveness of the tumour, and with consequent poor prognosis for the patient. From many immunocytochemical studies of brain tumours it appears that the marker antigens present in the normal cell type from which the tumour arose may be retained within the tumour cells or lost from them. In some cases, marker antigens not present in the normal cells of origin may appear within tumour cells.

Astrocytic Tumours

Astrocytic tumours comprise some 40% of primary intracranial neoplasms in adults and approximately 45% in children. Most of the astrocytomas in young people are well differentiated whereas the majority of cerebral astrocytic tumours in older adults are anaplastic. Immunocytochemical staining for the astrocyte marker GFAP is very valuable for the firm identification of astrocytic tumours. In well-differentiated astrocytomas the processes of most of the cells, particularly in the fibrillary astrocytomas, are positive for this marker, whereas in poorly differentiated anaplastic astrocytomas and in glioblastoma multiforme only a proportion of the cells may express GFAP and many may be completely negative. Fig. 2.1 shows an area of an anaplastic astrocytoma composed of cells with pleomorphic nuclei and only a small proportion of the tumour cells expressing GFAP in the cytoplasm. There are several advantages in the use of immunostaining for GFAP in the study of astrocytic tumours. The cell type can be identified by the presence of GFAP in the cytoplasm and the shape of the cell defined. This technique can also be applied to frozen, cryostat sections and to tissue smears when the diagnosis is not immediately apparent using routine methods. The immunoperoxidase technique can be completed within 30–40 minutes of tumour biopsy, allowing an accurate intra-operative diagnosis to be made. Poorly differentiated astrocytoma cells usually exhibit fewer GFAP-containing processes than the reactive astrocytes surrounding or admixed with the tumour. Although this is not always a firm rule, it may allow the distinction to be made between reactive and tumour astrocytes in small biopsies taken near the edge of the tumour.

Anaplastic astrocytomas arise in association with well-differentiated astrocytic tumours and tend to infiltrate the brain in a rather diffuse pattern. Glioblastoma multiforme, on the other hand, has a great diversity of histological pattern which may sometimes resemble an astrocytic tumour and sometimes an oligodendroglioma: the two patterns not infrequently coexist in the same tumour. The margin of invasion at the edge of a glioblastoma is usually relatively narrow although the anaplastic tumour cells still insinuate themselves between the elements of normal brain. Fig. 2.2 shows the infiltrating edge of a glioblastoma; the small tumour cells are not stained for the astrocytic marker, GFAP, but the astrocytes

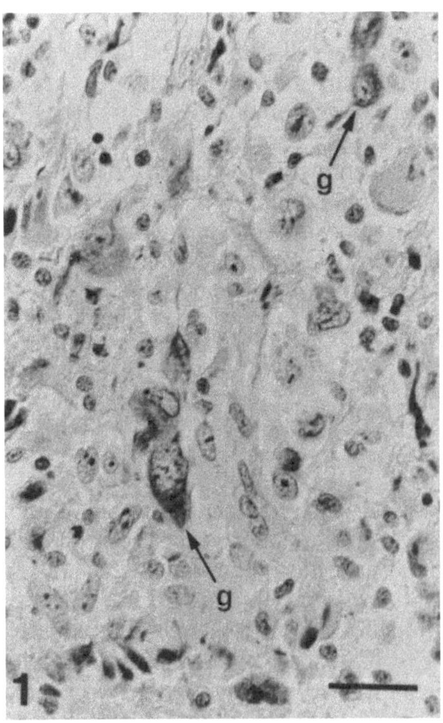

Fig. 2.1. Anaplastic astrocytoma with staining for GFAP (g) in the cytoplasm of only a few cells. Immunoperoxidase technique. Bar represents 30 μm.

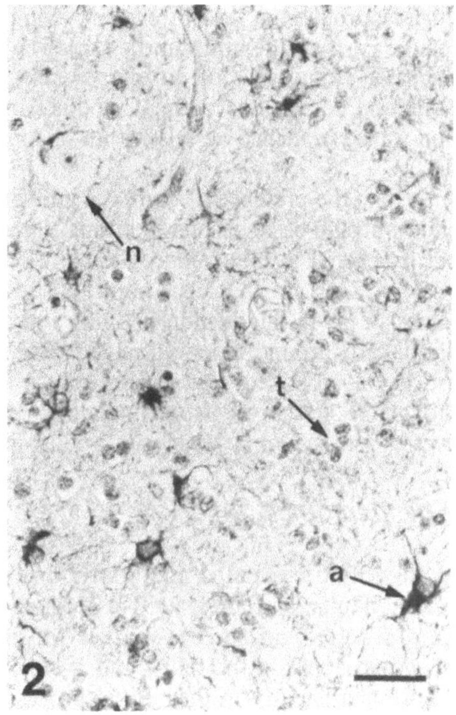

Fig. 2.2. Glioblastoma multiforme tumour cells (t) infiltrating cortex are unstained. A neuron (n) can also be seen. Reactive astrocytes (a) are well stained. Immunoperoxidase technique for GFAP. Bar represents 30 μm.

reacting to the presence of the tumour are stained. A surviving neuron is also present in this field of tumour invasion. Immunocytochemistry has been used to identify various non-glial tissue elements which are present within well-differentiated and anaplastic astrocytic tumours. A small proportion of anaplastic astrocytomas contain a spindle cell element which is not glial in origin.They form a group of well-circumscribed tumours: the gliosarcomas. The astrocytic component of these tumours may be small but the identification of tumour cells containing GFAP is a valuable indicator of diagnosis of gliosarcoma.

Blood vessel proliferation with capillary endothelial proliferation is a prominent feature in many glioblastomas and anaplastic astrocytomas. Immunocytochemistry for factor-VIII-related antigen allows the endothelial cells of the blood vessels to be identified within the tumour. Such staining reveals how the tufts of capillary endothelial cells proliferate around the central core of non-endothelial cells to form glomeruloid structures (Weller et al. 1981).

Oligodendrogliomas

Oligodendrogliomas are much less common than astrocytic tumours and often contain a mixture of astrocytic elements. They occur mainly in the cerebral hemispheres of adults but can be present as small tumours in children. Well differentiated oligodendrogliomas are often very compact and do not necessarily spread into remote parts of the brain in the same way as do astrocytomas. In adults, however, the small round cells of an oligodendroglioma may extend diffusely through the brain and accumulate as small nodules on the surface of the cerebral cortex. The thin-walled branched vessels within oligodendrogliomas are often a useful diagnostic aid.

Despite the presence of carbonic anhydrase C in normal adult oligodendrocytes, and of myelin basic protein in infant oligodendrocytes, neither of these markers has been reported in oligodendrogliomas (Bonnin and Rubinstein 1984, Weller et al. 1985). GFAP, on the other hand, is present in the cytoplasm of a proportion of tumour cells in oligodendrogliomas and is also seen in reactive astrocytes located particularly around blood vessels in these tumours. GFAP is present too in tumour astrocytes in mixed oligoastrocytomas. Thus, although oligodendrogliomas are thought to be derived from oligodendrocytes (Zülch 1979), the tumour cells may express astrocytic markers but have lost markers for normal oligodendrocytes.

Ependymomas

Both well-differentiated and poorly differentiated ependymomas occur in children and in adults, and are usually associated with the ventricular system or the spinal cord. There is no specific marker for ependymal cells in routine use, but many ependymal cells in the fetus, and a minority of such cells in the adult, do contain GFAP particularly in their basal processes. A high proportion of ependymomas, even poorly differentiated tumours, also contain GFAP particularly in the delicate processes that form the characteristic halos or pseudo-rosettes around blood vessels. The pattern of GFAP staining, rather than its specificity, is useful for the diagnosis of ependymomas. In subependymomas there is a profusion of glial fibrils forming a matted network of GFAP-positive material surrounding small islands of cuboidal tumour cells. These tumours usually present as firm nodules growing slowly into the ventricles of older patients, but they do occasionally become anaplastic.

Neuronal Tumours

Neuronal tumours in the cerebral hemispheres often have a sufficiently distinctive histological pattern to establish the diagnosis of gangliocytoma or ganglioglioma. Many of the more mature cells contain NSE, but this enzyme is not specific for neuronal tumours; it is present in many other types of tumour cells and even within reactive astrocytes in damaged brain (Vinores et al. 1984). Staining for GFAP in these tumours is often valuable as the astrocytes within the tumour are outlined and their processes may be seen weaving between the GFAP-negative tumour cells. The differentiation between neuronal tumours and astrocytic tumours may have implications for the planning of treatment.

Medulloblastomas

Medulloblastomas are one of the commonest tumours of childhood, and together with astrocytomas of the cerebellum and pons form a substantial proportion of primary intracranial tumours in younger patients. Recently, medulloblastomas have been grouped with primary tumours of similar morphology in the cerebral hemispheres and with neuroblastomas elsewhere in the body under the general heading of primitive neuroectodermal tumours (PNET) (Rorke 1983). Immunocytochemistry has shown that a variety of marker proteins may be present within different PNET or within the same PNET. Such markers include GFAP, neurofilament protein and NSE; myoglobin is present in the striated muscle cells of some PNET (medullomyoblastoma) (Weller 1984). Fig. 2.3 shows a PNET (medulloblastoma) stained for GFAP. A proportion of the tumour cells express this marker antigen and can be distinguished by their nuclear morphology and by their shape from reactive astrocytes which are scattered throughout the tumour.

In addition to the biological interest raised by the presence of a number of different marker antigens in PNET, preliminary clinical studies suggest that the presence of such markers may give some indication of prognosis. In a study of 38 medulloblastomas of childhood, Packer et al. (1984) showed that in the 20 tumours which expressed neither cellular differentiation nor marker antigens, there was a 70% 4-year survival rate. In those patients with tumours exhibiting glial, ependymal or neuronal differentiation, however, there was only a 32% 4-year survival rate. This particular study illustrates the sort of prognostic index which may be valuable in the future when the results of larger series of immunocytochemical studies of tumours are available.

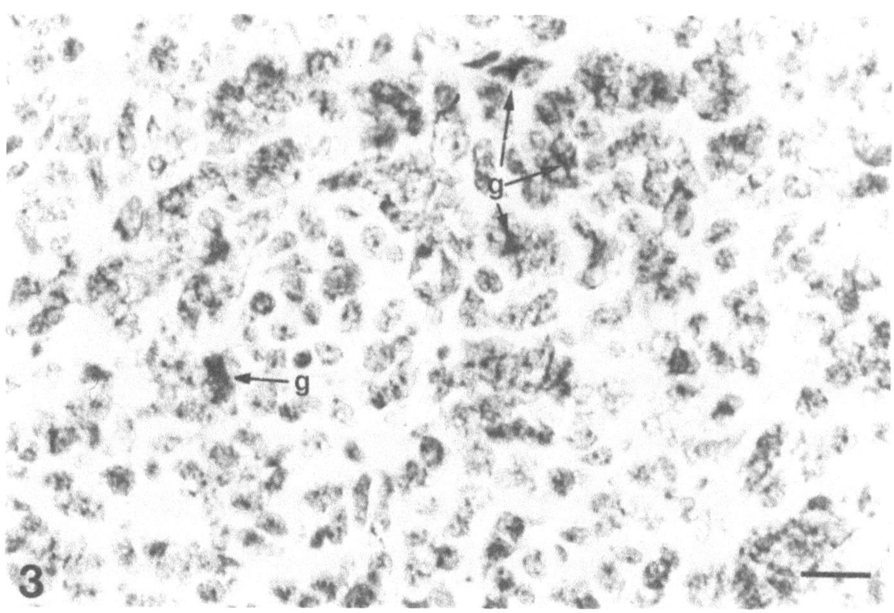

Fig. 2.3. Medulloblastoma: primitive neuroectodermal tumour showing groups of cells (g) with cytoplasm stained for GFAP. Immunoperoxidase technique. Bar represents 15 μm.

Other Tumours

Diagnostic difficulties in differentiating between glial tumours and metastatic carcinomas in the brain are usually resolved by the use of routine connective tissue stains or by staining the tissue with antibodies to GFAP. However, choroid plexus papillomas may, on occasion, be difficult to distinguish with routine histological stains from metastatic adenocarcinomas. Immunocytochemistry for marker proteins facilitates the differential diagnosis. Choroid plexus papillomas arise in the cerebral ventricles or the fourth ventricle as frond-like growths with epithelial cells mounted upon a connective tissue stroma. Although such a histological pattern resembles an adenocarcinoma, the diagnostic picture may be clarified by immunocytochemistry. Normal choroid plexus epithelium contains carbonic anhydrase C, an enzyme concerned with the hydration of carbon dioxide and the dehydration of carbonic acid. This enzyme appears to be associated with the formation of cerebrospinal fluid. Carbonic anhydrase C is not present in ependyma and, although it is present in normal stomach and colon epithelium and in renal tubular epithelium, it has not been identified in carcinomas arising from these tissues. Immunocytochemistry of choroid plexus papillomas (Weller et al. 1985), however, has shown that they contain carbonic anhydrase C (Fig. 2.4), GFAP (Fig. 2.5) and S-100 protein. Staining for GFAP may be rather patchy within the epithelium or may be confined to portions of the stroma. None of the metastatic carcinomas examined exhibited any of these three markers.

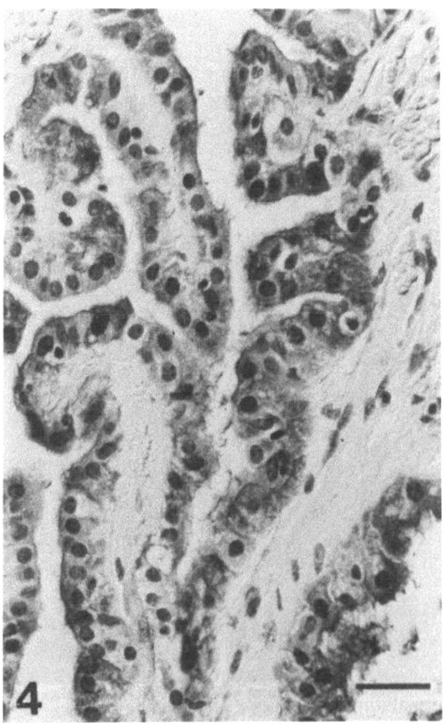

Fig. 2.4. Choroid plexus papilloma showing epithelium darkly stained for carbonic anhydrase C. Immunoperoxidase technique. Bar represents 30 μm.

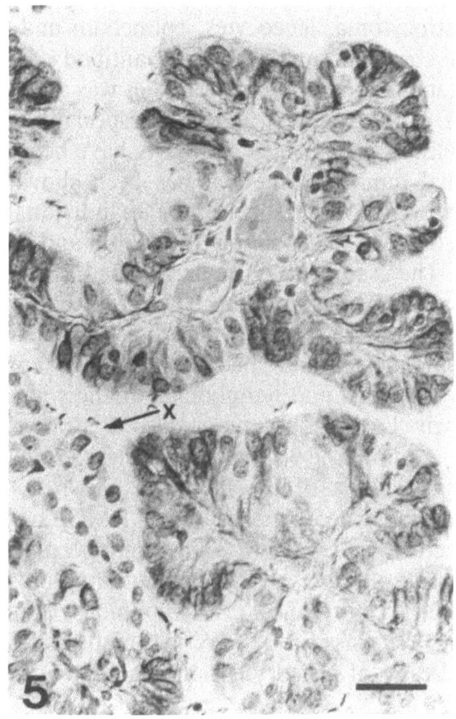

Fig. 2.5. Choroid plexus papilloma. Most of the epithelial cells in this area are stained for GFAP, but some are negative (x). Immunoperoxidase technique. Bar represents 30 μm.

Monoclonal Antibodies and the Diagnosis of Intracranial Tumours

Polyclonal antibodies (PCAs) are raised by the injection of purified marker proteins into rabbits etc.; the animal's serum thus contains antibodies which can be used with the peroxidase-antiperoxidase immunocytochemical method (Sternberger 1979). One of the advantages of PCAs is that they recognise various antigenic determinants on the marker molecule, which increases their sensitivity and makes them more suitable for use with paraffin sections in routine laboratory work. Monoclonal antibodies (MCAs), on the other hand, are directed against a single determinant on the antigen molecule for which they are specific. They are not necessarily more useful than PCAs as an increase in specificity does not always imply increased sensitivity (Bonnin and Rubinstein 1984). The majority of MCAs can only be used with cryostat, frozen sections or with isolated cells; this means that many cannot be employed to study formalin-fixed histological material in the pathology laboratory. MCAs are ideal for recognising antigenic determinants on cell surfaces.

A large number of MCAs have been raised against gliomas but, as yet, no glioma-specific antigen has been produced. Glioma-associated antigens have been produced but these antigens are also expressed by normal fetal cells, especially brain, or by normal and neoplastic lymphoid cells (McComb and Bigner 1984). Coakham et al.

(1985) assembled a panel of seven MCAs prepared from human fetal brain, astrocytoma, leucocytes, epithelium and chick retina and studied 164 spinal and cerebral tumours with each antibody. They found that the observed pattern of staining by the seven antibodies was a valuable adjunct to routine histology in 20% of cases examined and most especially in the tumours composed of small round cells. Similar panels of MCAs have been very usful in the study of the biology of glial tumours, where it has been shown that there is variation in the antigens expressed on cell surfaces within individual tumours and even within a single tumour cell line in tissue culture (McComb and Bigner 1984).

The use of MCAs in diagnostic tumour pathology is probably most advanced in the field of lymphomas. Different lymphocyte subsets can be identified by their surface antigens such that T cells and their subsets can be differentiated from B lymphocytes and macrophages. The application of MCAs to primary cerebral lymphomas and lymphomas of the spinal extradural compartment has facilitated their classification and enabled accurate characterisation of their pathology.

Although it was becoming clear from morphological criteria that the so-called microglioma of the brain was, in fact, not a tumour of microglial cells but a lymphoid neoplasm, the use of MCAs has considerably clarified the pathological picture. In a study of four primary cerebral lymphomas presenting in adult patients during the last 4 years in Southampton (Grant and Jones 1984) all proved to be follicle centre cell B cell lymphomas, centroblastic/centrocytic diffuse according to the Kiel classification (Wright and Isaacson 1983). In a clinicopathological study of 22 cases of primary lymphoma from Stanford, Helle et al. (1984) used histological

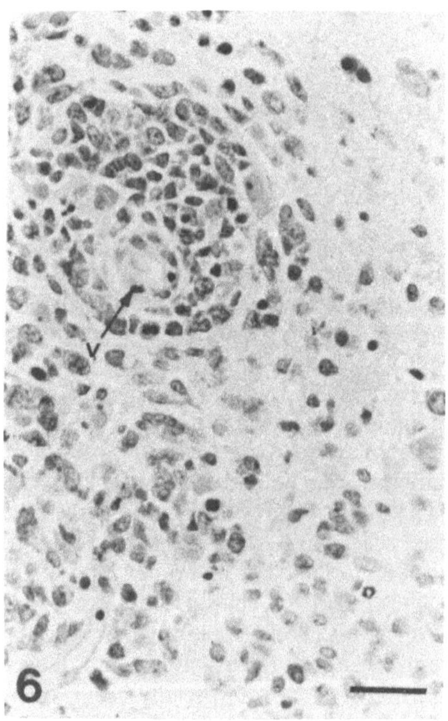

Fig. 2.6. Primary cerebral lymphoma showing tumour cells gathered around a vessel (v) at the edge of the tumour and diffusely invading surrounding brain (right). Haematoxylin and eosin. Bar represents 30 μm.

criteria for the diagnosis and did not employ immunocytochemistry. These authors found that the most common types of primary cerebral lymphoma, according to the Rappaport and Working Formulation System, were diffuse histiocytic lymphoma and immunoblastic lymphoma. Helle's cases would correspond broadly to those of Grant and Jones (1984).

Microglial cells derived from blood monocytes are indeed present within primary lymphomas but they appear to be reactive as are the reactive astrocytes. Fig. 2.6 shows the infiltrating edge of a primary lymphoma of the central nervous system. Many tumour cells have accumulated around a blood vessel but are also distributed in small groups or singly within the brain tissue. A number of reactive astrocytes are present within the infiltrated brain. MCA techniques applied to cryostat sections of this tumour show that the tumour cells exhibit the B cell marker identified by the RFB4 MCA (Fig. 2.7a). Microglial cells and monocytes within the tumour can be identified by using anti-monocyte-macrophage MCAs, in this case C7 (Fig. 2.7b); the tumour cells are negative for this marker but perivascular monocyte-macrophage-microglial cells do express the marker. Much of the confusion with the nomenclature of this tumour as a microglioma appears to have arisen from the histological identification of the reactive microglial cells. It was thus assumed that the tumour cells were also derived from microglial cells.

As the prognosis and treatment of primary lymphomas of the central nervous system differ from those of anaplastic gliomas or metastatic tumours with which they may be confused histologically, their accurate diagnosis may well significantly influence the management of the patient. A similar situation exists with regard to

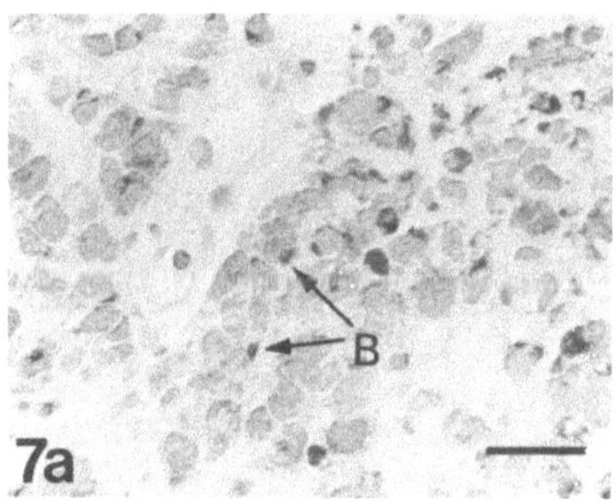

Fig. 2.7a. Primary cerebral lymphoma showing tumour cell cytoplasm positively stained (B) with the monoclonal anti-B lymphocyte marker RFB4. Immunoperoxidase technique on cryostat section. Bar represents 30 μm.

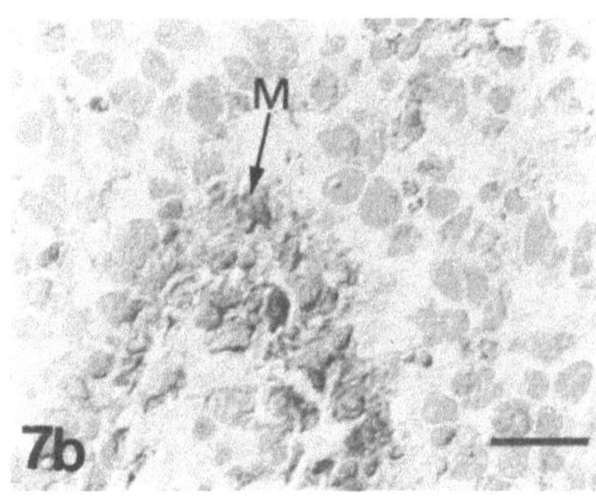

Fig. 2.7b. Primary cerebral lymphoma showing monocyte-macrophages and microglia (M) around a blood vessel (bottom) stained by the monoclonal macrophage marker C7. Lymphoma cells in the rest of the field are unstained. Immunoperoxidase technique on cryostat section Bar represents 30 μm.

spinal lymphomas. Of all the extradural tumours which present with spinal cord compression and no evidence of a primary tumour elsewhere in the body, lymphomas form a very significant proportion. In Southampton, 14 spinal lymphomas in the extradural space, presenting initially with spinal cord compression, were characterised by the use of MCAs (Grant and Jones 1985). There was a wider range of histological type than seen in the brain but most were follicle centre cell lymphomas. True histiocytic lymphomas and T cell lymphomas were also found. As there is a significant difference between lymphomas and metastatic carcinomas in their response to treatment, it is important to characterise such tumours fully, particularly those occurring in the spinal extradural space. Initial diagnosis of lymphoma is usually made just after the surgical operation has started by the use of rapid touch preparations made from the tumour tissue. MCA studies can be performed immediately on frozen tissue, or completed at a later date.

Immunological Responses Against Brain Tumours

The majority of patients with astrocytic tumours produce a specific humoral immune response to their own tumours (Gately et al. 1982). Antibodies are formed against factors present in normal and neoplastic cells, and against glioma-specific antigens. However, the cellular immune response is impaired. The decline in

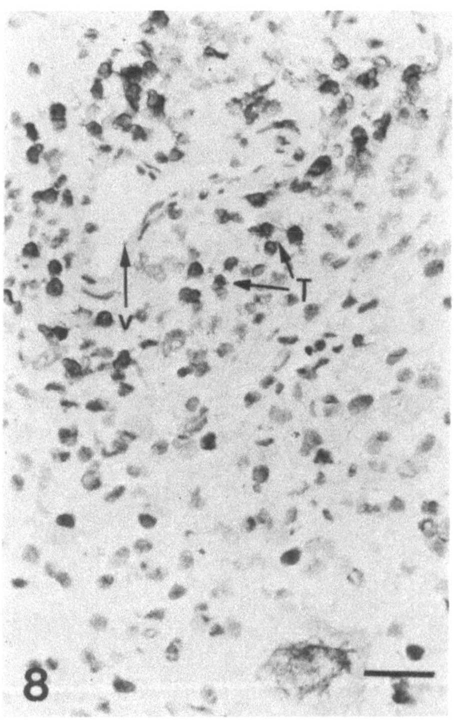

Fig. 2.8. Anaplastic astrocytoma showing a blood vessel (v) surrounded by T lymphocytes (T) stained for the monoclonal T cell marker T28. Unstained cells in the rest of the field are tumour cells. Immunoperoxidase technique on cryostat section. Bar represents 30 μm.

patients' immunocompetence (Brooks and Roszman 1980) is reflected in cutaneous anergy to common skin test antigens, impaired lymphocyte responsiveness, a reduction in T lymphocytes in the peripheral blood and the presence of humoral and cellular suppressor factors in patients with clinically significant tumour masses. Upon removal of the tumour mass, immunocompetence returns towards normal and suppressor factors in the system are reduced.

It has long been noted that cuffs of lymphocytes are present around blood vessels in some 60% of poorly differentiated gliomas, and it has been suggested that this may represent an immunological attack upon the tumour. However, immunocytochemical studies with MCAs have shown that lymphocytes in tumours are mainly T cells and the majority are T suppressor–cytotoxic cells (von Hanwehr et al. 1984). In Fig. 2.8, lymphocytes within an anaplastic astrocytoma have been stained with the monoclonal antibody T28 which identifies T cells. Although most of the stained cells are around a blood vessel at the top of the picture, T cells are also scattered throughout the tumour. It is these T cells which are mainly suppressor–cytotoxic cells. Very few B lymphocytes are present within anaplastic astrocytomas or glioblastoma multiforme. Numerous macrophages are present in poorly differentiated astrocytic tumours and can be identified by immunocytochemistry in regions of necrosis, around blood vessels and throughout the tumour tissue (Fig. 2.9). The presence of suppressor–cytotoxic cells in brain tumours may reflect suppression of immunological activity within the tumour rather than a cytotoxic attack. Suppressive factors have been identified not only in the serum but also in cyst fluid from patients with cystic gliomas, especially glioblastoma multiforme (Kikuchi and

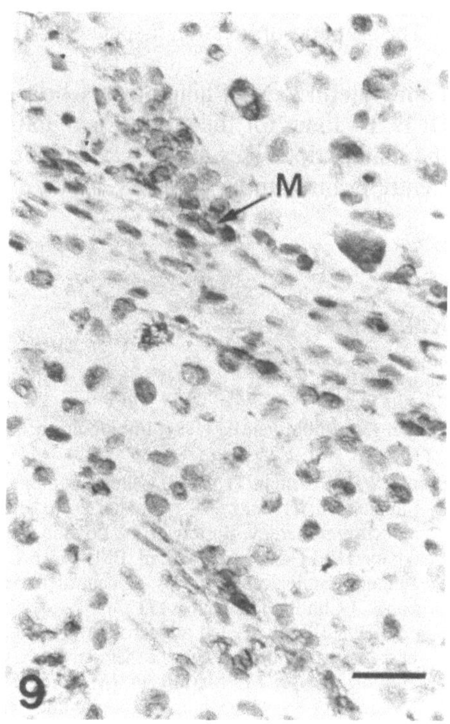

Fig. 2.9. Anaplastic astrocytoma showing macrophages (M) around a blood vessel stained by the monoclonal macrophage marker 3.9. Many unstained tumour cells are seen in this field. Immunoperoxidase technique on cryostat section. Bar represents 30 μm.

Neuwelt 1983). It appears also that human glioma cells may escape cellular immune attack through the presence of a mucopolysaccharide coat and through the failure to stimulate "helper" factors as well as through the production of immunosuppressive factors (Gately et al. 1982). The recognition that the cellular immune response is impaired in patients with gliomas is particularly significant as it is mainly the cellular immune response which is of primary importance for the eradication of solid tumours in vivo (Apuzzo and Mitchell 1981).

Summary

Immunocytochemical techniques are now widely used to identify specific proteins—marker antigens—in a number of cell types within the normal and tumorous nervous system. Antibodies to the astrocyte intermediate filament, glial fibrillary acidic protein (GFAP), can be used to characterise astrocytic and ependymal tumours. GFAP is also present in oligodendrogliomas and in primitive neuroectodermal tumours (medulloblastoma). Neuron-specific enolase is restricted to neurons in normal tissue but is present in a wide variety of tumours. Carbonic anhydrase C, on the other hand, is present in normal oligodendrocytes but not in oligodendrogliomas; this enzyme is a valuable marker for normal and neoplastic choroid plexus. S-100 protein is present in Schwann cells and other cells of neural crest origin; it is also found in tumours derived from these cells. Monoclonal antibodies to cell surface components are particularly valuable in the characterisation of cerebral and spinal lymphomas.

The immunosuppression associated with the presence of brain tumours is discussed.

I am grateful to Mr Philip Steart who performed the immunocytochemistry and to Dr D. B. Jones for the monoclonal antibodies. Miss Margaret Harris kindly typed the manuscript. This study was supported by the Wessex Regional Neurological Centre Brain Tumour Research Fund.

References

Apuzzo MLJ, Mitchell MS (1981) Immunological aspects of intrinsic glial tumours. J Neurosurg 55: 1-18

Bonnin JM, Rubinstein LJ (1984) Immunohistochemistry of central nervous system tumours. J Neurosurg 60: 1121-1133

Brooks WH, Roszman TL (1980) Cellular immune responsiveness of patients with primary intracranial tumours. In: Thomas DGT, Graham DI (eds) Brain tumours: Scientific basis, clinical investigation and current therapy. Butterworths, London, pp 121-132

Coakham HB, Garson JA, Allan PM, Harper EI, Brownell B, Kemshead JT, Lane EB (1985) Immunohistological diagnosis of central nervous system tumours using a monoclonal antibody panel. J Clin Pathol 38: 165-173

Eng LF (1980) Brain related antigens. In: Thomas DGT, Graham DI (eds) Brain tumours: Scientific basis, investigation and current therapy. Butterworths, London, pp 109-120

Gately MK, Glaser M, McCarron RM, Dick SJ, Dick MD, Mettetal RW, Kornblith PL (1982) Mechanisms by which human gliomas may escape cellular immune attack. Acta Neurochir 64: 175-197

Grant JW, Jones DB (1984) Immunohistochemistry of lymphomas affecting the nervous system. Neuropathol Appl Neurobiol 10: 310

Grant JW, Jones DB (1985) Spinal cord compression as first presentation of lymphoma. J Pathol 145: 92A

von Hanwehr RI, Hofman FM, Taylor CR, Apuzzo MLJ (1984) Mononuclear lymphoid populations infiltrating the microenvironment of primary CNS tumours. Characterisation of cell subsets with monoclonal antibodies. J Neurosurg 60: 1138–1147

Helle TL, Britt RH, Colby TV (1984) Primary lymphoma of the central nervous system. Clinicopathological study of experience at Stanford. J Neurosurg 60: 94–103

Kikuchi K, Neuwelt EA (1983) Presence of immunosuppressive factors in brain-tumor cyst fluid. J Neurosurg 59: 790–799

Martinez AJ, Lee H, Moossy J, Maroon JC (1980) Pituitary adenomas: Clinicopathological and immunohistochemical study. Ann Neurol 7: 24–36

McComb RD, Bigner DD (1984) The biology of malignant gliomas—a comprehensive survey. Clin Neuropathol 3: 93–106

Packer RJ, Sutton LN, Rorke LB, Littman PA, Sposto R, Rosenstock JG, Bruce DA, Schut L (1984) Prognostic importance of cellular differentiation in medulloblastoma of childhood. J Neurosurg 61: 296–301

Rorke LB (1983) The cerebellar medulloblastoma and its relationship to primitive neuroectodermal tumors. J Neuropathol Exp Neurol 42: 1–15

Schlaepfer WW, Lee V, Wu HL (1981) Assessment of immunological properties of neurofilaments' triplet proteins. Brain Res 226: 259–272

Schmechel D, Marangos PJ, Brightman M (1978) Neurone-specific enolase is a molecular marker for peripheral and central neuroendocrine cells. Nature (Lond) 276: 834–836

Schnitzer J, Franke WW, Schachner M (1981) Immunocytochemical demonstration of vimentin in astrocytes and ependymal cells of developing and adult mouse nervous system. J Cell Biol 90: 435–447

Sternberger LA (1979) Immunocytochemistry, 2nd edn. Wiley, New York

Vinores SA, Bonnin JM, Rubinstein LJ, Marangos PJ (1984) Immunohistochemical demonstration of neuron-specific enoclase in neoplasms of the CNS and other tissues. Arch Pathol Lab Med 108: 536–540

Weller RO (1984) Colour atlas of neuropathology. Harvey Miller/Oxford University Press, Oxford, p 77

Weller RO, Davis BE, Wilson POG, Mitchell J (1981) Capillary proliferation in cerebral infarction, gliomas, angioblastic meningiomas and haemangioblastomas. In: Cervós-Navarro J, Fritschka E (eds) Cerebral microcirculation and metabolism. Raven Press, New York, pp 41–48

Weller RO, Steart PV, Moore IE (1985) Carbonic anhydrase C as a marker antigen in the diagnosis of choroid plexus papillomas and other tumours: An immunoperoxidase study. J Neurooncol (in press)

Wright DH, Isaacson PG (1983) Biopsy pathology of the lymphoreticular system. Chapman and Hall, London, pp 119–127

Zülch KJ (ed) (1979) Histological typing of tumours of the central nervous system. International histological classification of tumours. World Health Organisation, Geneva

3 Imaging Techniques in the Investigation of Cerebral Tumours

Ivan Moseley

Introduction

Clinical findings, together with simple, non-invasive investigations such as the electroencephalogram, usually make it clear that the patient with a brain tumour does indeed have a structural lesion—although there is undoubtedly a large number of positive clinical diagnoses impossible to assess retrospectively. The data required of imaging investigations therefore include the following:

1) confirmation of the presence of an intracranial structural abnormality;
2) determination of its probable nature;
3) prediction of its degree of malignancy;
4) assessment of its extent and location relative to critical structures;
5) prediction of its internal structure and probable consistency; and
6) evaluation of the response to treatment.

It is evident that many of these characteristics are inter-related and that most are relevant not simply to diagnosis but to the therapeutic possibilities and to assessment of prognosis.

Other chapters in this book are devoted to recent developments in imaging, namely positron emission tomography and magnetic resonance imaging. While it is certain that both have enormous potential contributions, particularly as regards the biological characterisation of cerebral tumours in vivo, their practical utility is limited by economic considerations and by very restricted availability. This review is therefore concerned with the more conventional techniques based on X-rays (plain films, computerised tomography and angiography), radionuclides and ultrasound, and each will be reviewed for its suitability in producing the data listed above. The discussion will largely be restricted to the commoner supratentorial intra-axial tumours, i.e. gliomas, to avoid too diffuse an overview.

Plain Radiographs

Although skull radiographs have been a traditional investigation in the diagnostic assessment of patients suspected of harbouring a cerebral tumour, they have proved sufficiently unreliable to be discarded when other non-invasive tests are available. In a series of 200 patients with confirmed intracranial tumours seen in a German neurological centre, only 14% showed abnormalities on skull films. These abnormalities were often non-specific, and merely indicated raised intracranial pressure (Hillemacher 1982). Plain films of a similar group of 170 patients seen at the National Hospital for Nervous Diseases, London, with the clinical diagnosis of a posterior cranial fossa lesion (excluding unilateral deafness) yielded an almost identical proportion of abnormalities; but two thirds of these abnormalities did not affect management, and in two cases they were counterproductive (Du Boulay and Radue 1978). There are no pathognomonic plain film findings in cases of glioma, although the combination of signs of raised intracranial pressure (erosion of the lamina dura of the sella turcica in adults, splaying of the sutures in children, etc.) and amorphous intracerebral calcification is highly suggestive. Gliomas are the commonest cause of pathological calcification which appears, on multiple projections, to lie within the brain.

The chest radiograph is of more practical use, since it may reveal an inflammatory process or primary or secondary neoplasms, and thus facilitate differential diagnosis of intracranial lesions shown by more reliable techniques.

Conventional Radionuclide Studies

Conventional radionuclide studies have most frequently been performed with intravenous technetium. Recording the distribution of the radionuclide immediately after injection will indicate areas of relative hyper- or hypovascularity, while images obtained 30–45 minutes later show areas in which the tracer has accumulated in the extracellular space because of an absent or defective blood–brain barrier. The latter technique has been the most widely used, sometimes supplemented by a tomographic method, analogous to that used in computerised X-ray tomography, to increase both spatial resolution and lesion detectability.

At the time of their most widespread use, i.e. around 1970–1973, radionuclide studies were by far the most reliable non-invasive means of detecting intracranial lesions. However, since altered vascularity and disturbances of the blood–brain barrier are not characteristic of low-grade gliomas, many tumours of this type were overlooked. The gamma camera sees essentially superficial lesions, generally those greater than 2 cm in diameter, so that small or deeply placed tumours are also problematic, as are those in the posterior cranial fossa. Studies conducted in the United States for the National Cancer Institute yielded negative results in at least one quarter of proven cases of malignant brain tumours (Baker et al. 1980). In the case of brain stem and cerebellar tumours the false negative rates can be as high as 60% and 30% respectively (Burrows 1976), and in one series of 18 confirmed gliomas in the brain stem only one produced a definite abnormality (Felgin et al. 1975).

In addition to problems of detection the value of conventional radionuclide studies is limited by the non-specific nature of the abnormalities shown, as well as the lack of information as to the internal structure of the lesion and its effects on the adjacent brain, etc. There is, therefore, little justification for continued conventional radionuclide scanning of the head, for either screening purposes or more definitive examinations, when less unsatisfactory non-invasive procedures are available. The use of radionuclide studies as a follow-up study after surgery is vitiated by abnormal uptake of radionuclides at the operation site, which can persist for months.

Ultrasound

Recent technical developments have made cranial ultrasound a very valuable tool in certain situations. Previously it gave only rather primitive information about midline displacements and other gross changes, and had largely fallen into disuse when superior methods were to hand. With the introdution of real-time grey-scale images and small probes its use has increased. However, because of marked attenuation of the ultrasonic waves by the bone of the skull it is still restricted to patients with naturally occurring defects in the vault, i.e. young children, or those with traumatic or iatrogenic defects.

The technique has become the procedure of choice for the initial exploration of suspected hydrocephalus, intracranial haemorrhage, or other neurological complications in neonates and infants. Intracranial tumours are readily detected, and considerable information as to their internal structure may be obtained, but recourse to other imaging modalities is usually necessary prior to treatment (Han et al. 1984).

A number of groups have used intra-operative sonography for localisation of subcortical lesions. After craniotomy a sterile probe is placed on the surface of the brain. A real-time probe 13 mm in diameter will show most of the underlying hemisphere and some of the contralateral side (Gooding et al. 1981). Since the sonographic images enable not only identification and localisation of a cystic area but also depth measurements, then aspiration, biopsy and even ventricular shunt placement, employing purpose-built guides, is relatively easy. Knake et al. (1982) reported successful biopsy of 16 intracerebral masses, 10 of which were less than 2.5 cm in diameter. The pulsatile nature of very vascular lesions is readily appreciated, so that biopsy of an arteriovenous malformation can be avoided (Fasano et al. 1983).

Limited post-operative assessment can be carried out via existing burr holes, using smaller probes.

X-ray Computerised Tomography (CT)

From its introduction to clinical neuroradiology in 1972, CT was seen to be superior not only to previously used non-invasive techniques but also to angiography and pneumoencephalography for the detection of intracranial tumours (Ambrose et al.

1975). Subsequent experience has shown it to be more satisfactory also for providing most of the data listed above as desirable for optimum management of cerebral gliomas.

Confirmation of the Presence of a Structural Lesion

The National Cancer Institute study mentioned previously revealed that virtually all of the 20% of cerebral tumours not detected by radionuclide examinations were seen on CT, and numerous other investigations have confirmed CT's superiority to radionuclide techniques in this context (Claveria et al. 1978, Tans and de Jongh 1978).

Parallel CT and radionuclide studies in cases of glioma have confirmed that concentration of iodinated contrast medium in the former correlates well with accumulation of tracers in the latter. It may therefore be attributed to the same factors of increased vascularity and disturbances of the blood-brain barrier (Butler et al. 1979). In an attempt to ensure that no tumour is overlooked, a number of workers have suggested that all patients suspected of having cerebral tumours should be given contrast medium. However, as will be seen later, low-grade infiltrating lesions rarely show a detectable increase in density with intravenous contrast medium, while glioblastomas are rarely visible without injection. A review of 1000 consecutive patients receiving contrast medium at the National Hospital for Nervous Diseases revealed none in whom cerebral tumours were shown following injection when the initial scans had been normal (Moseley 1977). Experience elsewhere has been similar (Thomson 1976, Barrington and Lewtas 1977, Butler and Kricheff 1978). Despite these findings, other groups have proposed that double the normal dose of intravenous contrast medium, containing 80 g instead of 40 g of iodine, should be used, and delayed images 1–2 hours after injection obtained in addition to immediate images, to increase tumour detection rates (Hayman et al. 1980). Neither the studies designed to prove the merits of this approach, nor others, have provided evidence that these measures (which increase the duration, cost and risk of the examination) achieve the desired aim (Kazner et al. 1982).

Specificity of Diagnosis

Claveria et al. (1978) reviewed cases in which glioma had been diagnosed on CT, or shown subsequently by other methods, among the first 6500 patients examined by the new techniques at the National Hospital for Nervous Diseases. In only 9% of cases had the correct diagnosis not been suggested (sometimes as part of a differential diagnosis) and in only one case was the examination wrongly considered normal. Metastases, radionecrosis and cerebral infarcts were the chief causes of false positive readings. The last often presented with a clinical history suggestive of a progressive abnormality, which adversely swayed the radiologist. In retrospective review of these patients' computerised tomograms, the correct diagnosis of glioma was possible in 70.7% without intravenous contrast medium and in 90% following injection.

Other workers have reported similarly high degrees of diagnostic accuracy. Tans and de Jongh (1978) found only one false negative and no false positive diagnoses of glioma in a series of 2500 patient examinations. Errors in predicting histology were made in eight patients.

Although the radiographic appearances may be confused with those of multiple metastases, CT is the most reliable conventional technique for demonstrating multifocal gliomas, which form 2.5%–10% of reported series. Location in the corpus callosum or basal ganglia is suggestive of a multifocal primary lesion rather than secondary deposits (Sundaresan et al. 1981).

Specificity of diagnosis is considered further in the section on angiography (p 46).

Assessment of the Degree of Malignancy

The results of CT in a large series of cerebral tumours were analysed by Kazner et al. (1982), with results which are summarised in Table 3.1. Contrast enhancement takes the form of a ring, usually thick and irregular in at least part of its periphery, in 85% of glioblastomas. It will be seen that grade 1 astrocytomas are typically of low density, and do not show either peritumoral vasogenic oedema or contrast enhance-

Table 3.1. CT characteristics of cerebral tumours (after Kazner et al. 1982)

(*a*) *Before contrast enhancement*

Tumour	*n*	Density compared with normal brain (%)			
		Reduced	Normal	Increased	Mixed
Astrocytoma I	15	86	7	0	7[a]
Astrocytoma II	157	43	1	12	44
Oligodendroglioma	174	26	5	14	55[b]
Glioblastoma	711	11	11	8	70[c]
Pilocytic astrocytoma	112	31	20	15	34
Ependymoma	54	13	9	41	37
Medulloblastoma	67	4	10	65	21

(*b*) *After contrast enhancement*

Tumour	Contrast enhancement (%)	Not seen before contrast (%)	Not seen (%)	Oedema (%)	
				+	+ +
Astrocytoma I	1[a]	0	0	1	1
Astrocytoma II	82	3	3	23	35
Oligodendroglioma	46	0	0	22	16
Glioblastoma	97[d]	2	0	23	68
Pilocytic astrocytoma	82	4	0	25[e]	2
Ependymoma	84	2[f]	0	26	17
Medulloblastoma	93	5[f]	1[f]	46	46

[a]Both gemistocytic.
[b]70% calcified.
[c]Calcification rare; haemorrhage more common.
[d]Ring configuration in 84%.
[e]Oedema less striking than with any other enhancing glioma.
[f]Posterior fossa lesions.

ment. These findings are similar to those in many other series and permit a rough guide as to the degree of malignancy, but differences between grade 2 gliomas and more malignant tumours are largely a matter of degree, and may not be reliable in individual cases. This radiographic pleomorphism led Silverman and Marks (1981) to postulate that grade 2 tumours might be usefully differentiated on the basis of CT appearances into those of greater or lesser malignant potential. However, in a rather small but well-matched series of adults with contrast-enhancing tumours, 4-year actuarial survival rates were insignificantly different, at 58% and 65% respectively; the tumours in the former group were, moreover, slightly larger at presentation than the remainder.

Calcification, as is well known, favours the diagnosis of oligodendroglioma (being observed in over 90% of some series), as does a predominantly frontal location, observed in about two thirds of cases (Marcu et al. 1980).

Lewander and his co-workers (1978) attempted to correlate the time course of changes in radiographic density with the results of stereotactic biopsy guided by CT. A recurrent problem in assessment of the histopathological significance of radiographic changes is uncertainty that the same tissue is being examined. Given the variability in grading of tumours in specimens taken from different sites, this is clearly of major concern. Nevertheless it was possible to confirm that gliomas of grade 1 and 2 showed no significant increase in density after injection, and that necrotic portions of more malignant tumours were similarly unchanged. However, while the apparently solid portions of glioblastomas showing marked contrast enhancement represented viable tumour, so too could non-enhancing areas, even in the most malignant lesions. Non-enhancing oligodendrogliomas may also show abundant mitotic figures (Marcu et al. 1980).

The increase in attenuation coefficients of the blood caused by intravenous contrast media shows a linear relationship to iodine concentration; one group, comparing CT and post-mortem histological studies, concluded that zones of marked contrast enhancement correspond to areas of vascular proliferation, rather than to cellularity or anaplasia. Even within grossly malignant tumours, zones in which vascular proliferation was absent were not observed to show striking contrast enhancement (Takeda et al. 1980). However, if all the increase in radiographic density seen in malignant gliomas were due to intravascular iodine, the blood pool should represent 50%–60% by volume of the tumour; histological examination shows this not to be the case. Furthermore, other workers have not found such a strong correlation between vascularity and intensity of contrast enhancement on routine CT (Butler et al. 1978).

Lewander (1979) proposed, on the basis of serial measurements made on different tumours, that leakage of the contrast medium into the extravascular component of the mass, as the result of a defect in the blood–brain barrier, could be fast or slow, depending on the histological type of the tumour. The density of the intensely enhancing portions of glioblastomas was observed to fall slowly during the first hour after injection, suggesting that leakage occurs relatively rapidly. Most contrast-enhanced tomograms are obtained sufficiently long after injection that only this late "washout" phase of contrast medium distribution is seen. It is, however, possible on a modern scanner unit to form a series of images, each reconstructed from an "incomplete" set of data, relatively rapidly. Thus, Dubois et al. (1981) obtained six images in 33 seconds in order to examine the changes in radiographic density immediately following injections. They studied 14 intracranial tumours, including nine gliomas. The time to peak increase in density (ΔHUmax) was identical for solid components of the tumour and normal cerebral cortex: 12–15 seconds after rapid intravenous injection. But by 33 seconds the residual increase in density (ΔHUres) of the cortex had fallen by 60%, whereas that in tumour tissue remained at 77% of ΔHUmax. This supported the concept of rapid egress into the extracellular fluid. Among the cases of glioma, although no correlation could be established between HUres and angiographic findings, there was excellent correlation between rapid increase in density and increased vascularity assessed by angiography. The ΔHUmax of five apparently "avascular" tumours was 2–5.5 (mean 3.4) Hounsfield units, while that for four "moderately hypervascular" lesions was 7–12 units, i.e. there was no overlap between the two groups. However, the technique of rapid serial scanning was less successful in distinguishing between tumours and inflammatory, vascular or traumatic lesions.

That the high ΔHUmax of cerebral tumours is related to leakage rather than to high blood flow is borne out by CT measurements of local cerebral blood flow and partition coefficients in patients with gliomas. Inhalation of stable gaseous xenon in 35% concentration during scanning permits correlation of variations in local flow with radiological and histological features in a manner impossible with other techniques, although earlier work with intra-arterial radioactive xenon had suggested reduced flow. CT flow studies against age-matched controls confirm that flow is reduced within the glioma, and in the remainder of the affected cerebral hemisphere, even at a considerable distance from the tumour. Reduction of both flow and partition coefficients is more marked and more uniform in low-grade tumours than in glioblastomas, although partition coefficients in the surrounding brain are most reduced with the latter, probably as a reflection of more intense oedema (Tachibana et al. 1984).

Most of the patients with gliomas examined by Lewander (1979) were receiving systemic corticosteroids, which are known to exert profound effects on the blood–brain barrier, and particularly on extravasation of contrast medium. Patients who had not been operated upon or treated with chemo- or radiotherapy were studied by Latchaw et al. (1980), who took a very sophisticated approach to the changes produced by intravenous contrast media. X-ray attenuation in CT is a function of effective atomic number (Z^*) and electron density, but Z^* also depends on the energy of the beam, since the relationship between X-ray energy and tissue absorption is not linear. Scanning of tumours before and after intravenous contrast medium with effective beam energies of 90 and 130 kVp enabled calculation of change in attenuation (%ΔZ^*) at each of the energy levels "μ shift" ($\Delta\mu$130%), "μ spread" (the relationship between $\Delta\mu$90 and $\Delta\mu$130), and finally in effective atomic number (%ΔZ^*).

It is immediately apparent from the results summarised in Table 3.2 that whereas the complex methodology and numerical analysis might considerably facilitate

Table 3.2. The effect of intravenous contrast medium on effective atomic number (Z^*) in intracranial tumours (after Latchaw et al. 1980)

	Mean μ90 (%)	Mean μ spread (%)	Mean ΔZ^* (%)
Astrocytomas			
Grades 1, 2	2.2	13.3	8.0
Grades 3, 4	1.8	13.4	7.8
Meningiomas	5.0	35.0	16.0
Metastases	3.8	45.0	22.0

distinction of gliomas from benign or secondary tumours, the way in which contrast medium leaks into the enhancing portions of astrocytomas is rather uniform, regardless of histological grading. Tapias et al. (1978), taking a more simplistic approach, confirmed what most experienced neurologists have suspected for some years: which is that statistical analysis of radiographic density before and after intravenous contrast medium enables distinction of tumours which do not superficially resemble each other but is non-contributory in cases presenting diagnostic problems. Analysis of attenuation coefficients before contrast medium administration has been found to be unhelpful for distinguishing tumour, brain invaded by tumour, anaplasia, necrosis or oedema (Takeda et al. 1980).

Pullicino et al. (1979) attempted a correlation of CT findings in cystic tumours with analysis of fluid aspirated at surgery. The constituents assayed, and their presumed pathophysiological significance were: protein as a product of breakdown of the blood–brain barrier; cholesterol as a product of tumour cells, or of destruction of neoplastic or brain cells; alkaline phosphatase as an indicator of cell activity; and lactic dehydrogenase and phosphohexose isomerase as measures of cell destruction.

Surprisingly, there was no correlation between the radiographic density and the protein content of the cyst contents, but alkaline phosphatase concentrations were significantly lower in cysts with dense walls, possibly because of a higher proportion of benign lesions in this group. However, the mean attenuation coefficients of the cyst in grossly malignant lesions (83% glioblastomas, 17% metastases), less malignant tumours (75% low-grade gliomas, the remainder haemangioblastomas) and benign neoplasms (50% craniopharyngiomas) were virtually identical at 17.4–19.6 EMI units. Cyst size did not correlate with malignancy or biochemical profile.

Although the capsule of the cyst in highly malignant tumours was more often thick and irregular than that of the other lesions, there was no significant correlation with these features and the cyst contents. Tumours showing dependent layering (see below) had no specific biochemical characteristics. Tumour cysts whose margins showed contrast enhancement contained significantly higher concentrations of lactose dehydrogenase and phosphohexose isomerase, and slightly increased levels of alkaline phosphatase. This presumably indicated more extensive necrosis and rapid turnover of the cells lining the cavity, and underlines the importance of contrast enhancement as an indicator of malignancy in cerebral tumours. However, although the anticipated general trends were observed there was no significant correlation between the extent of surrounding oedema—another CT correlate of malignancy—and the biochemical indices, probably because of marked individual variations.

Assessment of the Extent of the Lesion

In clinical neurology the practical significance of the degree of malignancy of cerebral tumours is largely prognostic, and a number of workers have related CT features to outcome rather than to histology, which, as noted above, may be misleading. Several studies have therefore been concerned with determination of the size of the tumour and the effect this has on prognosis. Survival has not been found to be related to the apparent cross-sectional area of the nidus of the tumour, nor to the extent of oedema, prior to operation (Reeves and Marks 1979), although the latter has repeatedly been found to correlate well with histological grading (Tchang et al, 1977, Weisberg 1980, Kazner et al. 1982).

It may be argued that volumetric measurements should be more relevant in assessing the extent of the tumour (McCullough et al. 1979) and, perhaps more importantly, that CT is very inadequate for detection of cellular infiltration. There is conflicting evidence, both clinical and laboratory, as to this latter point. On the other hand, studies with gliomas induced in monkeys by inoculation with human polyomavirus confirmed the familiar clinical observation that lesions were clearly identifiable by CT in animals who were apparently intact neurologically (Rieth et al. 1980). On the other hand there have been a number of case reports of normal CT examinations (often patients presenting with epilepsy) followed within a few months or even weeks by demonstrations of large, sometimes very large, gliomas (Wulff et al. 1982, Bolender et al. 1983). The tumours concerned were not always of high grade, although they often contained large cysts. However, repeated scans of unoperated glioblastomas in humans have suggested a very high growth rate, with a volume doubling time almost always shorter than 3 weeks, and occasionally as little as 2 weeks (Yamashita and Kawabara 1983), so that these "false negative" examinations are easily understood.

Evidence from positron emission tomography (PET) suggests that metabolic changes compatible with tumour spread are usually more extensive than abnormalities on CT. Correlative CT and post-mortem examinations in patients with glioblastomas have repeatedly revealed discrepancies in the apparent volume of the tumour, showing cellular infiltration not only in other lobes of the same hemisphere but also in the contralateral hemisphere, of which CT gave no clue. Some of the radiological studies were, however, several weeks ante-mortem (Burger et al. 1983), but similar examinations carried out as little as 3 days before death have also failed to demonstrate a CT correlate of widespread cellular infiltration (Takeda et al. 1980).

Tumours have also been demonstrated by magnetic resonance imaging (MRI) in symptomatic patients with normal CT, but Bradley et al. (1984) found the latter technique superior for differentiation of tumours from surrounding oedema. As pointed out by Taylor and Bore (1981), this may not be surprising in view of the first-order correlation of MR relaxation times with water density, and poses a theoretical question over the specificity of tissue diagnosis with this technique. Recent work with paramagnetic contrast media for MRI suggests that this shortcoming may, however, be resolved.

Correlative CT and histological studies in tumours recurring after radiotherapy have demonstrated no viable tumour cells outside an enhancing ring (Selker et al. 1982) and it has been claimed that in the large majority of tumours neoplastic cells cannot be found further than 2 cm from the apparent radiographic limits of the tumour (Hochberg and Pruitt 1980). Nevertheless, in even moderately large tumours, underestimating the radius by up to 2 cm may greatly decrease the apparent size of the lesions. Thus in the case of a rounded tumour which appeared to have a diameter of 5 cm, the error would be fivefold.

Despite these difficulties, the correlation of the apparent volume of residual tumour after initial treatment with prognosis is highly significant (Andreou et al. 1983). Both, however, can be affected by corticosteroids. Since intensity of enhancement also correlates with cellular pleomorphism and necrosis, although somewhat less well with cellularity and vascularity (Butler et al. 1978), these observations are not surprising.

Internal Structure and Consistency

It is very tempting to look at a lesion showing an obvious ring of enhancement and say that it should be cystic; however, Lewander et al. (1978) found this prediction to be fulfilled in only one third of cases. Serial studies up to 1 hour after intravenous contrast medium may show "filling in" of apparently cystic area (Norman et al. 1978). Areas confirmed at surgery as cysts within tumours have very similar attenuation coefficients to those of necrotic, non-cystic regions: in one study the ranges were 8–15 and 10–17 EMI units respectively. Cysts in recurrent gliomas tend to have thin, regular walls more like those of abscesses, whereas necrosis leaves a thick, irregular wall (Afra et al. 1980). Layering of debris or of contrast medium given intravenously within a low-density area is the only pathognomonic sign that a lesion is cystic rather than necrotic. Nevertheless, many lesions found to be cystic at surgery fail to show this sign, and in one series of cystic tumours of all histological types, 11% showed no evidence of their cystic nature on CT (Pullicino et al. 1979).

Radue and Kendall (1978) reported experimental clinical studies using prolonged inhalation of stable xenon gas (in 70% concentration) producing saturation, as a combined contrast medium and general anaesthetic agent for CT. Xenon diffuses freely in all tissues, and being lipophilic tends to be concentrated in the brain, to an extent proportional to lipid content and to blood flow. A decrease in focal flow has already been referred to; these saturation studies showed very low levels of xenon (around 10% of the concentration in normal brain) in cysts, with those in necrotic areas being generally somewhat higher. However, the cost and practical complexity of this method make it unsuitable for routine use.

Although there is some correlation between radiographic density before injection, intensity of enhancement and cellularity, low-density areas are not necessarily necrotic or even soft. In one small series of masses whose radiographic density was that of cerebrospinal fluid, more than half proved to be solid astrocytomas or metastases (Latchaw et al. 1977). It is also general experience that a small proportion of "low-density" tumours may be hard enough to merit sharp surgical dissection.

The Effects of Treatment

CT is an excellent method for assessing the beneficial and untoward effects of surgery and of chemo- or radiotherapy.

In order to reduce the diagnostic radiation dose to the eyes, examinations may be carried out only after intravenous contrast medium, unless there has been a sudden alteration in the patient's condition, which might indicate haemorrhage. In this latter situation pre-injection scans should also be obtained. There is a good correlation between clinical status and CT findings in the months following surgery. Thus about three quarters of patients deteriorating will show an increase in overall size of the lesion and/or a central low-density area, as opposed to less than one sixth of those whose status is stable or improving. Increase in contrast enhancement or oedema correlates somewhat less well (Norman et al. 1976).

However, although it provides a permanent objective record, CT is not actually superior to neurological assessment nor even, in some series, to serial radionuclide studies (Levin et al. 1977). Thus, Mahaley et al. (1983), following more than 40 patients with anaplastic gliomas, found CT to be the first indicator of treatment failure in only six, and in only three of the 26 whose relapse occurred in the first 6 months after surgery. They therefore felt unable to recommend routine follow-up CT. Transient enlargement, with increased central necrosis and contrast enhancement, suggesting progression of the tumour, can occur from 3 to 12 weeks after the termination of radiotherapy, so that repeat examinations during this period can be particularly misleading (Graeb et al. 1982).

This similarity in the radiographic appearances of recurrent tumour and radionecrosis also constitutes a troublesome shortcoming of CT in the longer term follow-up of patients treated by radiotherapy. Most workers have found that all of the characteristic features of the former, such as mixed density, mass effect, vasogenic oedema, contrast enhancement, and even haemorrhage and calcification, may be mimicked by the latter (Mikhael 1978, Burger et al. 1983). However, Selker et al. (1982), who carried out semi-stereotactic operations 3–11 months after the end of courses of cranial irradiation, found in every case that while a low-density central area represented necrotic tissue without mitoses, and surrounding low-density areas always showed changes of coagulation necrosis, a zone of ring enhancement separating these two contained viable tumour cells in every case. There was neovascular proliferation, giant cells, mitoses, bizarre nuclear hyperchromatism and, in four of seven cases, fibrosarcomatous changes.

It has been claimed that PET with [^{18}F]fluorodeoxyglucose is superior to CT for differentiation of necrosis and recurrent tumour (Patronas et al. 1982). Unfortunately, most neurological centres do not have access to this technique.

A persistent hindrance to the accurate comparison of abnormalities on serial imaging studies of any kind is the limited reproducibility of radiographic positioning. Numerous methods have been proposed, which will not be discussed here. With the increasing application of purpose-built stereotactic frames for use with CT, methods giving uniformity of positioning for a range of diagnostic and/or therapeutic manoeuvres would seem desirable. They include techniques such as the base plate with aluminium bars for head restraint, suitable for CT, angiography, pneumography, surgery and radiotherapy, described by the team at the Karolinska Sjukhuset in Stockholm (Boethius et al. 1980).

CT and Surgery

The cross-sectional data from CT have been used to facilitate biopsy of intracranial lesions, by techniques ranging from the essentially freehand (Moran et al. 1979) to formal stereotaxis (Rushworth 1980), by way of intermediate techniques using simple external markers placed on the skull (Maroon et al. 1977). Some surgeons have actually carried out craniotomies in the scanner room (Shalit et al. 1979), but the practical disadvantages of this procedure are self-evident.

The method used at the National Hospital for Nervous Diseases, described in detail by Anderson et al. (1983), has now been used successfully in 200 cases, predominantly hemisphere gliomas.

Cerebral Angiography

The period of almost 50 years during which angiography was used to diagnose cerebral tumours ended about 10 years ago, with the introduction of CT (Ambrose et al. 1975). Since then, angiography has been relegated to a supplementary role, confirming the diagnosis in problematic cases, occasionally resolving doubts as to the exact location of the tumour relative to the neuraxis, and demonstrating its blood supply and its relationship to major arteries and veins. More recently the possibilities of intra-arterial therapy have been explored (see below).

One of the first major reports on the use of angiography in the era of CT was that of Ambrose et al. (1975). Definite abnormalities were present in 89% of the tomograms of their patients with supratentorial gliomas, as compared with 75% of the angiograms. A comparison of the accuracy of clinical assessment, the electroencephalogram, CT and radionuclide studies with angiography in predicting the presence, the neoplastic nature and the specific diagnosis of supratentorial astrocytomas in a group of 40 patients also showed angiography still to be surpassed only by CT (Tans and de Jongh 1978). It may be argued that the demonstration of specific angiographic abnormalities may be of relevance to prediction of tumour type and grading. This aspect was investigated by Joyce et al. (1978). No astrocytomas of grades 1 and 2 showed abnormalities such as tumour vessels or early draining veins; an increased capillary blush (staining) was seen in only 10%. These abnormalities were also present in no more than one fifth of grade 2/3 tumours, but in 95% of glioblastomas at least one of these specific signs was present. However, the same proportion of these malignant gliomas were equally characteristic at CT.

These angiographic statistics are somewhat more polarised than those reported by other groups, probably because of the somewhat idiosyncratic categorisation of the tumours. Butler et al. (1979), for example, found pathological vascularity in 14% of grade 2 tumours, and in 78% of glioblastomas. Many workers have found angiography least useful when CT fails to give a definitive positive result. Thus, in a series of 250 cerebral gliomas seen at the National Hospital for Nervous Diseases, pathological circulation was visible in only one of the eight cases in which the non-invasive study failed to localise an infiltrating tumour (Claveria et al. 1978). In a subsequent review of 314 cases, 40 gliomas were found to have been misdiagnosed on initial CT data; angiography revealed the true nature of the lesion in less than one third of these, while in 30 patients with miscellaneous lesions misinterpreted as gliomas, angiography provided the answer in only seven (Kendall et al. 1979).

In a series of eight glioblastomas invisible (or overlooked) on CT examination, then revealed on follow-up studies from 3 to 9 months later, angiography was also negative in every case in which it was carried out at the time of the initial presentation. This was also true of radionuclide studies and, in four of five cases, the electroencephalogram (Bolender et al. 1983). These findings are in keeping with those of a review of all patients subjected to invasive neuroradiological procedures after normal CT (or a study showing generalised cerebral atrophy) during the first five years after introduction of this technique at the National Hospital for Nervous Diseases. No confirmed cerebral tumours were uncovered in this way (Tatler and Moseley 1982).

Most of the data relevant to diagnosis and treatment of cerebral tumours obtainable from conventional cerebral angiography are available from good-quality intravenous digital subtraction studies. Preliminary investigations indicate that more than half of suspected intracranial neoplasms can be examined in this way, with good or excellent results, and at greatly reduced discomfort, risk and cost to the patient (Takahash et al. 1983).

French workers have emphasised the desirability of stereotactic angiography for the precise pre-operative localisation of cerebral tumours.The methodology is rather complex, and the utility of the results *vis à vis* other stereotactic procedures, such as CT controlled biopsy, depends on very sophisticated computer manipulation of the three-dimensional data (Scarabin et al. 1975). As mentioned previously, the potential benefits to be derived from this approach entail all investigations and treatment being related to compatible stereotactic coordinates.

The use of angiography for the assessment of patients suspected of having recurrent cerebral tumours is complicated by the fact that the recurrence may have different angiographic characteristics from the original tumour. In one small series, in which tumours were classified simply as avascular or hypervascular, about one third failed to recur true to type; half of these were previously hypervascular lesions which recurred as avascular masses (Schreyer and Fueger 1978). This is clearly a potential source of diagnostic confusion.

Therapeutic Angiography

Intra-arterial methods of devascularising extracerebral tumours as a palliative, pre-operative or definitive therapeutic measure have been established for more than 10 years. Difficulties of access to the more distal cerebral vessels, together with the risks inherent in introduction of toxic or embolic materials into the vessels supplying normal brain, and uncertainty that devascularising gliomas would be useful, have combined to preclude treatment of intra-axial lesions.

Advances in catheterisation materials and techniques now permit fine, flow-guided catheters to be placed in second- or third-order branches of the cerebral arteries, offering the possibility of introducing chemotherapeutic agents (or even radioactive emboli) close to the tumour. Brismar et al. (1978) reported percutaneous intra-arterial chemotherapy (with mitomycin C) of lesions supplied by the external cartoid artery. Solid emboli of graduated size, fashioned from carnauba wax and capable of carrying and releasing similar agents, have been manufactured (Raziel et al. 1980). Trials of such methods in the treatment of gliomas are in progress, but their clinical utility has not yet been established.

Cerebral Pneumography

The introduction of CT sounded the death knell of ventriculography as a neuroradiological investigation. During one year following the installation of a scanner in a London regional neurosurgical centre, while the number of diagnostic angiograms was cut by 60%, that of pneumograms fell by 90% (Bartlett and Neil-Dywer 1978). With continued sophistication of the more modern technique, this trend has continued.

Certain indications for ventriculography in the assessment of cerebral tumours persisted: to obtain precise localisation of lesions near the ventricular system; information about attachment to or infiltration of the ventricular walls; clues as to their nature. Studies in Germany and Scandinavia, however, directed specifically at establishing the efficacy of ventriculography and CT in resolving these problems led to an identical conclusion: ventriculography no longer had a valid contribution (Wende et al. 1982, Nakstad et al. 1982).

Conclusions

X-ray computerised tomography, while not ideal, is more reliable than other conventional neuroradiological procedures for detection, characterisation, grading and management of cerebral tumours. Comparative studies with more sensitive or physiologically orientated techniques, although not feasible in routine management, may permit further refinement of the technique. The contribution of cerebral angiography is debatable.

References

Afra D, Norman D, Levin VA (1980) Cysts in malignant gliomas. J Neurosurg 53: 821-825

Ambrose J, Gooding MR, Richardson AE (1975) An assessment of the accuracy of computerised transverse axial scanning (EMIScanner) in the diagnosis of intracranial tumour. Brain 98: 569-582

Anderson RE, Thomas DGT, Du Boulay GH (1983) Radiological aspects of CT-guided stereotactic neurosurgical procedures. Neuroradiology 24: 163-166

Andreou J, George AE, Wise A, De Leon M, Kricheff II, Ransohoff J, Foo SH (1983) CT prognostic criteria of survival after malignant glioma surgery. AJNR 4: 488-490

Baker HL, Houser OW, Campbell JK (1980) National Cancer Institute study: evaluation of computed tomography in the diagnosis of intracranial neoplasms. I. Overall results. Radiology 136: 91-96

Barrington NA, Lewtas NA (1977) Indications for contrast medium enhancement in computed tomography of the brain. Clin Radiol 28: 535-537

Bartlett JR, Neil-Dwyer G (1978) A clinical study of the EMIScanner: Implications for provision of neuroradiological services. Br Med J ii: 813-815

Boethius J, Bergstrom M, Greitz T, Ribbe T (1980) CT localization in stereotaxic surgery. Appl Neurophysiol 43: 164-169

Bolender NF, Cromwell LD, Graves V, Margolis MT, Kerber CW, Wendling L (1983) Interval appearance of glioblastomas not evident on previous CT examination. J Comput Assist Tomogr 7: 599-605

Bradley WG, Waluch V, Yadley RA, Wycoff RR (1984) Comparison of CT and MR in 400 patients with suspected disease of the brain and cervical spinal cord. Radiology 152: 695-702

Brismar J, Bjorlund A, Elner A, Eneroth CM (1978) Selective intra-arterial cytostatic injection in malignant head and neck tumours. Neuroradiology 16: 434-437

Burger PC, Dubois PJ, Schold SC, Smith KR, Odom GL, Crafts DC, Giangaspero F (1983) Computerized tomographic and pathologic studies of the untreated, quiescent and recurrent glioblastoma multiforme. J Neurosurg 58: 159-169

Burrows EH (1976) Clinical reliability of posterior fossa scintigraphy. Clin Radiol 27: 473-481

Butler AR, Kricheff II (1978) Non-contrast CT scanning: Limited value in suspected brain tumour. Radiology 126: 689-693

Butler AR, Horii SC, Kricheff II, Shannon MB, Budzilovich GN (1978) Computed tomography in astrocytomas: A statistical analysis of the parameters of malignancy and the positive contrast-enhanced CT scan. Radiology 129: 433-439

Butler AR, Passalaqua AM, Bernstein A, Kricheff II (1979) Contrast enhanced CT scan and radionuclide brain scan in supratentorial gliomas. AJR 132: 607-611

Claveria LE, Du Boulay GH, Kendall BE (1978) The diagnostic limitations of computerised axial tomography in hemispheric tumours. In: Bories J (ed) The diagnostic limitations of computerised axial tomography. Springer-Verlag, Berlin, pp 2-16
Dubois PJ, Drayer BP, Heinz ER, Osborne D, Roberts L, Sage M (1981) Rapid serial cranial computed tomography for tumour diagnosis. Neuroradiology 21: 79-86
Du Boulay GH, Radue EW (1978) How should one investigate the posterior fossa? Neuroradiology 15: 253-261
Fasano VA, Ponzio RM, Liboni W, de Mattei M (1983) Preliminary experiences with 'real time' intraoperative ultrasonography associated to the laser and ultrasonic aspirator in neurosurgery. Surg Neurol 19: 318-323
Felgin DS, Welch DW, Siegel BA, James AE (1975) The efficacy of the brain scan in diagnosis of brain stem gliomas. Radiology 116: 117-120
Gooding GAW, Boggan JE, Bank WO, Beglin B, Edwards MSB (1981) Sonography of the adult brain through surgical defects. AJNR 2: 449-452
Graeb DA, Steinbok P, Robertson WD (1982) Transient early computed tomographic changes mimicking tumor irradiation. Radiology 144: 813-817
Han BK, Babcock DS, Oestreich AE (1984) Sonography of brain tumors in infants. AJR 143: 31-36
Hayman LA, Evans RA, Hinck VC (1980) Delayed high dose contrast computed tomography. Cranial neoplasms. Radiology: 677-684
Hillemacher A (1982) Der Wert amnestischer und klinischer Daten sowie apparativer Intersuchungsbefunde bei der Diagnose von Hirntumoren. Fortschr Neurol Psychiatr 50: 93-112
Hochberg FH, Pruitt A (1980) Assumptions in the radiotherapy of glioblastoma. Neurology 30: 907-911
Joyce P, Bentson J, Takahashi M, Winter J, Wilson G, Byrd S (1978) The accuracy of predicting histologic grades of supratentorial astrocytomas on the basis of computerized tomography and cerebral angiography. Neuroradiology 16: 346-348
Kazner E, Wende S, Grumme T, Lanksch W, Stochdorph O (1982) Computed tomography in intercranial tumours. Springer-Verlag, Berlin
Kendall BE, Jakubowski J, Pullicino P, Symon L (1979) Difficulties in diagnosis of supratentorial glioma by CAT scan. J Neurol Neurosurg Pyschiatr 42: 485-492
Knake JE, Chandler JE, McGillicuddy JE, Silver TM, Gabrielsen TO (1982) Intraoperative sonography for brain tumor localisation and ventricular shunt placement. AJR 139: 733-738
Latchaw RE, Gold LHA, Moore JS, Payne JT (1977) The nonspecificity of absorption coefficients in the differentiation of solid tumors and cystic lesions. Radiology 125: 141-145
Latchaw RE, Payne JT, Loewenstein RB (1980) Predicting brain tumor histology: Change of effective atomic number with contrast enhancement. AJR 135: 757-762
Levin VA, Crafts DC, Norman DM, Hoffer PB, Spire JP, Wilson CB (1977) Criteria for evaluating patients undergoing chemotherapy for malignant brain tumors. J Neurosurg 47: 329-335
Lewander R (1979) Contrast enhancement with time in gliomas. Acta Radiol [Diagn] 20: 689-702
Lewander R, Bergstrom M, Boethius J, Collins VP, Edner G, Greitz T, Willems J (1978) Stereotactic computer tomography for biopsy of gliomas. Acta Radiol [Diagn] 19: 867-888
Mahaley MS, Mitchell WG, Whaley R, Dudka L, Symons MJ (1983) The relative roles of neurological examination, functional abilities and computed tomography in the definition of treatment failure in patients with anaplastic gliomas. Surg Neurol 20: 297-300
Marcu H, Vonofakos D, Hacker H (1980) Characteristic CT signs in oligodendrogliomas. In Wackenheim A, Du Boulay GH (eds) Choices and characteristics in computerized tomography. Kugler, Amsterdam, pp 93-102
Maroon JC, Bank WO, Drayer BP, Rosenbaum AE (1977) Intracranial biopsy assisted by computerized tomography. J Neurosurg 46: 740-744
McCullough DC, Huang HK, De Michelle D, Manz HJ, Sinks LF (1979) Correlation between volumetric CT imaging and autopsy measurements of glioblastoma size. Comput Tomogr 3: 133-141
Mikhael MA (1978) Radiation necrosis of the brain: Correlation between computed tomography, pathology and dose distribution. J Comput Assist Tomogr 2: 71-80
Moran CJ, Naidich TP, Gado MH, Marchovsky JA (1979) Central nervous system lesions biopsied or treated by CT-guided needle placement. Radiology 131: 681-686
Moseley IF (1977) The use of contrast media as an adjunct to CT scanning. In Kuhler WJ (ed) Computer assisted tomography. Excerpta Medica, Amsterdam. pp 26-45
Nakstad P, Sortland O, Hovind K (1982) The evaluation of ventriculography as a supplement to computed tomography. Neuroradiology 23: 85-88
Norman D, Enzmann DR, Levin VA, Wilson CB, Newton TH (1976) Computed tomography in the evaluation of malignant glioma before and after therapy. Radiology 121: 85-88
Norman D, Stevens DA, Wing SD, Levin V, Newton TH (1978) Quantitative aspects of contrast

enhancement in cranial computed tomography. Radiology 129: 683–688
Patronas NJ, Di Chiro G, Brooks RA, De La Paz RL, Kornblith PL, Smith BH, Rizzoli HV, Kessler RM, Manning RG, Channing M, Wolf AP, O'Connor CM (1982) Work in progress: [^{18}F]fluoroxyglucose and positron emission tomography in the evaulation of radiation necrosis of the brain. Radiology 144: 885–889
Pullicino P, Thompson EJ, Moseley IF, Zilkha E, Shortman RC (1979) Cystic intracranial tumours. Cyst fluid, biochemical changes and computerised tomographic findings. J Neurol Sci 44: 77–85
Radue EW, Kendall BE (1978) Xenon enhancement in tumours and infarcts. Neuroradiology 16: 224–227
Raziel A, Puisieux F, Terracol D, Hoffman P, Cave G, Merland JJ, Bories J (1980) Wax microemboli tailored for therapeutic embolization. AJR 134: 404–405
Reeves GI, Marks JA (1979) Prognostic significance of lesion size for glioblastoma multiforme. Radiology 132: 469–471
Rieth KG, Di Chiro G, London WT, Sever JL, Houff SA, Kornblith PL, McKeever PE, Buonomo C, Padgett BL, Walker DL (1980) Experimental glioma in primates: A computed tomography model. J Comput Assist Tomogr 4: 285–290
Rushworth RG (1980) Stereotactic guided biopsy in the computerized tomographic scanner. Surg Neurol 13: 451–454
Scarabin JM, Pecker J, Simon J, Touzalain JC (1975) Stereotaxic angiography in cerebral tumors. In: Salamon G (ed) Advances in cerebral angiography. Inserm/Springer-Verlag, Berlin, pp 251–261
Schreyer H, Feuger GF (1978) Radiological detection of glioblastoma recurrence. Acta Neurochir 42: 127–132
Selker RG, Mendelow H, Walker M, Sheptak PE, Phillips JG (1982) Pathological correlation of CT ring in recurrent, previously treated gliomas. Surg Neurol 17: 251–254
Shalit MN, Israel Y, Matz S, Cohen ML (1979) Intra-operative computerized tomography. Surg Neurol 11: 382–384
Silverman C, Marks JE (1981) Prognostic significance of contrast enhancement in low-grade astrocytomas of the adult cerebrum. Radiology 139: 211–213
Sundaresan N, Galicich JH, Tomita T, Shapiro W, Krol G (1981) Computerized tomography findings in multifocal glioma. Acta Neurochir 59: 217–226
Tachibana H, Meyer JS, Rose JE, Prasab K (1984) Local cerebral blood flow and partition coefficients measured in cerebral astrocytomas of different grades of malignancy. Surg Neurol 21: 125–131
Takahash M, Hirota Y, Bussaka W, Tsuchigame T, Miyawaki M, Ueno S, Matsukado Y, Hirata Y (1983) Evaluation of prototype equipment for digital subtraction angiography in diagnosing intracranial lesions. AJNR 4: 259–262
Takeda N, Tanaka R, Yamakazi K (1980) Correlation of computed tomography with post-mortem histopathology of cerebral malignant glioma. Neurol Med Chir (Tokyo) 20: 603–611
Tans JTJ, de Jongh IE (1978) Computed tomography of supratentorial astrocytoma. Clin Neurol Neurosurg 80: 156–168
Tapias PL, Debaene A, Borrely P, Serrano R, Legré J (1978) An attempt at improvement of tissue diagnosis in brain tumours by the study of densities at CAT. In: Bories J (ed) The diagnostic limitations of computerised axial tomography. Springer-Verlag. Berlin, pp 29–39
Tatler GLV, Moseley IF (1982) Use of invasive neuroradiological investigations in patients with normal computerised tomography. Br Med J ii: 1026–1028
Taylor DG, Bore CF (1981) A review of the magnetic resonance responses of biological tissue and its applicability to the diagnosis of cancer by NMR radiology. CT: J Comput Tomogr 5: 122–134
Tchang S, Scotti G, Terbrugge K, Melançon D, Belanger G, Milner C, Ethier R (1977) Computerized tomography as a possible aid to histological grading of supratentorial gliomas. J Neurosurg 46: 735–739
Thomson JLG (1976) Computerised axial tomography and the diagnosis of glioma: A study of 100 consecutive histologically proven cases. Clin Radiol 27: 431–441
Weisberg LA (1980) Cerebral computer tomography in the diagnosis of supratentorial astrocytoma. Comput Tomogr 4: 87–105
Wende S, Kishikawa T, Heuwel N, Kazner E, Grumme T, Lanksch W (1982) Do we need ventriculography in the era of computed tomography? Neuroradiology 23: 89–90
Wulff JD, Proffitt PQ, Panszi JG, Ziegler DK (1982) False-negative CTs in astrocytomas: The value of repeat scanning. Neurology 32: 766–769
Yamashita T, Kawabara T (1983) Estimation of rate of growth of malignant brain tumours by computed tomography scanning. Surg Neurol 20: 464–470

4 Central Nervous System Tumours: Recent Developments in Magnetic Resonance Imaging

Graeme M. Bydder

Introduction

Interest in the use of magnetic resonance imaging (MRI) for the diagnosis of tumours was first stimulated over a decade ago by the in vitro observation of abnormal MR properties in rat tumours (Damadian 1971). The necessary concept for MRI was proposed soon afterwards in 1973 (Lauterbur 1973) and the appearance of tumours were first described in 1980 (Hawkes et al. 1980).

For many reasons the initial clinical emphasis on MRI in many centres has focused on the brain. A high level of grey/white matter contrast can be obtained with MRI which provides anatomical detail previously unavailable with other techniques. Coronal and sagittal imaging is particularly applicable to the brain and the absence of bone artefact in the posterior fossa is a major advantage over X-ray computerised tomography (CT). Flow effects are well demonstrated and the technique is sensitive to a variety of pathological changes within the brain (Bydder et al. 1982, Brant-Zawadski et al. 1983, Zimmerman et al. 1983, Bradley et al. 1984). The convergence of these two streams of thought—changes seen in vitro in tumours and the amenability of the brain to MRI—has stimulated considerable interest in the MR diagnosis of cerebral tumours. There has been great progress in this area over the last three years.

Both the general articles on MRI quoted above and recent more specific articles (McGinnis et al. 1983, Brant-Zawadski et al. 1984, Bydder et al. 1984) have covered the diagnosis of cerebral tumours in considerable detail and it is clear that MRI is likely to have an important role in this area. Rather than review all the last four years' work the emphasis here will be on the most recent developments. With a rapidly evolving field such as MRI obsolescence is a problem; for example the technique used to demonstrate tumours in 1980 was no longer being used in 1982.

Nevertheless certain patterns are emerging and many of the recent improvements in technique appear to be here to stay—although there is still a worry that a new sequence or some other technical advance will render obsolete everything to date. First the basic physics of MRI will be summarised and then the significant developments in the last year reviewed.

Instrumentation

All MRI machines are constructed around a large magnet which provides a uniform static magnetic field (Fig. 4.1). In the presence of this field hydrogen nuclei behave like tiny bar magnets. Their magnetisation is aligned with the static magnetic field producing a net proton magnetisation in the long axis of the patient. Additional perpendicular magnetic pulses are applied by means of a coil surrounding the patient. These pulses are used to rotate the nuclear magnetisation, following which it recovers or relaxes back to its original position. During this recovery or relaxation phase the component of the magnetisation in the long axis of the patient recovers exponentially to its original magnitude. This recovery is called longitudinal or spin-lattice relaxation and is characterised by the time constant T_1. Relaxation of the magnetisation in the transverse direction back to its original value of zero is termed tranverse relaxation or spin-spin relaxation and is characterised by the time constant

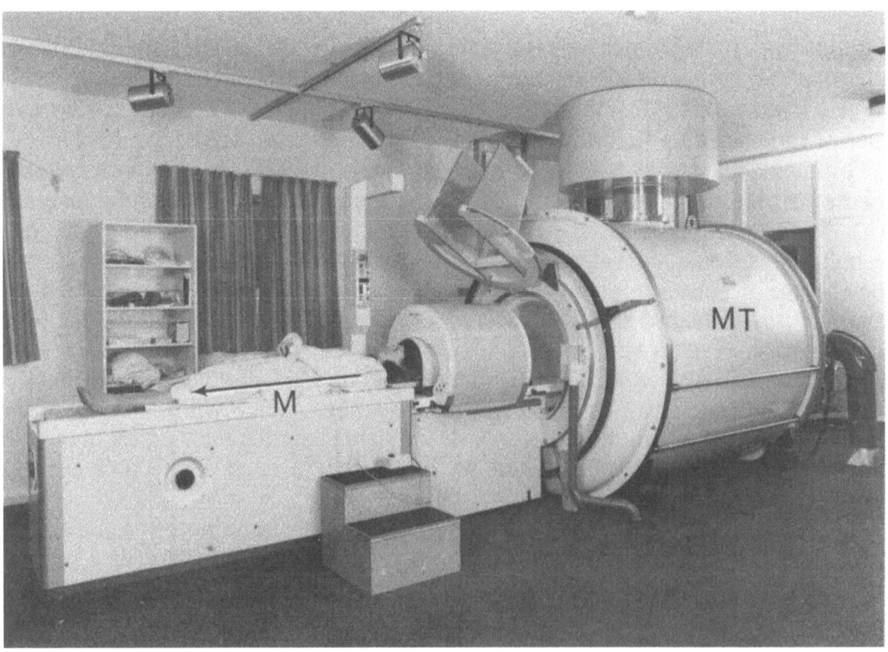

Fig. 4.1. An MR imaging machine. The machine is constructed around a large magnet (MT) which induces a net magnetisation (M) in the long axis of the patient.

T_2. As the magnetisation recovers it induces an electrical signal in a receiver coil which surrounds the patient. The electrical signal detected by this coil is known as the free induction decay and it is this signal which is used to reconstruct the image.

Longitudinal relaxation (T_1) depends on the interaction of protons with surrounding nuclei and molecules (the "lattice"), whereas transverse relaxation (T_2) depends on the interaction of protons with each other. Both T_1 and T_2 are sensitive indices of the local nuclear and molecular environment. NMR images are obtained using short magnetic pulses to perturb the patient's nuclear magnetisation, after which the electrical signal is detected: these pulse sequences are derived from classical spectroscopy and produce images with varying dependence on proton density (ϱ), T_1 and T_2.

Image Interpretation

Image interpretation has largely proceeded on an empirical basis. Increases in T_1 and T_2 are seen in a variety of pathological processes in which the water content of the lesion is increased, such as inflammation, oedema and many tumours. In contrast, a relative decrease in T_1 is seen in such conditions as acute haemorrhage, fatty lesions, fibrosis and pleural thickening. The change in T_1 or T_2 may be 200%–300% but is relatively non-specific. Specificity is usually derived from localisation and the clinical context.

The three sequences listed in Table 4.1 produce images with varying dependence on ϱ, T_1 and T_2. Saturation-recovery (SR) pulse sequences produce images whose contrast depends on proton density and T_1. An increase in proton density produces a lighter appearance on the grey scale, whereas an increase in T_1 produces a decrease in pixel values. Hence a lesion with a long T_1 has a dark appearance. Inversion-recovery (IR) pulse sequences also produce images whose contrast depends on proton density and T_1, but there is a stronger dependence on T_1. As with SR sequences an increase in T_1 produces a dark appearance. Spin-echo (SE) pulse sequences are more complex. Pixel values depend on proton density as with SR and IR sequences. They decrease with increasing T_1 but in addition increase with increasing T_2. In practice it is usual to choose SE sequences where the T_2 dependence

Table 4.1. Typical MRI pulse sequences

Pulse sequence	Duration of scan cycle (ms)	TI (ms)	TE[a] (ms)
Saturation-recovery (SR)			
SR_{1000}	1000		
SR_{2000}	200		
Inversion-recovery (IR)			
$IR_{n1400/400}$	1400	400	
$IR_{1500/500/44}$	1500	500	44
Spin-echo (SE)			
$SE_{544/44}$	544	44	
$SE_{1500/80}$	1500	80	

[a]TE, echo time.

is dominant. Hence lesions with a long T_2 appear lighter than surrounding tissue. The multivariable nature of MR images obtained with SR, IR and SE sequences means that it is not possible to use a simple grey scale as with CT images. It is possible to calculate T_1 and T_2 values for tissues and display these as T_1 and T_2 maps. These images are noisier than those from which they are derived but do not have the advantage that T_1 and T_2 values can be read off directly.

High-Resolution Imaging

Initial MR images were reconstructed onto a 64×64 or 128×128 matrix, but with improvements in machine design and coil design most manufacturers are now operating at 256×256 resolution. This provides the possibility of sub-millimetre resolution and makes available detail which previously appeared unattainable. This advance has been achieved by many small improvements rather than any radical change in concept or design.

Paramagnetic Contrast Agents

Most of the contrast apparent in MR images is a result of differences in the tissue relaxation times T_1 and T_2. Paramagnetic contrast agents offer the possibility of changing the T_1 and T_2 of tissues. The agents usually contain unpaired electrons of

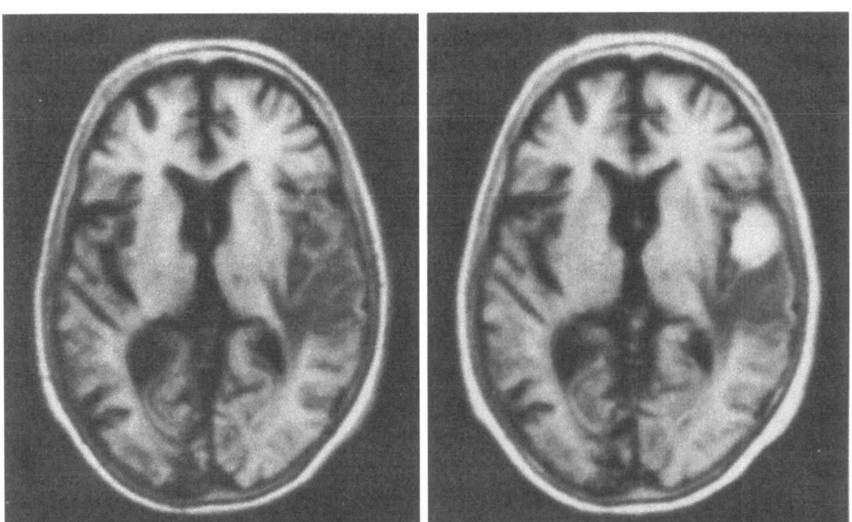

a b

Fig. 4.2. Breast metastasis before (**a**) and after (**b**) intravenous Gd-DTPA. There is marked enhancement of the tumour.

the metallic ions manganese, gadolinium or iron. The ions are chelated in order to reduce their toxicity. The first such compound used in clinical practice has been gadolinium-DTPA (Gd-DTPA) produced by Schering. It is injected intravenously, circulates in the vascular system and is excreted unchanged through the kidneys. It crosses the blood–brain barrier and then produces a decrease in T_1 and T_2 (Fig. 4.2). Its initial application has been in defining the abnormal blood–brain barrier in order to depict the margin between tumour and oedema (Carr et al. 1984). The results have been similar to those presently available with X-ray CT using iodinated contrast agents and so far no significant toxicity has been encountered. Prior to the use of this contrast agent lack of differentiation between tumour and oedema was a disadvantage of MRI in relation to contrast-enhanced CT (Bydder et al. 1982), although improved results have been obtained by using slower variants of the SE sequence. Gd-DTPA has produced enhancement in areas of apparent oedema surrounding tumour in 4 of 17 cases of malignant tumour (Graif et al. 1985). This sign may indicate more extensive tumour infiltration than shown on the unenhanced scans.

Recognition of Short T_1, Short T_2 Tumours

Although Damadian initially drew attention to the increased T_1 and T_2 of animal tumours (Damadian 1971), in a later paper (Damadian et al. 1973) he also noted that malignant melanoma metastases may produce a decrease in T_1 relative to normal tissue (Fig. 4.3). Since that time a much wider variety of circumstances have been recognised in which the T_1 and T_2 of tumours are not elevated. This has been important in establishing diagnostic strategies and in the choice of sequences both for screening purposes and in order to provide more specific information about the tumour.

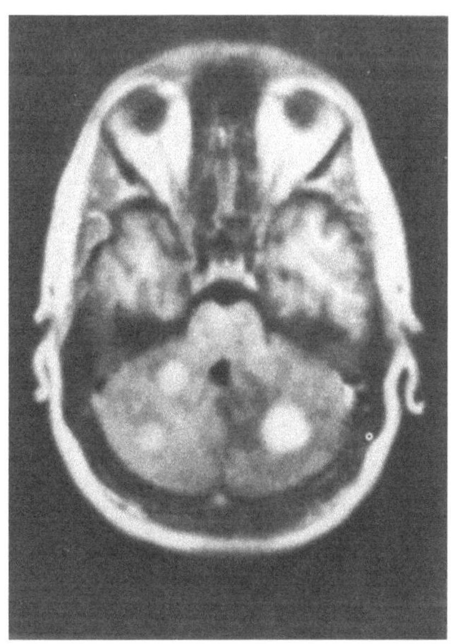

Fig. 4.3. Malignant melanoma. The tumour has a short T_1 with the signal intensity greater than that of white matter.

In some circumstances, such as in lipomas and dermoid tumours, the presence of fat would reasonably be expected to produce a short T_1 and this has been noted by several authors (Fig. 4.4). Following radiotherapy we have seen the T_1 of a tumour shorten to within normal range for grey matter (Fig. 4.5).

The reason why malignant melanomas have a short T_1 is uncertain. This may be due to the presence of melanin or haemorrhage within the tumour. In other tumours, such as metastases from carcinoma of the breast, haemorrhage can be associated with a decreased T_1. A number of benign tumours, including meningiomas and acoustic neuromas, may also have T_1 and T_2 values within the normal range.

There is also a group of tumours where the reason for the decreased T_1 and T_2 is unclear. In our experience the most striking example of this phenomenon was a metastatic carcinoma of the rectum. Histology of this lesion showed no distinctive features accounting for the MR appearance.

If such tumours are associated with oedema the latter may indicate the margin of the tumour, but with benign tumours oedema is not always obvious. Two groups have so far reported that contrast-enhanced X-ray CT generally demonstrated meningiomas better than unenhanced MR (Bradley et al. 1984, Zimmerman 1984). The use of IR sequences may improve results since short T_1, short T_2 tumours frequently have a decreased proton density and the small contribution to difference in contrast produced by the slightly increased T_1 is additive with the IR sequence.

The other approach to this problem is the use of Gd-DTPA, and initial results in meningioma with this agent demonstrate a high level of contrast enhancement (Fig. 4.6).

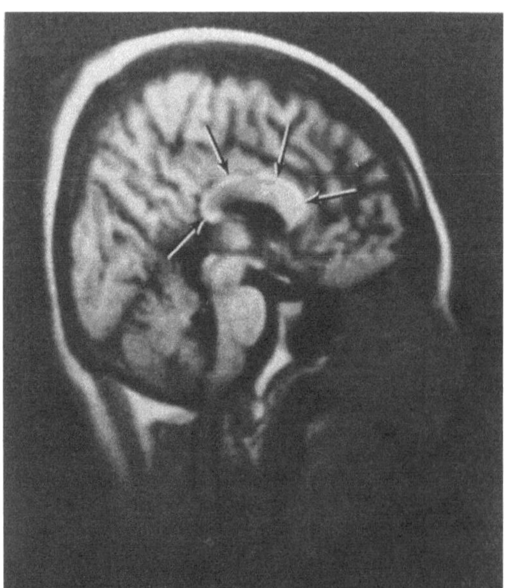

Fig. 4.4. Lipoma of the corpus callosum. The tumour (arrows) surrounds the partially atrophic corpus callosum.

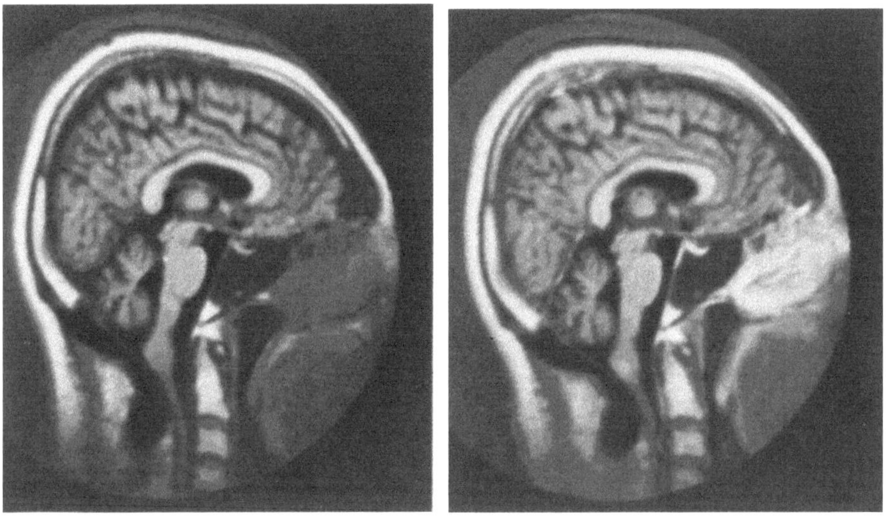

a b

Fig. 4.5. Astrocytoma grade I before **(a)** and after **(b)** Gd-DTPA. The tumour shows slight enhancement (grey).

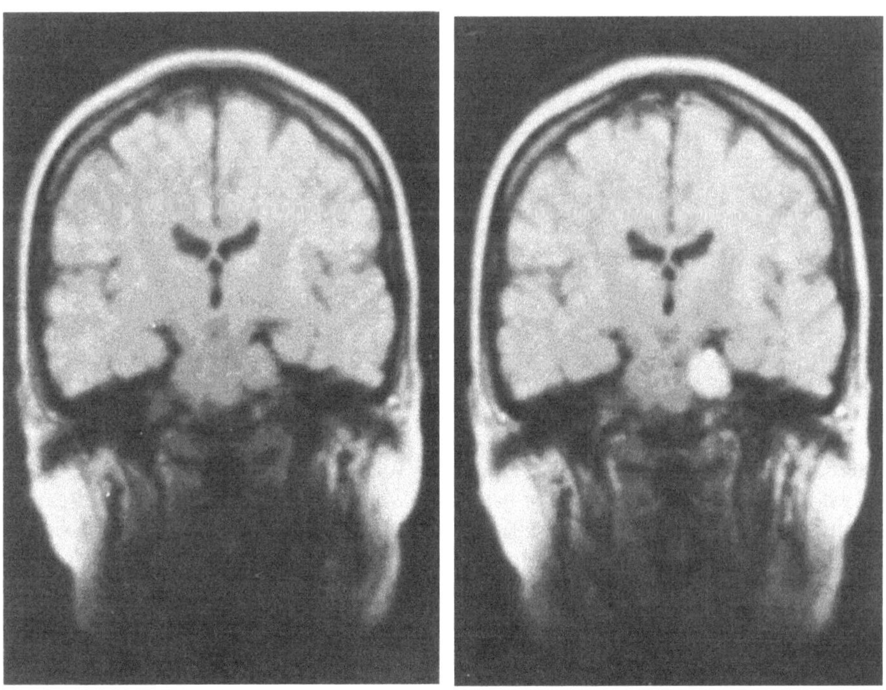

a b

Fig. 4.6. Meningioma before **(a)** and after **(b)** intravenous Gd-DTPA. The tumour is well seen and there is marked contrast enhancement.

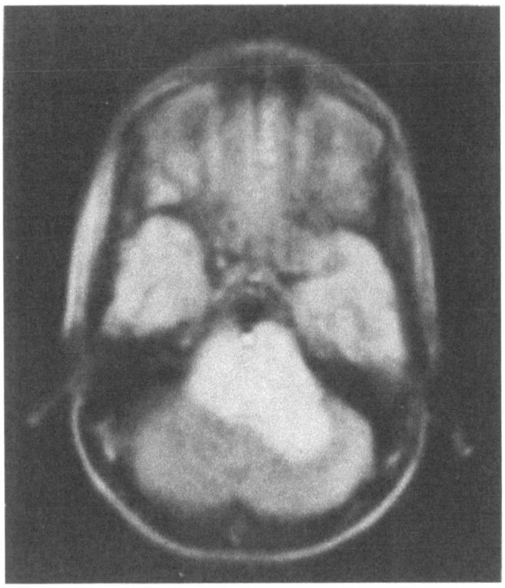

Fig. 4.7. Brain stem glioma in a one-year-old child.

Paediatric Tumours

The normal neonatal and infant brain is notable for its increased water content which produces an increase in T_1 and T_2 relative to the values found in adults. Over the first two years of life the water content of the brain drops and this is associated with a decrease in T_1. Another important change during this period is the process of myelination; this is most active during the first two years of life and then plateaus, but continues into the second decade.

The pattern of tumours seen in infants is different from adults and so is the appearance of the surrounding brain. Nevertheless it has so far proved possible to use MRI to detect tumours in this age group with a high degree of accuracy (Peterman et al. 1984) (Fig. 4.7).

Stereotactic Biopsy

A stereotactic frame suitable for use in biopsy has recently been described (Leksell et al. 1985). Frames of this type have been used with CT for several years and can be modified for use with MRI by suitable substitution of all ferromagnetic components; avoiding closed conducting loops which may have currents induced in them; and using appropriate materials (such as Gd-DTPA solution) for the marking artefacts.

We have used such a system modified from the Brown–Trent–Wells CT system and have been able to perform stereotactic MRI-guided biopsies (Fig. 4.8). This system promises to be useful in performing MRI-guided biopsies on lesions not seen with X-ray CT.

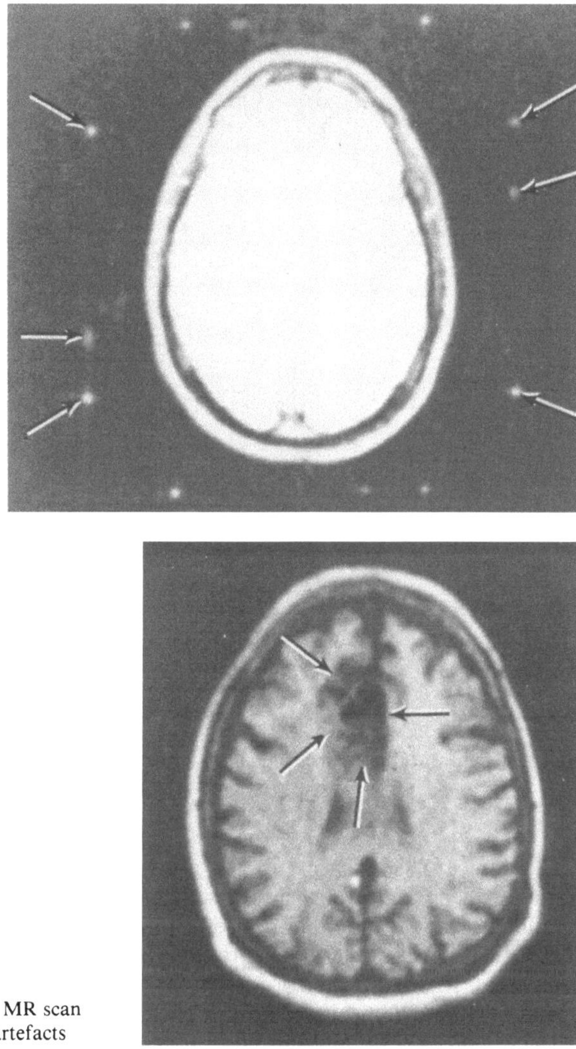

a

b

Fig. 4.8. Low-grade astrocytoma: MR scan displayed to show: (**a**) stereotactic artefacts (arrows) and (**b**) tumour (arrows).

Spinal Cord

Over the last year surface coils have been used for imaging of the spinal cord with a useful improvement in image quality. They have previously been used extensively in spectroscopy but their introduction into imaging has been recent. The images produced by surface coils are restricted to a smaller area than those obtained with full-size coils and usually display a gradient in signal intensity making them more difficult to interpret than the standard images. Nevertheless they are useful for a small number of applications involving fairly superficial structures. Fortunately the spinal cord is within their range and the results in the cervical cord have been good, although there is not such a pronounced advantage in the thoracic cord.

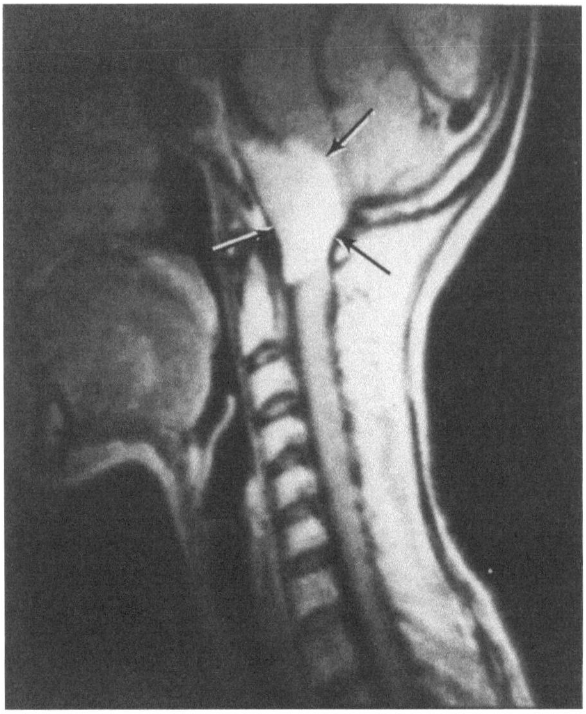

Fig. 4.9. Contrast-enhanced meningioma at the foramen magnum. The tumour is highlighted (arrows).

The choice of sequences for the cord is different from that for the brain. For example, using relatively simple sequences to demonstrate whether the cord is expanded or not is much more useful than the corresponding exercise in the brain. There are also techniques to ensure that the signal from cerebrospinal fluid is greater or less than that from the cord itself.

Another important consideration is that the alternative to MRI is myelography (with or without CT), and this latter investigation cannot really be classified as non-invasive. The situation is different from that in the brain where X-ray CT and MRI are usually regarded as about equally invasive. MRI also provides a technique for recognising intramedullary disease where the spinal cord is not expanded. Image quality is now satisfactory and the demonstration of tumours in the cervical and thoracic cord has been good. All eight spinal cord tumours we have so far imaged before and after use of Gd-DTPA have shown enhancement (Fig. 4.9).

The Orbit

Surface coils have been useful in demonstrating the orbit (Fig. 4.10) and conventional techniques are useful in demonstrating lesions in the optic nerve and optic tract (Fig. 4.11).

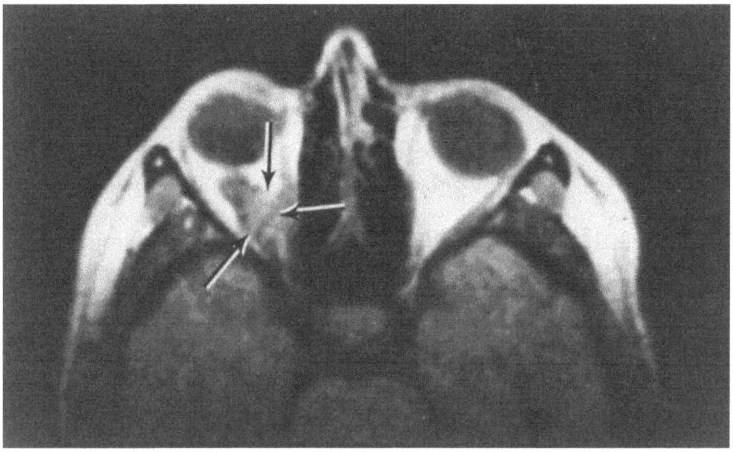

Fig. 4.10. Meningioma of the optic nerve. The tumour is well displayed (arrow).

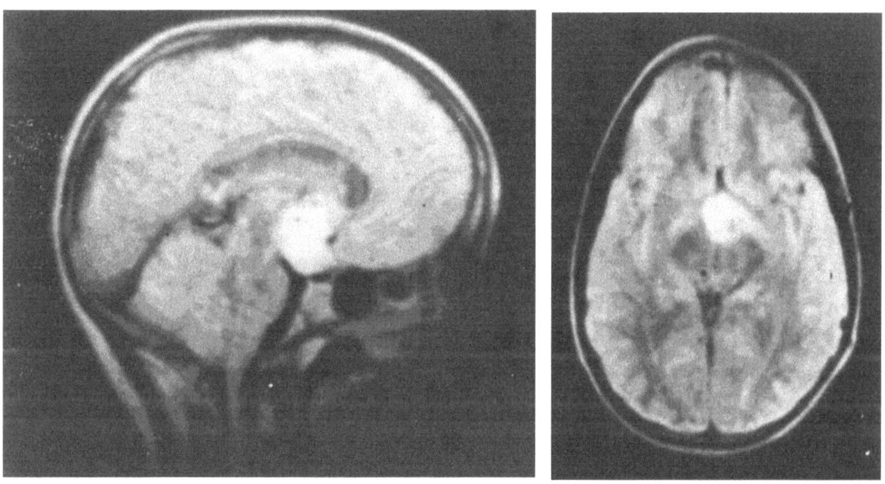

a b

Fig. 4.11. Optic nerve glioma. The tumour is seen in the sagittal plane **(a)** and extends along the optic tract **(b)**.

Future Developments and Summary

The advantages of MRI of posterior fossa tumours have been recognised relatively quickly, but even in the supratentorial compartment it has a useful role in showing the extent of pathological change and in locating tumours where only the mass effect or hydrocephalus is seen with X-ray CT.

The paramagnetic contrast agent gadolinium-DPTA (Gd-DTPA) has been used in clinical practice over the last year with useful results, particularly in distinguishing tumour from oedema. More clinical situations are now being recognised in which relaxation times of tumours are not increased. The use of closely coupled coils has resulted in improved image quality particularly with the spinal cord. Stereotactic frames suitable for MRI are now being used in clinical practice. MRI continues to evolve rapidly although how long the present rate of development can continue remains an open question.
There remains a great deal of work to be done in establishing optimum dose, sequence and time of administration of Gd-DTPA and it will be some years before its efficacy as an MRI contrast agent becomes clear.

References

Bradley WG, Waluch V, Yadley RA, Wycoff RR (1984) Comparison of CT and MRI in 400 patients with suspected disease of the brain and cervical spinal cord. Radiology 152: 695–702
Brant-Zawadski M, Davis PL, Crooks LE et al. (1983) NMR demonstration of cerebral abnormalities: Comparison with CT. AJR 140: 847–854
Brant-Zawadski M, Badami JP, Mills CM, Norman D, Newton TH (1984) Primary intracranial tumour imaging: A comparison of magnetic resonance and CT. Radiology 150: 435–440
Bydder GM, Steiner RE, Young IR, Hall AS, Thomas DJ, Marshall J, Pallis CA, Legg NJ (1982) Clinical NMR imaging of the brain: 140 cases AJR 139: 215–236
Bydder GM, Pennock JM, Steiner RE et al. (1984) The NMR diagnosis of cerebral tumors. J Mag Res Med 1: 5–29
Carr DH, Brown J, Bydder GM et al. (1984) Intravenous chelated gadolinium as a contrast agent in NMR imaging of cerebral tumours. Lancet I: 484–486
Damadian R (1971) Tumour detection by nuclear magnetic resonance. Science 171: 1151–1153
Damadian R, Zaner K, Hor D (1973) Brain tumours by NMR. Physiol Chem 5: 381–402
Graif M, Bydder GM, Niendorf H-P, Thomas DGT, Young IR (1985) Magnetic resonance imaging of malignant tumours with contrast enhancement. AJR (in press)
Hawkes RC, Holland GN, Moore WS, Worthington BS (1980) Nuclear magnetic resonance (NMR) tomography of the brain: A preliminary clinical assessment with demonstration of pathology. J Comput Assist Tomogr 4: 577–586
Lauterbur P (1973) Image formation by induced local interactions: Examples employing nuclear magnetic resonance. Nature 242: 190–191
Leksell L, Leksell D, Schwekel J (1985) Stereotaxis and nuclear magnetic resonance. J Neurol Neurosurg Psychiatr 48: 14–18
McGinnis BD, Brady TJ, New PFJ et al. (1983) Nuclear magnetic resonance (NMR) imaging of tumours in the posterior fossa. J Comput Assist Tomogr 7: 575–582
Peterman SB, Steiner RE, Bydder GM (1984) MR imaging of intracranial tumours in children and adolescents. AJNR 5: 703–709
Zimmerman RA, Bilaniuk LT, Goldberg HI et al. (1983) Cerebral NMR imaging: Early results with a 0.12T resistive system. AJR 141: 1187–1198
Zimmerman RA (1984) MRI in intracranial meningiomas (Abstr). Society of Magnetic Resonance in Medicine Abstracts, p. 779 (Presented at the Third Annual Meeting, New York, 15–17 August 1984)

5 Functional Aspects of Human Brain Tumours as Studied by Positron Emission Tomography

Ronald P. Beaney

Introduction

Positron emission tomography (PET) is not just another imaging device; it provides us with a unique opportunity to measure regional cerebral function in a virtually non-invasive fashion. PET does not compete with conventional computerised tomography (CT) or magnetic resonance imaging (MRI) for the anatomical localisation of a lesion but rather complements these other techniques by providing additional information on regional tissue blood flow and a variety of physiological and metabolic processes.

The whole concept of PET is based on two requirements. The first is the administration of biological tracers labelled with short-lived, cyclotron-produced, positron-emitting radionuclides. The second prerequisite is a detector system or imaging device: the positron computed tomograph.

Some of the radionuclides employed, along with their tracer forms and applications, are given in Table 5.1. The radionuclides used are those of the common biological elements (carbon, nitrogen and oxygen). There is no positron-emitting isotope of hydrogen so fluorine-18, which behaves in a similar fashion, is used in its place. These radionuclides decay by emitting positrons (positive electrons) that travel a few millimetres in soft tissue before being captured by a negative electron; both particles then disappear and are replaced by two 0.51 MeV photons (annihilation radiation) given off at approximately 180° to each other. It is the coincidence detection of these paired photons, if and when they are emitted from the body, that forms the basis of PET. An important fact that separates PET from other radionuclide imaging procedures is the ability to correct for the loss of signal caused by tissue attenuation. The PET system collects the data, sorts it, and processes it through a reconstruction algorithm. This then ultimately provides us with the true spatial distribution of the radioactive tracer in a transaxial slice of the brain in

Table 5.1. Some of the radionuclides used in PET and their applications

Radionuclide	Physical half-life (min)	Labelled tracer	Application
Oxygen-15	2.07	$C^{15}O_2$	Blood flow
		$H_2{}^{15}O$	Blood flow
		$N_2{}^{15}O$	Blood flow
		$^{15}O_2$	Oxygen utilisation
		$C^{15}O$	Blood volume
Carbon-11	20.4	^{11}CO	Blood volume
		2-[^{11}C]deoxyglucose	Glucose utilisation
		[^{11}C]glucose	Glucose utilisation
		[^{11}C]methylglucose	Glucose transport
		^{11}C-labelled amino acids	Amino acid uptake/protein incorporation
		$^{11}CO_2$	Cerebral pH
Nitrogen-13	10.00	$^{13}NH_3$	$^{11}NH_3$ uptake/blood flow
		^{13}N-labelled amino acids	Amino acid uptake/protein synthesis
Rubidium-82	1.25	$^{82}RbCl$	Blood–brain barrier integrity
Fluorine-18	110.00	^{18}F-labelled 2-deoxy-D-glucose	Glucose utilisation

absolute units (Bq/ml). The patient set-up and details of the PET scanner in both emission mode (i.e. detecting the paired photons given off from the tracer in the tissues) and transmission mode (i.e. measuring the regional tissue attenuation coefficients by employing an external ring of the positron emitter, germanium-68) are given in Fig. 5.1. The regional tissue attenuation coefficients are derived by performing a transmission scan first with nothing but air between the detectors and then with the patient positioned on the scanner. The transmission data are required to correct for the effects of tissue attenuation.

Fig. 5.1. a The patient set-up for PET, showing the cyclotron, radiochemist, scanner and on-line computer.

b The PET in emmission mode, showing the principle of PET data collection. Two opposing sodium iodide detectors are arranged so that the annihilation radiation can be registered (coincidence detection). The sources of background noise arising from random and scattered coincidences are shown. Each detector is in possible coincidence with 11 detectors in the opposite face of the hexagonal array. A total of 363 coincidence line pairs can be accepted at any one time.

c This diagram shows how, as a result of the fan beam geometry of the recording coincidence line pairs, increased data sampling is obtained within the thickest part of the object being scanned relative to its edge. This design feature ensures that the maximal statistical recording is achieved in the part of the tissue where superimposition of signal and tissue attenuation is greatest.

d Diagram showing the PET scanner in transmission mode. The ring source of the long-lived positron-emitting isotope (germanium/gallium-68) which is housed in the machine head is exposed during the transmission scan. The data obtained are then used to correct for the loss of signal brought about by tissue attenuation.

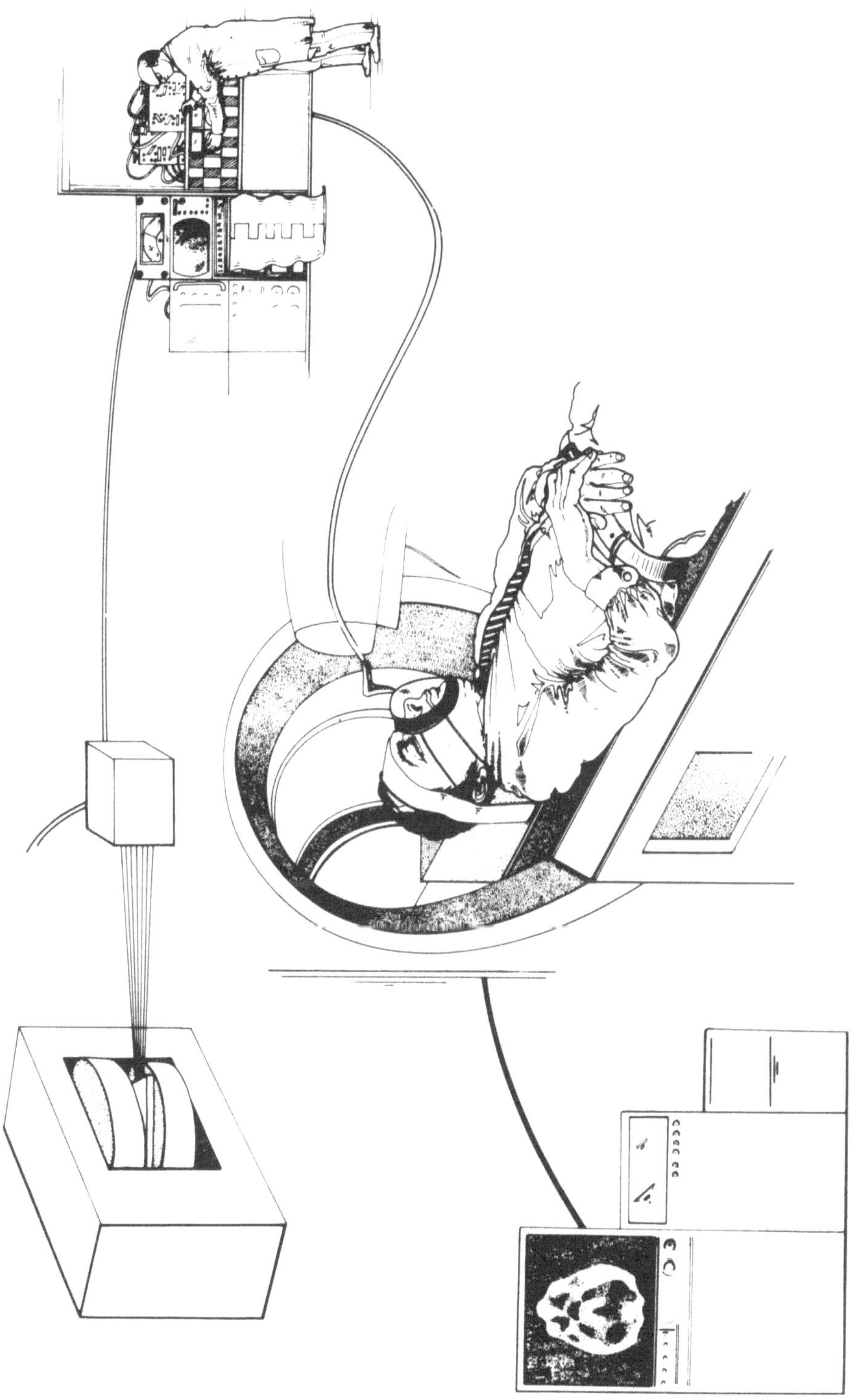

Fig. 5.1. a

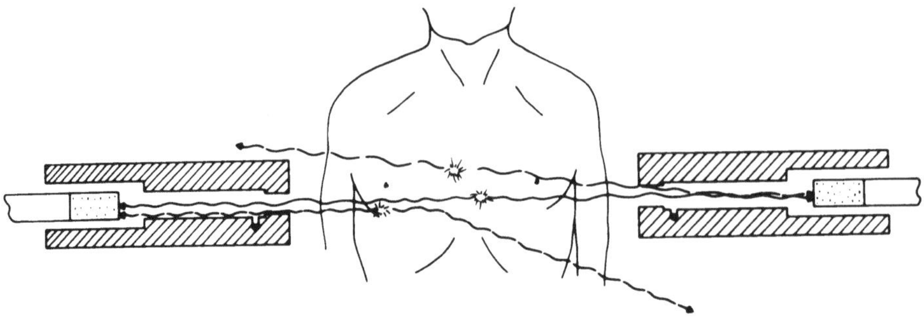

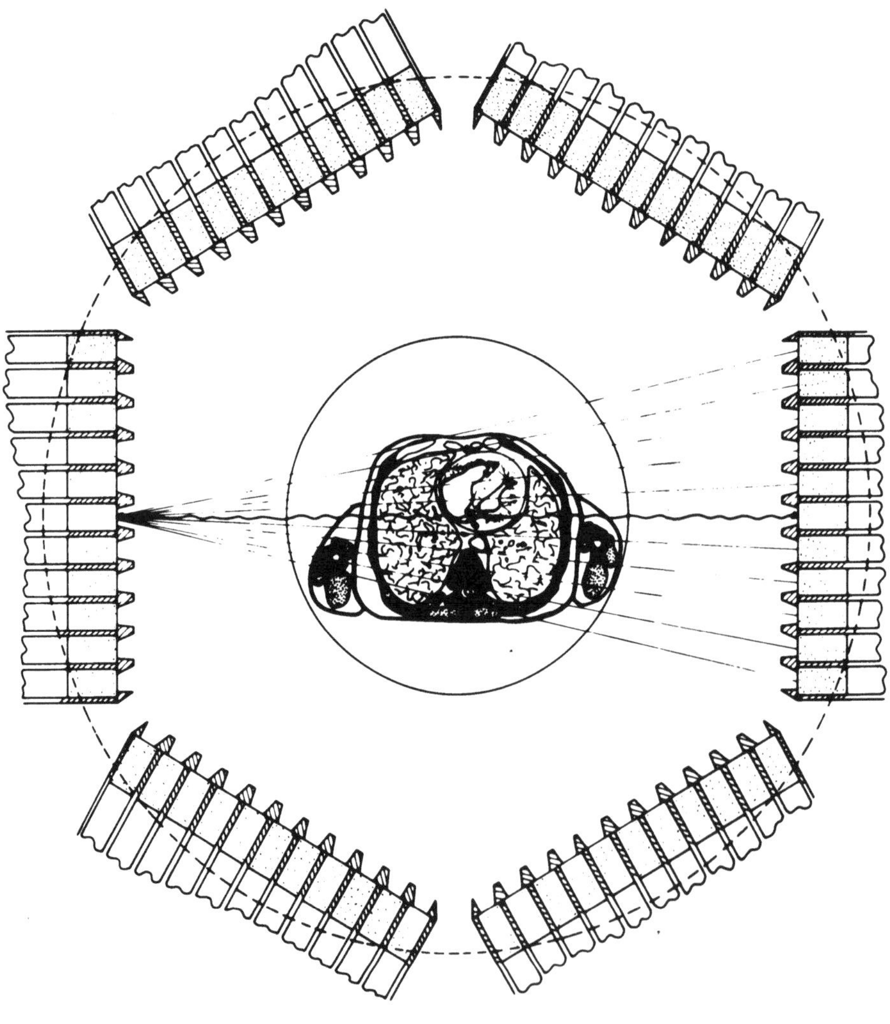

Fig. 5.1. b

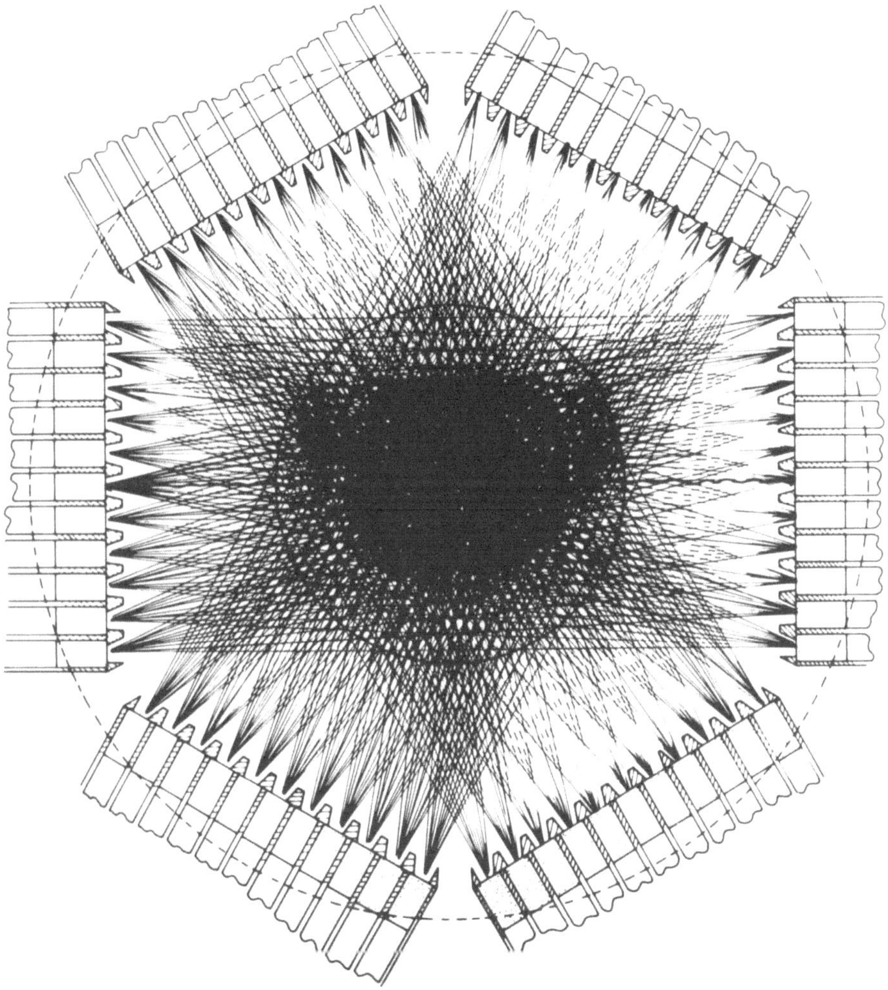

Fig. 5.1. c

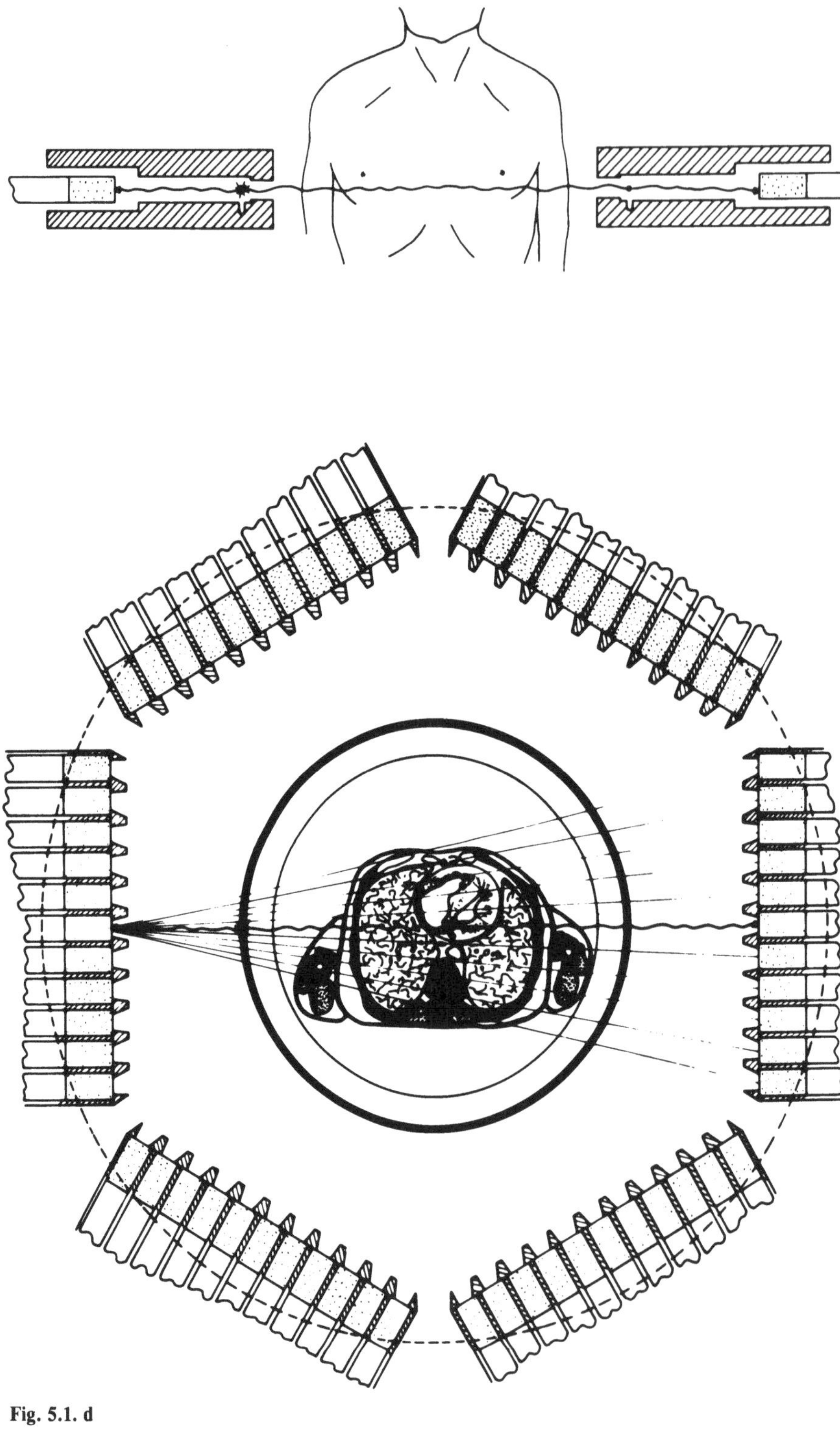

Fig. 5.1. d

Tracer kinetic models that accurately describe the fate of a tracer provide the basis for the derivation of operational equations. To solve these tracer equations knowledge of the regional tissue concentration of the tracer (using PET) and the concentration of the tracer in the blood is necessary. To measure the latter, blood is withdrawn during the scan and tracer concentration measured in a cross-calibrated well counter. This in turn allows the physiological process under investigation to be measured in absolute units and displayed in a tomographic fashion. PET has rather accurately been described as in vivo quantitative autoradiography. A general review article on the use of PET in the study of cerebral function has been written by Phelps et al. (1982). It is important to remember that due to the resolution of the scanner used, the values given for tissue function are really mean values for a volume of tissue no less than 5 cm^3. With the new generation of scanners becoming available it is now realistic to talk in terms of a volume of 1 cm^3. The data presented here were obtained using an ECAT II scanner (EG and G Ortec, Oakridge, Tennessee) (Williams et al. 1979). The resolution of this scanner is 17 mm × 17 mm × 17 mm (full width half maximum).

The values quoted for tissue function then, are mean values for all the cells lying within a volume of several cubic centimetres. If one remembers that some brain tumours have quite marked heterogeneity and that the grade of the tumour is classified with respect to its most anaplastic part, then the limitation of the technique is evident. The values given for "cortex" are lower than one would expect from pure grey matter. This is due principally to the unavoidable inclusion of some white matter in the "cortical" region of interest.

Cerebral Blood Flow and Oxygen Metabolism

The data on cerebral blood flow and oxygen utilisation in this chapter were obtained using the oxygen-15 steady-state inhalation technique. This was originally described by Jones et al. (1976), extended by Frackowiak et al. (1980) and adapted by Lammertsma (Lammertsma and Jones 1983, Lammertsma et al. 1983a). In brief the sequential inhalation of $C^{15}O_2$ and $^{15}O_2$ allows the measurement of regional cerebral blood flow (rCBF), regional cerebral oxygen utilisation ($rCMRO_2$), and the relationship between the two, called the regional oxygen extraction ratio (rOER). Inhalation of a tracer amount of ^{11}CO, which labels the red cell mass, permits measurement of cerebral blood volume (rCBV).

Normal Brain

In the normal brain, rCBF and $rCMRO_2$ are higher in grey matter than in white matter (Fig. 5.2). The fractional extraction of oxygen (OER) is normally similar in grey and white matter (normal range 0.35–0.48). In other words, about 40% of the oxygen delivered to the normal brain is extracted. If one looks upon $rCMRO_2$ as the demand for oxygen and rCBF as oxygen supply, then in normal brain there is a close coupling or matching between supply and demand. This relationship is reflected in a featureless OER image. Table 5.2 gives mean values for CBF, OER and $CMRO_2$ for

Table 5.2. Normal values for cerebral blood flow and oxygen utilisation determined by PET in normal volunteers

	Grey matter	White matter
Blood flow, CBF (ml/100 ml per min)	41.8 ± 4.5	23.7 ± 9.0
Oxygen extraction ratio, OER	0.423 ± 0.078	0.399 ± 0.007
Oxygen utilisation, $CMRO_2$ (ml O_2/100 ml per min)	3.03 ± 0.04	1.63 ± 0.31
Blood volume, CBV (ml/100 ml)	3.75 ± 0.47	2.49 ± 0.27

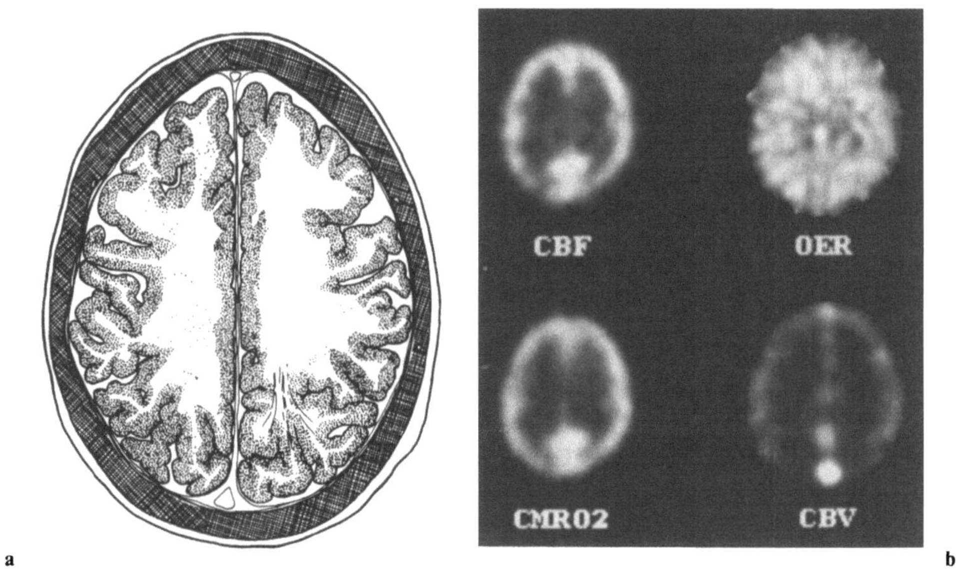

Fig. 5.2. a Diagram of normal brain 6.5 cm above and parallel to the orbitomeatal line, showing the ribbon of cortex and white matter of the centrum semiovale.
b All PET images in this chapter are represented by a grey scale where white is the high value and black lowest. PET images taken through the same plane showing the close matching between rCBF and $rCMRO_2$. The rOER image is homogeneous, indicating that the fraction of oxygen being extracted from the blood supplying the cortex is the same as that supplying white matter. The sagittal sinus is clearly visible on the CBV image.

a group of normal volunteers whose ages ranged from 25 to 75 years. There is evidence to suggest that cortical rCBF declines with age. Some workers have also found a gradual decrease in cortical $rCMRO_2$ with age but this has not been confirmed by other groups (Frackowiak et al. 1984).

Ischaemic Brain

In underperfused, but otherwise normal brain where rCBF (oxygen supply) is low but $rCMRO_2$ (demand for oxygen) is normal a raised OER is found. In ischaemic

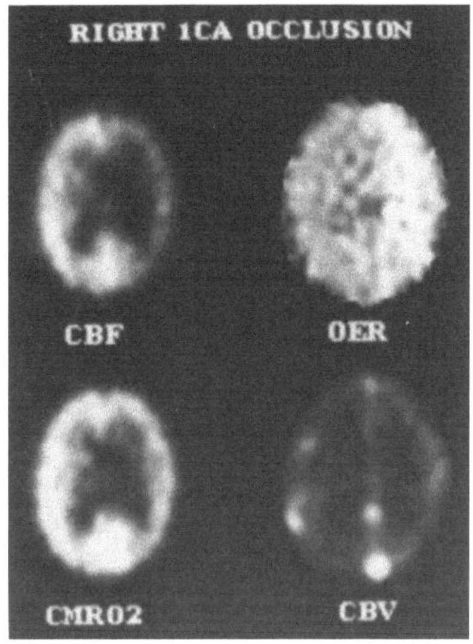

Fig. 5.3. PET rCBF, rOER, $rCMRO_2$ and rCBV images of a patient with right internal carotid occlusion. In spite of the raised OER, the reduction in rCBF has been severe enough to cause cellular death in the affected cortex with a resultant fall in $rCMRO_2$.

brain where blood flow is insufficient to meet local metabolic demands the raised OER will still not deliver enough oxygen to the tissues and cell death occurs with a resultant fall in oxygen demand ($rCMRO_2$). This is shown in Fig. 5.3.

Primary Cerebral Tumours

Figure 5.4(a) shows an X-ray CT scan of a patient with a grade 3 astrocytoma of the left frontal region, and Fig. 5.4(b) the CBF, OER, $CMRO_2$ and CBV PET images taken through the same plane. It shows that both blood flow and oxygen utilisation in the tumour were lower than in the corresponding region of the contralateral brain. This low demand for oxygen, which has characterised every brain tumour studied, is reflected in a low rOER.

Fig. 5.5 shows both CT and PET images of a patient with an enormous grade 4 astrocytoma of the left frontal region. From the PET images it can be seen that blood flow in this tumour was considerably higher than that in the normal surrounding brain. Oxygen utilisation in the tumour, however, was lower than that in contralateral brain.

Quantitative data from a group of 12 patients are given in Fig. 5.6. It can be seen that rCBF in tumour tissue is variable; the mean value for this group of patients lay close to the mean value for contralateral white matter. Within some very large high-grade tumours, however, rCBF may vary from virtually zero (in cystic and necrotic regions) to values in excess of that for normal grey matter. Oxygen utilisation by cerebral tumours is normally lower than that of normal brain.

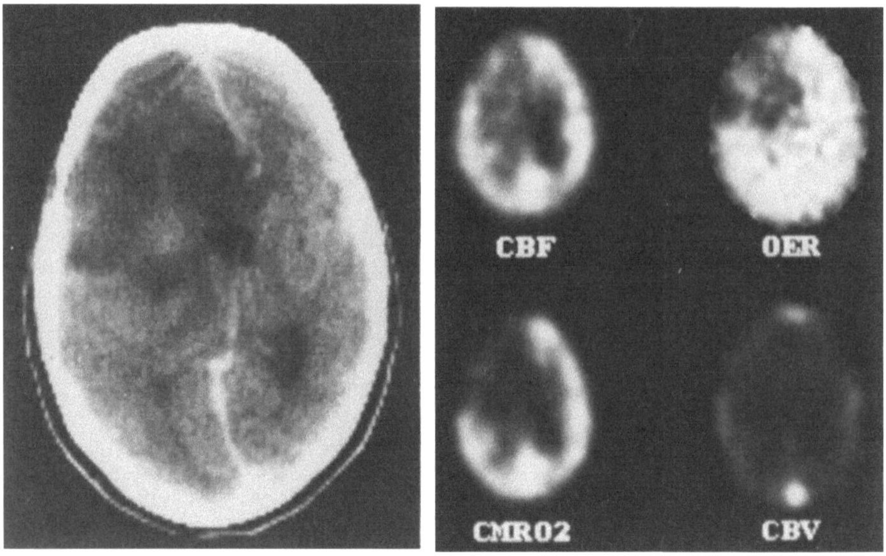

a b

Fig. 5.4. a X-ray CT scan of a patient with a grade 3 astrocytoma of the left frontal region. **b** PET CBF, OER, $CMRO_2$ and CBV images through the same plane as in **a** showing the lower CBF and $CMRO_2$ in the region of the tumour.

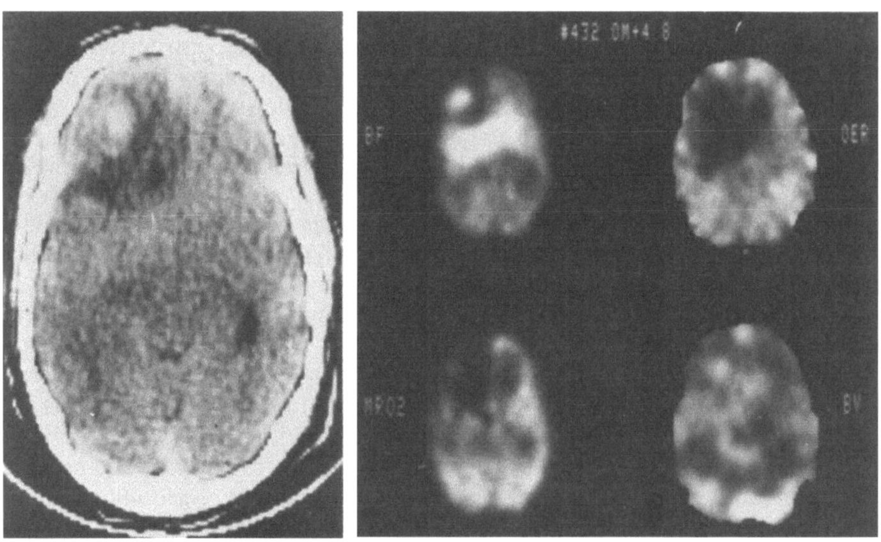

a b

Fig. 5.5. a CT scan of a patient with an enormous grade 4 astrocytoma of the left frontal region. **b** PET CBF, OER, $CMRO_2$ and CBV images taken through the same plane as in **a** showing an increased blood flow through the tumour but low oxygen utilisation.

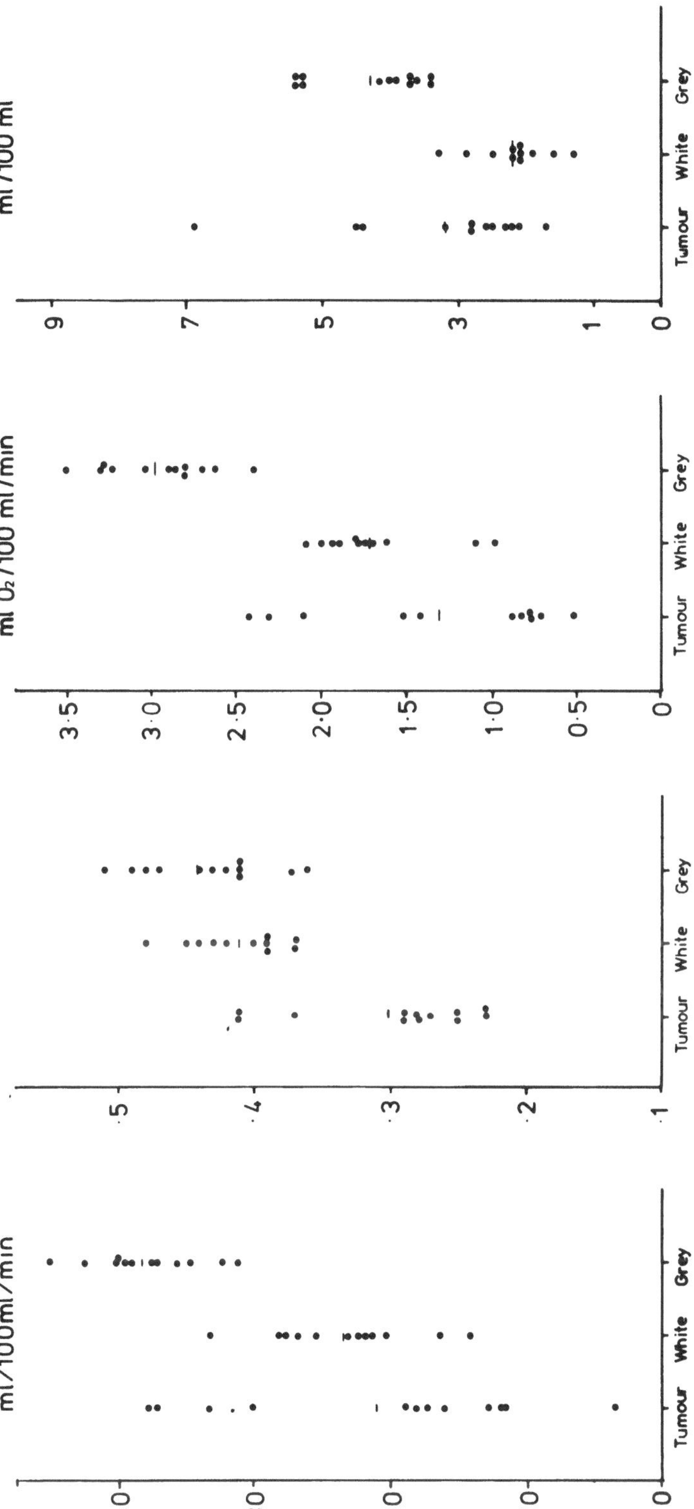

Fig. 5.6. Quantitative data from a group of 12 brain tumour patients. CBF, OER, $CMRO_2$ and CBV values for the tumour were compared with representative values for contralateral white and grey matter. In one patient an area of representative white matter was not obtainable.

The Remote Effects of an Intracranial Neoplasm

Intracranial tumours may profoundly affect the physiology of both near and distant parts of the brain. Thus a reduction in both rCBF and $rCMRO_2$ has been recorded in areas of peritumour oedema (Lammertsma et al. 1984). Physiological changes have also been recorded in areas of cortex remote from the tumour (Lammertsma et al. 1983b, 1984). Ito et al (1982) demonstrated a depression of both rCBF and $rCMRO_2$ in the ipsilateral cortex compared with the contralateral cortex. Other workers found that in brain tumour patients with symptoms and signs of increased intracranial pressure, both CBF and $CMRO_2$ in the contralateral cortex were significantly lower than cortical values found in normal volunteers (Beaney et al. 1985). A depression in glucose utilisation has also been noted in areas of peritumour oedema and cortical regions that were adjacent to the tumour or neuronally connected. The latter findings have been explained in terms of deafferentation (De La Paz et al. 1983a). K. L. Leenders (pers. comm.) has noted that some patients with meningiomas in the anteromedial aspect of the frontal lobe have a marked depression in CBF and $CMRO_2$ in the ipsilateral basal ganglia. Clinically these patients have hemi-Parkinson's disease that usually disappears after removal of the meningioma. PET has also revealed the phenomenon of crossed cerebellar diaschisis. Baron clearly demonstrated a reduction in glucose metabolism in the cerebellar hemisphere contralateral to a supratentorial infarct (Baron et al. 1981), but other workers have shown the same phenomenon with supratentorial tumours (De La Paz et al. 1983b).

Glucose Utilisation

Many workers have tried to identify differences between normal and neoplastic tissue in terms of aberrant carbohydrate metabolism. There is considerable experimental evidence to suggest increased glycolysis in tumours (Weber 1977a, b) and an attempt was made to exploit this increased glucose demand in the radiodiagnosis of tumours. The most commonly used tracer in PET work is the glucose analogue ^{18}F-labelled 2-deoxy-D-glucose (^{18}F-DG). The method for determining regional cerebral glucose utilisation (rCMRGlu) in man was based on the [^{14}C]deoxyglucose (DG) autoradiographic model developed by Sokoloff to measure rCMRGlu in rats (Sokoloff et al. 1977). Deoxyglucose competes with glucose for facilitated transport at both endothelial and cell membranes. Once inside the cell it competes with glucose for hexokinase-mediated phosphorylation to deoxyglucose-6-phosphate. This phosphorylated product is essentially trapped in the cell and is not metabolised further. This simplifies the modelling and allows the reaction to be described by a series of first-order membrane transport and enzyme kinetic processes. The [^{14}C]deoxyglucose autoradiographic technique was adapted and extended for clinical use with ^{18}F-DG and PET by several workers (Phelps et al. 1979, Huang et al. 1980).

Several investigators have attempted to characterise cerebral tumours by way of their abnormal glucose metabolism. Di Chiro et al. found a correlation between glucose utilisation and tumour grade (Di Chiro et al. 1984): glucose utilisation was higher in grade 3 and 4 astrocytomas than in grade 1 and 2 tumours. These workers extended their studies to include patients with radiation-induced cerebral necrosis and were able to differentiate regions of tumour recurrence, where there was high glucose utilisation, from those of necrosis, which showed low glucose utilisation.

Abnormalities in the oxidative metabolism of glucose in human cerebral gliomas were studied by Rhodes et al. (1983). These workers used the oxygen-15 steady-state inhalation technique to measure rCBF and oxygen utilisation and then ^{18}F-DG (with a simplified version of the Sokoloff method) to measure rCMRGlu in seven patients with gliomas. Unlike Di Chiro, they did not take the peak value for rCMRGlu within the tumour volume as the rCMRGlu value, but took the mean value for a region of interest no smaller than 2.6 cm^2. Rhodes found that tumour rCBF was comparable to that of contralateral cortex. Oxygen utilisation in the tumour tissue was depressed. This low demand for oxygen by the tumour resulted in a rOER lower than that for normal brain. In contrast, the rCMRGlu in the tumour was not significantly different from that in normal contralateral cortex. This virtually normal demand for glucose resulted in glucose extraction ratios (rGER) that were similar for tumour and normal brain tissue. Rhodes indicated that in normal brain there is close coupling between oxygen and glucose consumption and expressed this relationship in the form of the metabolic ratio (MR), i.e. $rCMRO_2$/rCMRGlu. In cerebral tumours this ratio was lower than in contralateral normal brain, indicating an increase in the non-oxidative metabolism of glucose. Fig. 5.7 illustrates the PET rCBF, rOER, $rCMRO_2$, rCMRGlu, rGER and MR images of a patient with a glioma in the right parieto-occipital region. It shows that rCBF in the tumour was slightly lower than that of contralateral grey matter. The rOER and $rCMRO_2$ were

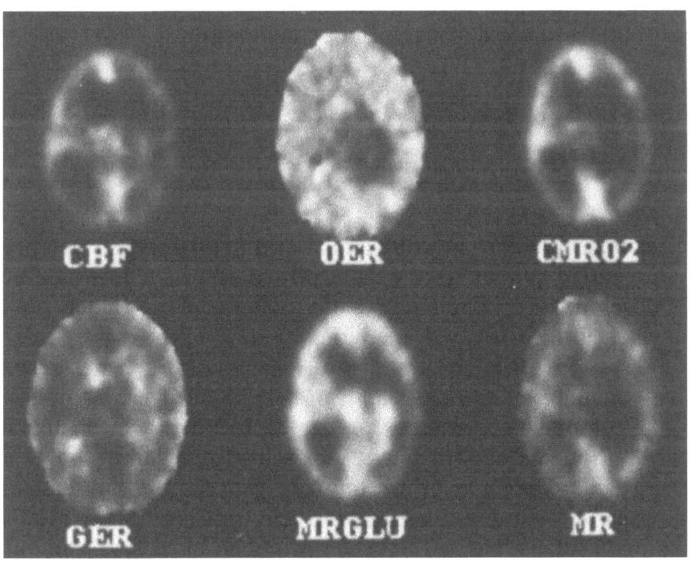

Fig. 5.7. The PET rCBF, rOER, $rCMRO_2$ and rCMRGlu, rGER, and MR images of a patient with a recurrent right hemisphere glioma. The region of the tumour can be most easily seen in the rOER image. Of special interest is the marked imbalance between oxygen consumption ($rCMRO_2$) and glucose consumption (rCMRGlu) relative to surrounding normal brain, which results in a low tumour metabolic ratio (MR).

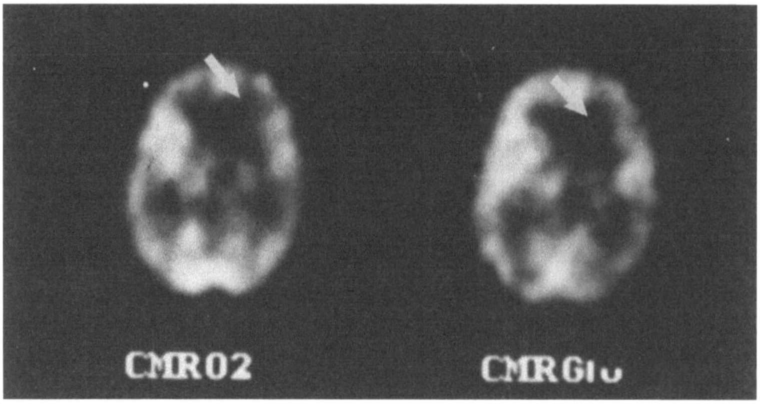

Fig. 5.8. The PET $rCMRO_2$ and rCMRGlu images of a brain. The arrowed region was later proven histologically to be necrotic. The matched reduction in both oxygen and glucose utilisation is indicative of a region of hypometabolism.

lower in the tumour tissue compared with the corresponding part of the contralateral brain. The rCMRGlu and rGER, however, were slightly higher than those of the corresponding region in the contralateral hemisphere. The MR was low in the tumour, indicating an increase in the non-oxidative metabolism of glucose.

Fig. 5.8 shows the functional images of oxygen and glucose utilisation in a patient with a biopsy-proven necrotic lesion in the frontal region (arrowed) who had been treated with a combination of post-biopsy radiotherapy and chemotherapy. Unlike tumour, this necrotic region showed a significant decrease in both oxygen and glucose utilisation indicating a marked degree of hypometabolism.

Amino Acid Utilisation

PET provides us with an opportunity to measure amino acid uptake and its incorporation into protein. Qualitative studies have been reported for L-[^{14}C]methionine. Bustany et al. (1983) developed a three-compartment model (cerebral blood pool, free methionine and protein-incorporated methionine) that relies on an intact blood–brain barrier and has been used in the study of schizophrenia, dementia and normal volunteers. The oncological work to date can best be described as tumour imaging. The concept of tumour detection seeks to exploit metabolic differences in the uptake and incorporation of labelled amino acids into neoplastic and non-neoplastic tissue. Amino acid uptake may be greater in cancer cells as a consequence of cell membrane changes that permit increased amino acid transport (Holley 1972). An increase in uptake of DL[^{11}C]valine and DL[^{11}C]tryptophan in cerebral tumours was demonstrated by Hübner et al. (1982). On the basis of their essentially qualitative studies these workers were uncertain whether this increased uptake was indeed representative of increased amino acid utilisation or simply a consequence of disruption of the blood–brain barrier. Bergström and co-workers (1983) have shown increased [^{11}C]methionine uptake in cerebral tumours. In one case, [^{11}C]methionine uptake revealed extension of a tumour into adjacent brain that was judged normal by conventional enhanced CT scanning and PET imaging with both ^{68}Ga-labelled EDTA and [^{11}C]glucose and where presumably there would have been minimal, if any, disruption of the blood-brain barrier (Bergström et al. 1983). These workers pointed out the possible usefulness of this technique in accurately estimating the extent of a cerebral tumour.

Blood-Brain Barrier Integrity

In normal brain, the blood-brain barrier is highly impermeable to potassium ions (K^+), their transport being controlled by ATPases situated in the endothelial cell membranes. Rubidium-82 ($^{82}Rb^+$) is a positron-emitting analogue of K^+ with a half-life of 75 seconds. Using a steady-state model and PET, quantitative extraction data for $^{82}Rb^+$ transport across the blood-brain barrier have been obtained both in normal human subjects and in a variety of pathological conditions of the brain (Brooks et al. 1984a). A mean cerebral Rb extraction of 2.1% was found for normal volunteers which corresponds to a mean value of 1.1×10^6 cm/s for $^{82}Rb^+$ cation permeability across the blood-brain barrier. Cerebral tumours that demonstrated contrast enhancement on X-ray CT scanning showed an increase in local $^{82}Rb^+$ uptake. No correlation between tumour size or grade of glioma and $^{82}Rb^+$ extraction was found. A mean tumour $^{82}Rb^+$ extraction of 29.3% was recorded for 11 patients with a variety of intracranial neoplasms (Brooks et al. 1984a). Fig. 5.9 shows the increased $^{82}Rb^+$ uptake into a metastatic lesion in the left hemisphere. Preliminary studies have been performed in patients undergoing cranial irradiation. One serial

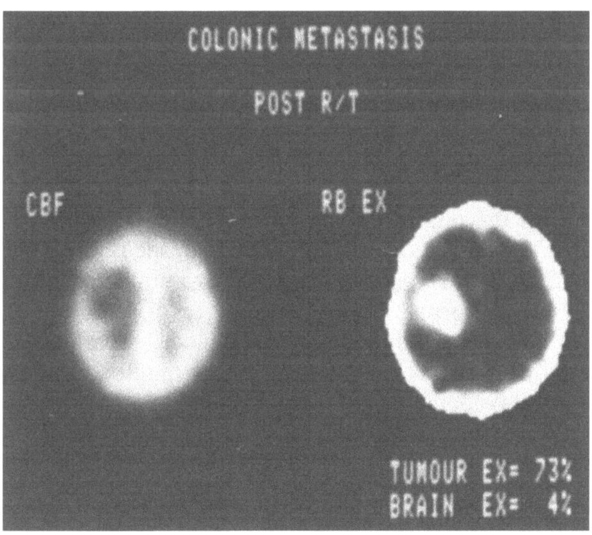

Fig. 5.9. $^{82}Rb^+$ extraction (RBEx) and regional blood flow (CBF) PET images from a patient with a left parietal metastasis. CBF is low in the region of tumour and perifocal oedema. $^{82}Rb^+$ extraction is high in the tumour region.

study suggested that tumour $^{82}Rb^+$ extraction can be acutely increased following radiation with no demonstrable increase in $^{82}Rb^+$ extraction in the normal brain.

Regional Cerebral pH

The potential use of $^{11}CO_2$ and PET for the measurement of regional cerebral pH in human subjects has already been reported (Raichle et al. 1979). $^{11}CO_2$ but not $H^{11}CO_3$ readily diffuses across the blood–brain barrier. As a consequence, the relative uptake of ^{11}C by arterial plasma and cerebral tissue during inhalation of $^{11}CO_2$ reflects the pH difference between the two compartments. Buxton and co-workers (1984) developed a model for the measurement of cerebral pH that enables the metabolic fixation of ^{11}C during $^{11}CO_2$ inhalation to be estimated. By administering $^{11}CO_2$ continuously rather than as a bolus the problems associated with ^{11}C fixation can be minimised. Other workers have used this method in man and found whole-brain pH values to be in the range 6.96 – 7.05 (Brooks et al. 1984b). Preliminary work on tumours indicates that in those tumours that are not enhanced on X-ray CT scanning, the pH is similar to or slightly higher than that of surrounding normal brain (Beaney et al. unpubl. data).

Receptor Binding and Drug Uptake Studies

Growing interest is being shown in the use of PET scanning in receptor binding and drug uptake studies. Most of the receptor work to date has dealt with dopaminergic receptors using ^{11}C-labelled ligands such as [^{11}C]methylspiperone (Wagner et al. 1983). This tracer crosses the blood–brain barrier and shows high affinity and selectivity for dopaminergic receptors. It is hoped that studies like this will help in unravelling some of the pathophysiological problems of movement disorders, in particular Parkinson's disease. Work is in progress studying not only the pharmacokinetics of analgesics in man but also specific opiate receptor binding in the brain (A.K.P. Jones pers. comm.).

Yamamoto et al. (1983) studied the pharmacokinetics of ^{11}C- and ^{13}N-labelled BCNU. They showed that the initial uptake of ^{11}C radioactivity in the tumour was related to rCBF and that [^{11}C]BCNU breakdown compounds accumulated in the tumour to a greater degree than in normal brain. The degree of later uptake appeared to be proportional to the degree of disruption of the blood–brain barrier, which could be locally enhanced by intravenous infusion of 20% mannitol. Cerebral uptake of [^{11}C]BCNU given by intravenous injection has been compared with the cerebral uptake after intracarotid injection. Although more drug is taken up by the tumour after intracarotid injection, the normal brain also takes up a considerably increased amount and the therapeutic ratio is somewhat reduced.

The Physiological Effects of Tumour Treatment

Dexamethasone

Leenders et al. (1985) measured rCBF, OER, $CMRO_2$ and CBV in brain tumour patients before and after the administration of dexamethasone. Dexamethasone treatment resulted in a significant decrease in CBF and CBV and a significant increase in fractional extraction of oxygen throughout the brain without a change in oxygen utilisation. It was suggested that dexamethasone causes a direct constriction of cerebral blood vessels.

Decompressive Surgery

As mentioned earlier, patients with symptoms and signs of increased intracranial pressure may have a depression of CBF and $CMRO_2$ in the contralateral normal brain. Decompressive surgery leads to a partial reversal of this cerebral hypofunction (Beaney et al. 1985). Data from seven patients are shown in Fig. 5.10.

Whole-Brain Irradiation

A group of patients with intracranial metastases was studied before, immediately after, and 3–4 months after a fractionated course of whole-brain radiotherapy. In the contralateral cortex, CBF and CBV were found to have risen at the end of the fractionated course of radiotherapy; oxygen utilisation, however, remained essentially unchanged. Four months later CBF and CBV had fallen again. It was unclear whether these changes in CBF were entirely due to the effects of the radiation on the normal brain tissue or partly due to the decompressive effect of the radiation-induced reduction in tumour volume. The later progressive fall in CBF and $CMRO_2$ may have been indicative of tumour regrowth rather than vascular damage. In tumour tissue on the other hand, $CMRO_2$ and CBV gradually declined indicating progressive cellular death.

External Beam Radiotherapy in Acromegaly

Twelve acromegalic patients were treated with external beam radiotherapy in either a two- or three-field arrangement. This resulted in the patients receiving either approximately 40 Gy or 20 Gy respectively to the temporal lobes, given over a period of approximately 4 weeks—a dose commonly accepted as well within brain tolerance. They were scanned by PET between 3 and 14 years after treatment and the values for CBF, OER and $CMRO_2$ compared with those obtained from normal volunteers. There was no demonstrable impairment in temporal lobe function (Beaney et al. unpubl. data)

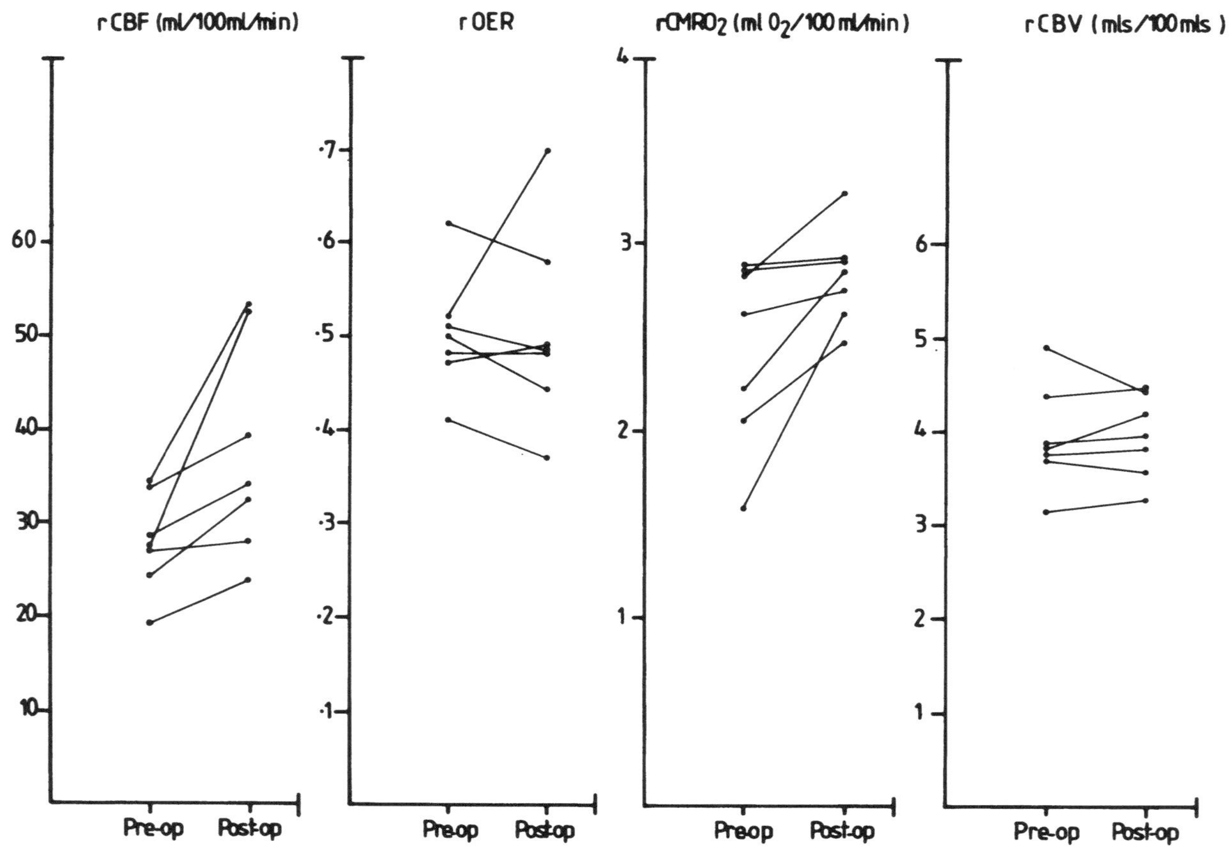

Fig. 5.10. Measurements of rCBF, rOER, rCMRO$_2$ and rCBV taken before and after operation in seven patients. The significant changes were an increase in rCMRO$_2$ and rCBF after craniotomy.

Summary

Positron emission tomography (PET) has been shown to be an important investigative tool in the study of the basic pathophysiology of human tumours in vivo. Their response to treatment, along with that of normal surrounding tissue, may be studied in both the acute and late stages after therapy.

I wish to thank Mr D. D. Vonberg, Dr C. G. McKenzie, Dr K. E. Halnan and Mr T. Jones and staff of the MRC Cyclotron Unit, in particular the Neurology and Radiochemistry Sections, for their invaluable support and technical help, and Mr F. Paice and Ms R. Jackson for their help in preparing the manuscript.

References

Baron JC, Bousser MG, Comar D, Duquesnoy N, Sastre J, Castaigne P (1981) Crossed cerebellar diaschisis: A remote functional depression secondary to supratentorial infarction of man. J Cereb Blood Flow Metabol 1 [Suppl 1]: S500–S501

Beaney RP, Brooks DJ, Leenders KL, Thomas DGT, Jones T, Halnan KE (1985) Blood flow and oxygen utilisation in the contralateral cerebral cortex of patients with untreated intracranial tumours as studied by positron emission tomography, with observations on the effect of decompressive surgery. J Neurol Neurosurg Psychiatr 48: 310–319

Bergström M, Collins P, Ehrin E, Ericson K, Eriksson L, Greitz T, Halldin C, Holst HV, Langström B, Lilja A, Lundqvist H, Nagren K (1983) Discrepancies in brain tumour extent as shown by computed tomography and positron emission tomography using [^{68}Ga]EDTA, [^{11}C]Glucose, and [^{11}C]Methionine. J Comput Assist Tomogr 7: 1062–1066

Brooks DJ, Beaney RP, Lammertsma AA, Leenders KL, Horlock PL, Kensett MJ, Marshall J, Thomas DG, Jones T (1984a) Quantitative measurement of blood-brain-barrier permeability using ^{82}Rb and positron emission tomography. J Cereb Blood Flow Metabol 4: 535–545

Brooks DJ, Lammertsma AA, Beaney RP, Leenders KL, Buckingham PD, Marshall J, Jones T (1984b) Measurement of regional cerebral pH in human subjects using continuous inhalation of $^{11}CO_2$ and positron emission tomography. J Cereb Blood Flow Metabol 4: 458–465

Bustany P, Henry JF, Sargent T, Zarifian E, Cabanis E, Collard P, Comar D (1983) Local brain metabolism in dementia and schizophrenia: In vivo studies with ^{11}C-L-methionine and positron emission tomography. In: Heiss W-D, Phelps ME (eds) Positron emission tomography of the brain. Springer-Verlag, Berlin, pp 208–211

Buxton RB, Wechsler LR, Alpert NM, Ackerman RH, Elmaleh DR, Correia JA (1984) Measurement of brain pH using $^{11}CO_2$ and positron emission tomography. J Cereb Blood Flow Metabol 4: 8–16

De La Paz RL, Patronas NJ, Brooks RA, Smith BH, Kornblith PL, Milam H, Di Chiro G (1983a) A PET study of suppression of glucose utilisation in cerebral grey matter associated with brain tumour. J Cereb Blood Flow Metabol 3 [Suppl 1]: S21–S22

De La Paz RL, Patronas NJ, Brooks RA, Smith BH, Kornblith PL, Milam H, Di Chiro G (1983b) Positron emission tomography study of suppression of gray-matter glucose utilisation by brain tumours. AJNR 4: 826–829

Di Chiro G, Brooks RA, Patronas NJ, Bairamian D, Kornblith PL, Smith BH, Mansi L, Barker J (1984) Issues in the in vivo measurement of glucose metabolism of human central nervous system tumours. Ann Neurol 15 [Suppl]: S138–S146

Frackowiak RSJ, Lenzi G-L, Jones T, Heather JD (1980) Quantitative measurements of regional cerebral blood flow and oxygen metabolism in man using ^{15}O and positron emission tomography: Theory, procedure and normal values. J Comput Assist Tomogr 4: 727–736

Frackowiak RSJ, Wise RJS, Gibbs JM, Jones T (1984) Positron emission tomographic studies in ageing and cerebrovascular disease at Hammersmith Hospital. Ann Neurol 15 [Suppl]: S112–S118

Holley RW (1972) A unifying hypothesis concerning the nature of malignant growth. Proc Natl Acad Sci USA 69: 2840–2841

Huang S-C, Phelps ME, Hoffman EJ, Sideris K, Selin CJ, Kuhl DE (1980) Noninvasive determination of local cerebral metabolic rate of glucose in man. Am J Physiol 238: E69–E82

Hübner KF, Purvis JR, Mahaley SM, Robertson JT, Rogers S, Gibbs WD, King P, Partain CL (1982) Brain tumour imaging by positron emission computed tomography using ^{11}C-labelled amino acids. J Comput Assist Tomogr 6: 544–550

Ito M, Lammertsma AA, Wise RJS, Bernardi S, Frackowiak RSJ, Heather JD, McKenzie CG, Thomas DGT, Jones T (1982) Measurement of regional cerebral blood flow and oxygen utilisation in patients with cerebral tumours using ^{15}O and positron emission tomography: Analytical techniques and preliminary results. Neuroradiology 23: 63–74

Jones T, Chesler DA, Ter-Pogossian MM (1976) The continuous inhalation of oxygen-15 for assessing regional oxygen extraction in the brain of man. Br J Radiol 49: 339–343

Lammertsma AA, Jones T (1983) Correction for the presence of intravascular oxygen-15 in the steady-state technique for measuring regional oxygen extraction ratio in the brain. I. Description of the method. J Cereb Blood Flow Metabol 3: 416–424

Lammertsma AA, Wise RJS, Heather JD, Gibbs JM, Leenders KL, Frackowiak RSJ, Rhodes CG, Jones T (1983a) Correction for the presence of intravascular oxygen-15 in the steady-state technique for measuring regional oxygen extraction ratio in the brain. II. Results in normal subjects and brain tumour and stroke patients. J Cereb Blood Flow Metabol 3: 425–431

Lammertsma A, Wise R, Gibbs J, Thomas D, Jones T (1983b) The pathophysiology of human cerebral tumours and surrounding white matter and remote cortex. J Cereb Blood Flow Metabol 3 [Suppl 1] S9–S10

Lammertsma AA, Wise RJS, Jones T (1984) Regional cerebral blood flow and oxygen utilisation in edema associated with cerebral tumours. In: Go KG, Baethmann A (eds) Recent progress in the study and therapy of brain edema. Plenum Press, New York, pp 331–344

Leenders KL, Beaney RP, Brooks DJ, Heather JD, McKenzie CG, Jones T (1985) Dexamethasone treatment of brain tumour patients: Effects on regional cerebral blood flow, blood volume and oxygen utilisation. Neurology (in press)

Phelps ME, Huang SC, Hoffman EJ, Selin C, Sokoloff L, Kuhl DE (1979) Tomographic measurement of local cerebral glucose metabolic rate in humans with (F-18)2-fluoro-2-deoxy-D-glucose: Validation of method. Ann Neurol 6: 321–388

Phelps ME, Mazziotta JC, Huang S-C (1982) Study of cerebral function with positron computed tomography. J Cereb Blood Flow Metabol 2: 113–162

Raichle ME, Grubb RL, Higgins CS (1979) Measurement of brain tissue carbon dioxide content in vivo by emission tomography. Brain Res 166: 413–417

Rhodes CG, Wise RJS, Gibbs JM, Frackowiak RSJ, Hatazawa J, Palmer AJ, Thomas DGT, Jones T (1983) In vivo disturbance of the oxidative metabolism of glucose in human cerebral gliomas. Ann Neurol 14: 614–626

Sokoloff L, Reivich M, Kennedy C, Des Rosiers MH, Patlak CS, Pettigrew KD, Sakurada D, Shinohara M (1977) The [^{14}C]Deoxyglucose method for the measurement of local cerebral glucose utilization: Theory, procedure and normal values in the conscious and anaesthetised albino rat. J Neurochem 28: 897–916

Wagner HN, Burns HD, Dannals RF et al. (1983) Imaging dopamine receptors in the human brain by positron tomography. Science 221: 1264–1266

Weber G (1977a) Enzymology of cancer cells: I. N Engl J Med 296: 486–493

Weber G (1977b) Enzymology of cancer cells: II. N Engl J Med 296: 541–555

Williams CW, Crabtree MC, Burgiss SG (1979) Design and performance characteristics of a positron emission computed axial tomograph ECAT-II. IEEE Trans Nucl Sci [NS]26: 619–627

Yamamoto YL, Diksic M, Sako K (1983) Pharmacokinetic and metabolic studies in human malignant glioma. In: Magistretti PL (ed) Functional radionuclide imaging of the brain. Raven Press, New York, pp 327–335

6 Immunolocalisation of Human Brain Tumours

A. Geraint Davies, Richard B. Richardson, Stephen P. Bourne,
John T. Kemshead and Hugh B. Coakham

Introduction

The specific targeting of radiolabelled antibody to human brain tumours for purposes of diagnosis or therapy is a most attractive concept. The ability to diagnose accurately the histological nature of a cerebral lesion with an immunological marker using scintigraphic imaging would be invaluable, and antibody targeting of therapeutic agents would offer another useful modality of treatment in this most refractory group of neoplasms.

Since the technique of radioimmunolocalisation is relatively new, we shall describe the development of radiolabelled antibody imaging of tumours. This is followed by a brief summary of the relevant technical considerations and a review of the current status of radioimmunolocalisation of brain tumours.

The idea of specifically targeting antibodies to tumour cells in vivo has provoked interest since the turn of the century when Paul Ehrlich's "magic bullet" hypothesis was soon followed by an appreciation of the properties of antibodies. The technique of delivering radiolabelled antibodies to tissue in vivo (radioimmunolocalisation, RIL) was pioneered by Pressman and Keighley (1948) over 30 years ago. Its application to man became possible with the characterisation of human tumour-associated antigens such as human chorionic gonadotrophin (HCG), carcino-embryonic antigen (CEA) (Gold and Freedman 1965) and alphafetoprotein (AFP).

Purified antisera against CEA, radiolabelled with ^{131}I, were first used to image gastrointestinal and ovarian tumours by Goldenberg et al. (1978). This approach was extended, using a range of heteroantisera, to include renal (Belitsky et al. 1978), testicular (Goldenberg et al. 1981), prostatic (Goldenberg et al. 1983) and germ cell tumours (Goldenberg et al. 1980, Halsall et al. 1981) and choriocarcinoma (Begent et al. 1980). It is pertinent to note that the first attempt at RIL of human brain tumours was a study of gliomas by Day, Mahaley and colleagues (1965), using a purified rabbit antiserum raised against preparations of glioma.

Monoclonal Antibodies

The introduction of monoclonal antibodies (MCAs) by Kohler and Milstein in 1975 was met with enthusiasm since these reagents had the considerable advantages of purity, specificity and unlimited supply. Application of this technology has also resulted in the detection of new tumour-associated antigens, which are suitable targets for RIL, and has produced better probes for the existing antigens. This has extended the range of tumours studied to thyroid carcinomas (Berche et al. 1982), melanomas (Larson et al. 1983) and neuroblastomas (Goldman et al. 1984). It has also improved results of imaging ovarian and gastrointestinal malignancies (Epenetos et al. 1982, Berche et al. 1982).

The field of RIL is moving rapidly at present. Objectives include the demonstration of tumour deposits not shown by other imaging techniques and investigation of the possibilities of antibody-targeted therapy in which antibody is conjugated with a toxin, chemotherapeutic agent or radionuclide.

The Target Molecules for Radioimmunolocalisation

The widespread production of MCAs against tumour cells has led to the identification of new types of antigens. Some of these have been used for antibody targeting in vivo and are shown, together with other previously described antibodies, in Table 6.1. These are all expressed on the cell surface and are thus accessible for antibody binding. The ideal antigen would be one which was truly tumour-specific. Unfortunately these are rare and may only be represented by the B cell lymphoma idiotype against which successful antibody therapy has been directed (Stevenson and Stevenson 1975). Although an MCA specifically recognises one antigenic site, the molecule bearing this binding site is generally not tumour-specific but may be distributed on normal tissues, or might occur on other unrelated tumours. The finding that MCAs can have unexpected cross-reactivities by recognising antigenic sites on unrelated molecules means that these reagents should be used in vivo only after extensive histological screening on normal tissues (Lane and Koprowski 1982, Garson et al. 1982).

Table 6.1. Tumour-associated antigens useful in human antibody targeting studies

Category	Example	Tumours imaged
Oncofetal	CEA	Gastrointestinal, breast, ovary, thyroid
Oncofetal	AFP	Germ cell neoplasms
Oncofetal	UJ181.4	Pineocytoma
Hormone	HCG	Choriocarcinoma
Epithelial proliferation antigen	Milk fat protein	Ovary, breast
Differentiation antigen	UJ13A	Gliomas, meningiomas
Receptors	Epidermal growth factor receptor	Glioma

The concept of operational specificity is becoming increasingly important, and means that antibodies can be used for a variety of diagnostic and therapeutic procedures in vivo without having exclusive tumour reactivity. This operational specificity is partly attributable to the restriction of antibody access to normal tissues by natural barriers such as epithelial basement membranes and capillary endothelial tight junctions. The blood-brain barrier is a relevant example in this context. This approach will be described below in our use of the MCA UJ13A, which will operationally image human brain tumours.

The Agents for Radioimmunolocalisation

Affinity purified antisera have produced excellent results in RIL but suffer the disadvantage of batch-to-batch variation. This is overcome by the use of MCAs, which are available in virtually infinite amounts. This ensures reproducibility, which is important when large quantities of antibody are needed for the production of fragments (see below) and also for radiolabelling for therapy.

The majority of MCAs used are murine, but some rat antibodies are now being produced. The use of the reagents in humans is limited by the human immune reaction which will take place after multiple injections. The most desirable reagents are human MCAs made by harvesting lymphocytes from resected tumours and immortalising them by fusion with a human myeloma cell line. The HuMy 2 cell line from the Ludwig Institute, London (Edwards et al. 1982) is one such example. However, results of human hybridoma production have been less successful than with the mouse system. Furthermore, it is possible that animal MCAs will recognise antigenic markers on the human tumour cell not recognised by the host, so that tumour antigens which are poorly immunogenic in man could be identified and targeted against. The fragments of antibody produced by enzymic cleavage may be better agents in vivo than whole antibody (see Fig. 6.1). This is because the Fc portion of the molecule may bind non-specifically in vivo to numerous cell types and consequently reduce the amount available for specific binding to the tumour target. It will also result in non-specific scintillation images. The smaller size of the immunoglobulin fragments means that their half-life in the circulation is reduced. This helps to reduce background activity. A further advantage is the reduced immunogenicity resulting from loss of the Fc fragment. This means multiple antibody administration given as part of diagnostic or treatment protocols may be better tolerated.

Choice of Radiolabel

There are a number of variables which govern the choice of radionuclide for antibody imaging techniques. These are: photon energy, half-life, ease and efficiency of labelling, and image quality (see Table 6.2).

Iodine-131 (^{131}I). This isotope emits rather a high γ energy which results in a sub-optimal scintillation image. However, the significant advantages of an 8 day half-life and easy, efficient labelling by the chloramine-T or lactoperoxidase methods make this the isotope of choice for many workers (Goldenberg et al. 1978, Begent et al. 1980, Baldwin et al. 1984). The β emission, however, contributes to a high radiation dose.

Iodine-123 (^{123}I). The image quality resulting from the lower γ energy of ^{123}I is

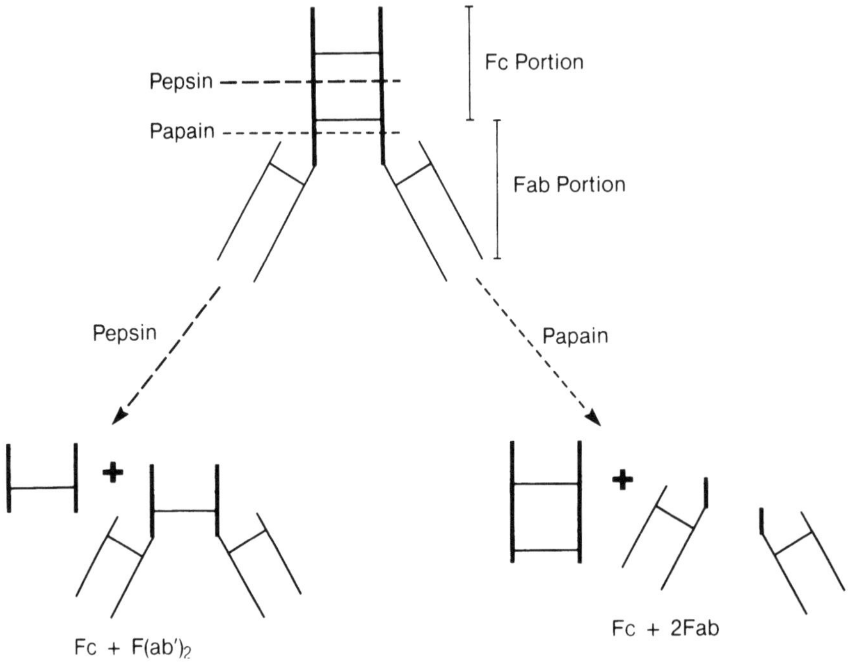

Fig. 6.1. Diagram of the sites of cleavage of gamma globulin molecules by the enzymes pepsin and papain in the production of antibody fragments.

Table 6.2. Radiolabels used with monoclonal antibodies

Radionuclide	Principal γ energies (keV)	β emissions	Half-life	Ease/efficiency of labelling	Image quality
^{131}I	364	+	8 days	+ +	+
^{123}I	160	–	13 hours	+	+ +
^{99m}Tc	140	–	6 hours	+/–	+ +
^{111}In	171 237	–	67 hours	+	+ +
^{67}Ga	92 185	–	78 hours	+	+ +

much better but the 13 hour half-life means that early imaging must take place when blood:tissue background activity is relatively high. This is favoured by some groups (Epenetos et al. 1982) who then use background subtraction techniques (see below). Subtraction using ^{99m}Tc cannot be employed, however, since the γ energies are too similar. It is thought by some that free iodine levels in vivo are higher than when ^{131}I is used, and for this reason some workers prefer enzymic iodination by lactoperoxidase.

Technetium-99m (^{99m}Tc). Although image quality with ^{99m}Tc is excellent, radiolabelling results are often not satisfactory and high levels of free ^{99m}Tc are found. Furthermore, the short half-life of 6 hours may not be sufficient for maximal localisation of antibody-conjugate to occur within the target tissue.

Indium-111 (^{111}In). This agent has been recommended on the grounds that the γ energies are suitable for good imaging with conventional equipment, and the half-life of 67 hours is reasonable for antibody imaging. Radiolabelling is achieved by the use of bifunctional chelating agents but has been met with variable success by different laboratories. Another problem is the high uptake by the liver due to the affinity of ^{111}In for transferrin.

Gallium-67 (^{67}Ga). The chief role of ^{67}Ga has been as a partner for ^{111}In in double-antibody subtraction techniques (see below).

Image Enhancement

Only a small fraction of an intravenously administered radiolabelled antibody localises in the tumour. The majority of the conjugate remains in the circulation and extravascular spaces and then contributes to the background "blood pool" effect seen on all RIL scans (Deland et al. 1980). This is a major problem when target tumours lie in the mediastinum or upper abdomen. It is not so important in the brain where the blood pool background of the cranium is lower. The background activity can be removed by subtraction techniques using non-specific vascular (and extravascular) markers or by subtracting the early image (usually 10 minutes post-injection) from a late image. This is possible since the maximal tumour uptake of antibody-conjugate takes several hours. However, subtraction techniques have their limitations (Ott et al. 1983) and may give rise to false positive artefacts.

The use of double-antibody technique using paired label analysis in an imaging system is attractive. This employs the high photon peak of ^{111}In linked to a specific MCA and the low photon peak of ^{67}Ga linked to a control MCA. This has been used successfully in an animal model (Haisma et al. 1984).

The use of $F(ab')_2$ or Fab antibody fragments may also improve localisation within the tumour for a number of reasons already cited.

Radioimmunolocalisation of Neuroectodermal Tumours

Initial trials of antibody delivery to human neural tumours have been carried out in animal systems, the most commonly employed being nude mice bearing subcutaneous or intracerebral xenografts. These studies have shown that satisfactory ratios of tumour to normal tissue activity can be obtained, with high specificity indices when both relevant and irrelevant (control) antibody is used and has been described for xenografts of neuroblastoma (Goldman et al. 1984) and glioma (Bourdon et al. 1984). In these two groups of experiments localisation indices (ratio of specific to control MCA) in the range 10–20 were obtained. Preliminary work indicates that the use of $F(ab')_2$ fragments results in improved tumour:tissue ratios, and also improved images (Ghose et al. 1982, J. T. Kemshead and D. H. Jones unpublished data).

Studies are at present under way in animals bearing intracerebral xenografts to investigate the role played by the blood–brain barrier and to compare intravenous with intracarotid routes of delivery. When considering the RIL of intracranial tumours in humans a number of conditions must be fulfilled. The antibody must be of sufficient specificity, the antigen must be accessible to circulating antibodies and the kinetics of the antibody in vivo must be such that specific localisation can be demonstrated (Kemshead et al. 1984).

The Specificity of Monoclonal Antibodies for Human Brain Tumours

Monoclonal Antibodies

The ideal MCA for RIL of brain tumours is one which binds only to malignant cells. Unfortunately such reagents do not exist. However, because of their operational specificity antibodies can be used successfully for a variety of diagnostic and therapeutic procedures both in vivo and in vitro without exclusive tumour reactivity (Miller et al. 1982, Ritz et al. 1982, Treleaven et al. 1984). Candidate antibodies which may give sufficient specificity for RIL of brain tumours certainly exist (Coakham et al. 1984). These can be divided into several classes according to the selective nature of their reactivity.

One essential prerequisite is that the target antigen is expressed on the tumour cell surface and is thus available for binding in vivo. The antigens most suitable are often carbohydrate moieties and are components of membrane glycoproteins or glycolipids (Feizi 1985). Extracellular matrix proteins are also an important group.

The most broadly reacting reagents are those which bind to either all or most neuroectodermally derived tumours or tissues. An example of this type of antibody is UJ13A, made following immunisation of mice with 16-week human fetal brain (Allan et al. 1983). Indirect immunofluorescence studies of frozen sections of fetal, paediatric and adult tissues indicate that the only neuroectodermally derived tissues or tumours which do not bind UJ13A are melanocytes and melanomas. UJ13A binds to both neural and glial cells in the brain. First considerations suggest that this type of reactivity is too broad to be useful for RIL studies.

Other antibodies with a more restricted pattern of binding to neural tissues and tumours have also been produced. UJ127.11 is an MCA binding to neural rather than glial cells in brain (Kemshead et al. 1983). Studies of frozen sections of neuronal tumours indicate that the reagent binds to medulloblastomas and neuroblastomas but not to gliomas. The antigen recognised by this MCA is a glycoprotein of molecular weight 220 000–240 000 found in the membrane of neural cells. Conversely, FD19.9 is an MCA binding only to glial rather than neural cells and recognises a 55 000 molecular weight intracellular antigen, glial fibrillary acidic protein. This reagent was raised following immunisation of mice with a low-grade astrocytoma.

MCAs with even greater specificity to cell types found in the brain have been described. For example UCHT1, whilst binding a membrane antigen on T lymphocytes, also cross-reacts with an intracellular antigen found only in Purkinje cells (Garson et al. 1982). However, all these antibodies, whilst sharing restricted specificity for different neuronal cell types, are not capable of distinguishing malignant cells from their normal counterparts.

A group of reagents which begin to satisfy this requirement are those with an oncofetal type of specificity. These are antibodies binding to differentiation antigens expressed on fetal and malignant neuronal cells. They are lost as cells differentiate to a more mature cell type. Examples of antibodies with this type of specificity are UJ181.4 and M340 (unpubl. data) made following immunisation of mice with human fetal brain and fresh human medulloblastoma respectively. Both these reagents bind to frozen sections of fetal brain, medulloblastoma, neuroblastoma and retinoblastoma, but not to paediatric or adult brain as assessed by indirect immunofluorescence studies

Finally, several antibodies have been produced which, on initial characterisation, appeared to bind only to malignant cells and not to normal fetal or adult neuronal tissues. FD32.3, made by immunising mice with low-grade human astrocytoma, was thought initially to bind to gliomas but not to normal glial cells from fetal or adult brain. However, extensive characterisation of the binding of this antibody showed that activated glial cells found at sites of inflammation also express the FD32.3 antigen. This antibody binds to an extracellular matrix protein found in gliomas. Other reagents with similar specifications have also now been produced (Bourdon et al. 1983). FD32.3 has additionally been found to bind to a series of non-neuroectodermally derived tumour outside the brain, such as rhabdomyosarcoma and Ewing's tumours.

The antibodies which are immediate candidates for human immunotargeting studies are shown in Table 6.3. Two of these, UJ13A and UJ181.4, have already been in use and results will be described below. Other MCAs have been reported which have specificity sufficient for consideration of use in vivo (Schnegg et al. 1981).

When the precise specifications of MCAs are established they are often found to bind to completely unrelated tissues. FD32.3 demonstrates this, as does UCHT1 (Beverley and Callard 1981). The antibody A_2B_5, thought to bind only to neural cells, has been shown to react with 26 of 40 secondary adenocarcinomas (H. B. Coakham et al. unpubl. obs.). Whether these rather unexpected cross-reactions are due to shared antigens between distinct cell types or to shared epitopes on biochemically dissimilar antigens remains to be determined in many cases. Whatever the

Table 6.3. Antibodies suitable for radioimmunolocalisation of human neural tumours

Monoclonal antibody	Antigen	Cell surface	Target neoplasm	Reference
UJ13A	Pan-neuroectoderm normal and neoplastic cells[a], ? glycolipid	+	All neuroectodermal tumours[b]	Allan et al. (1983)
UJ181.4	Embryonic and neoplastic neuronal cells	+	Neuroblastomas, medulloblastomas	Garson (1982)
M340	Neuronal cells	+	Primary pineal tumours	H.B. Coakham and J.T. Kemshead (unpubl. data)
FD32.3	Glioma-mesenchymal extracellular matrix	+	Glial neoplasms	Garson (1982)
81C6		+	Glial neoplasms	Bourdon et al. (1983)

[a]Except melanocytes.
[b]Except melanomas.

explanation for such cross-reactivities, the observation stresses the need for extensive studies on sections of tissues and tumours before reagents may be considered for RIL studies.

The Accessibility of Antibodies to Brain Tumour Antigens

The factors influencing accessibility of antibody-conjugates to solid tumours in vivo are still poorly understood but it seems that three major factors are involved:
a) The extent of vascularisation of the tumour and the dynamics of blood flow;
b) vascular permeability;
c) the extracellular fluid space.
Accessibility is particularly important when considering brain tumours because the blood–brain barrier (BBB) is capable of excluding macromolecules from the brain parenchyma. The evidence from ultrastructural (Reese and Karnovsky 1967) and permeability studies using horseradish peroxidase (Groothius et al. 1982, Deane et al. 1984) indicates that the BBB is largely disrupted in experimental and human brain tumours, especially those of higher malignancy. It is important to know the extent to which the BBB within tumours is permeable to immunoglobulins and to study any possible heterogeneity of vascular permeability which might limit the access of diagnostic or therapeutic probes. In addition, both low blood flow rates and limited diffusion into and out of the tumour tissue could interfere with the delivery of antibody-conjugates. In an attempt to address some of these problems, we have studied the behaviour in vivo of a radiolabelled MCA in a series of patients with primary brain tumours. The antibody selected was UJ13A which recognises both normal and neoplastic neuroectodermal tissue. Following initial use in a mouse xenograft model, and biodistribution studies in marmosets, UJ13A was used successfully to radioimmunolocalise deposits of disseminated neuroblastoma in children (Goldman et al. 1984). In the course of these studies no significant uptake of radiolabelled antibody into normal brain tissue was observed. The antibody labelled with ^{131}I was therefore used to investigate the integrity of the BBB within a small series of patients with tumours which included malignant gliomas (grades 3 and 4), an oligoastrocytoma and a meningioma (Table 6.4) (Richardson et al. 1985).

All patients were evaluated clinically and with computerised tomographic scans. Imaging with ^{99m}Tc-labelled glucoheptonate was performed in order to assess the BBB with respect to this molecule. Purified antibody was labelled with ^{131}I by the chloramine T method, sterilised by Millipore filtration and administered by intravenous injection as 250 μg protein carrying 1.5–2.0 mCi ^{131}I. Scintigraphic imaging

Table 6.4. Immunolocalisation of intracranial tumours. First series: [^{131}I]UJ13A alone

Patient no.	Tumour	MCA image	Subtraction
1	Meningioma	Good	No
2	Malignant glioma	Good	No
3	Malignant glioma	Good	No
4	Malignant glioma	Poor	Yes; improved localisation
5	Oligoastrocytoma	None	Yes; no image

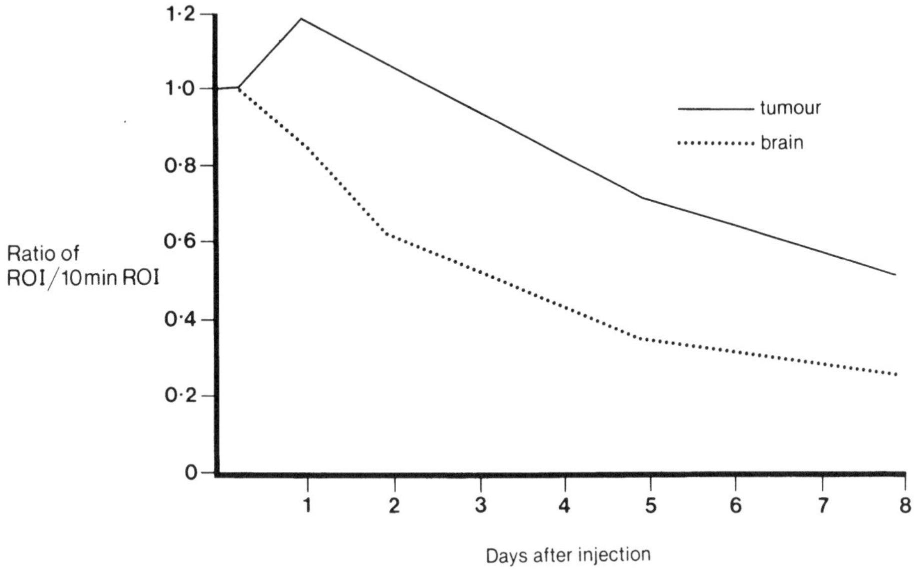

Fig. 6.2. [^{131}I]UJ13A activity in RO1 over the tumour and normal brain in the same patient as in Plate 1. Counts are expressed as a ratio to the counts obtained in the first (10 minute) scan. Scans were performed at 10 minutes, 4 hours, 24 hours, and thence daily. Note the peak of ^{131}I uptake at 24 hours. However, the best images were obtained later at 5 days when tumour:brain ratios of ^{131}I counts/minute were 2:1.

was carried out at regular intervals for up to 16 days and levels of ^{131}I activity in blood and urine were monitored. Operative samples of tumour and normal brain were obtained from three patients and ^{131}I activity was measured directly. In the majority of cases tumour images were obtained without the need for subtraction. Images of tumour uptake first appeared 4 and 24 hours after injection and improved subjectively between 24 and 48 hours. Many were subjectively optimal at about 5 days (Plate 1). Images often persisted until 6 days and in one case a good image remained at 12 days post injection of the radiolabel.

Using a cursor on the image analysis computer, selected regions of interest in tumour and normal brain could be compared (Plate 2). This objective method showed that maximum radionuclide uptake occurs between 4 hours and 24 hours. Progressive decrease in activity then occurs with clearance from the tumour proceeding at a slower rate than that of normal brain. During this time the tumour image becomes subjectively clearer despite the fall in activity, since the ratio of counts per

Table 6.5. ^{131}I activity in resected samples expressed in ratios

Patient no.	Day of operation post-injection	Neoplasm:brain ratio			Tissue:blood ratio	
		Tumour	Cyst	Necrosis	Tumour	Brain
1	6	3.4	5.2	—	0.48	0.21
2	16	12.8	14.9	19.3	5.14	0.40
3	16	3.1	10.5	11.5	0.64	0.20

minute from the tumour is improving with respect to that from brain (Fig. 6.2). In the three cases where resected tissue was examined, tumour:normal brain ratios of between 3.1:1 and 12.8:1 were obtained (Table 6.5). These ratios are comparable to those found in similar post-injection tissue analyses in other malignant tumours (Farrands et al. 1982, Mach et al. 1983). Increased amounts of radiolabel were consistently detected in regions of the tumours that were necrotic or cystic, suggesting perhaps that passive accumulation is taking place. In all studies the level of free iodide was low, being less than 2% in blood.

Blood-Brain Barrier Permeability to Monoclonal Antibody

In two of five cases the BBB interfered with satisfactory immunolocalisation. One case required use of a subtraction technique in order to produce a tumour image (Plate 3) but in the second case there was no detectable uptake of labelled antibody (mol. wt. 150 000), despite part of the tumour being permeable to [^{99m}Tc]glucoheptonate (mol. wt. 700) and to Conray (mol. wt. 630) (Fig. 6.3 and Plate 4). This case illustrates the two forms of BBB variability which have been shown in animal experiments, namely regional variation and qualitative variation (Giacomelli et al. 1979, Groothuis et al. 1982). This difficulty of access which we have demonstrated could theoretically be overcome by the use of a technique for BBB opening such as hyperosmolar intra-arterial mannitol infusion, as pioneered in humans by Neuwelt et al. (1980). It would then of course be necessary to employ a more tumour-specific carrier antibody.

The various factors influencing the accessibility of intravenously administered antibody to tumour conspire to limit antibody delivery quite markedly.

In our study the absolute amount of antibody-conjugate which reaches a glioma is very small. When expressed as per cent of injected dose per gram of tissue, it is in the order of 0.001. This may have important implications for targeted radiation therapy: for example, an intravenous injection of 50 mCi ^{131}I-conjugate would result in only 0.5 mCi reaching 1 g of the tumour. Thus a tumour weighing 100 g would receive a dose of only 50 mCi.

Plate 1. Positive [^{131}I]UJ13A scan of a malignant glioma 5 days post-injection of reagent in patient no. 2.

Plate 2. Cursors on the scintillation image over an area of increased uptake of ^{131}I and over normal brain in the same patient as in Plate 1. Objective measurements of counts within these selected areas are then obtained for Regions of Interest (ROI) Analysis.

Plate 3. A positive [^{131}I]UJ13A image of malignant glioma in patient no. 4 using subtraction techniques (early from late image).

Plate 4. Patient 5. The image on the right is a ^{99m}Tc glucoheptonate scan showing ^{99m}Tc uptake in a small area of the tumour which corresponds to the region of Conray enhancement shown in Fig. 6.3b. Both are small molecules with a molecular weight of less than 1000. The [^{131}I]UJ13A scintigram is on the left. No tumour uptake of radiolabelled antibody was seen at any time, even with the use of subtraction. This demonstrates the impermeability of the BBB to the larger immunoglobin molecule and regional permeability to the smaller molelcules. Conray and glucoheptonate.

Plate 5. Positive [^{131}I]HMFG2 (control MCA) scan 6 days post-injection in patient no. 10 with a gliosarcoma.

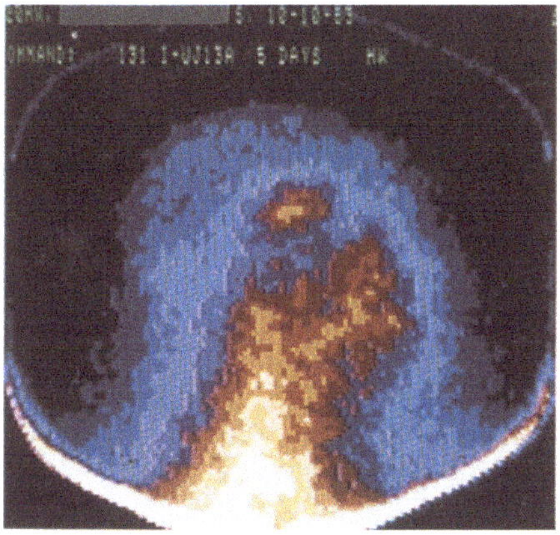

Plate 1

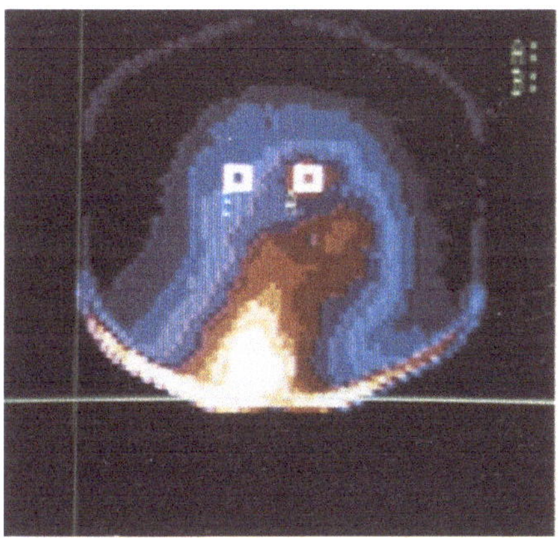

Plate 2

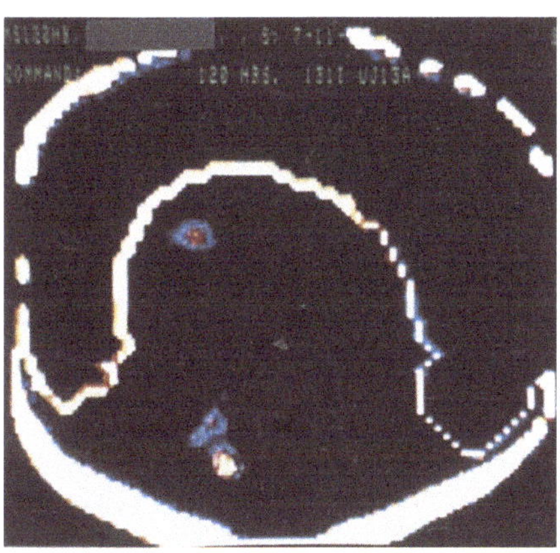

Plate 3

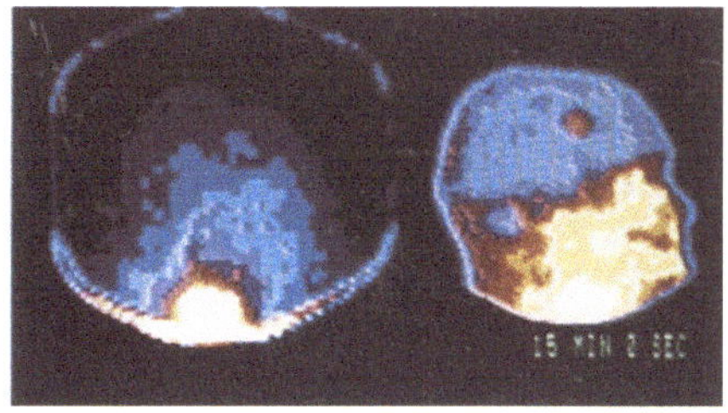

Plate 4

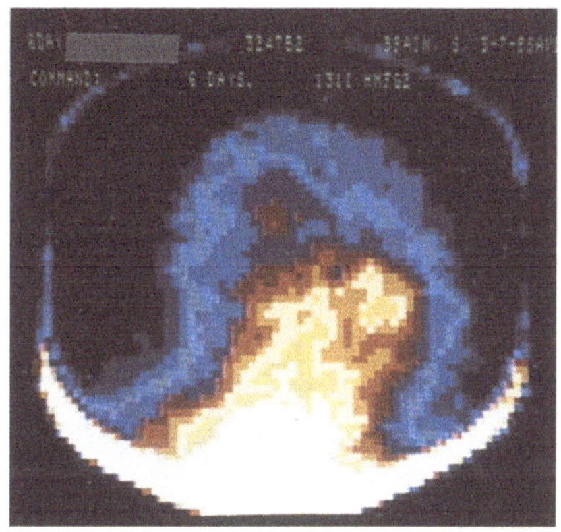

Plate 5

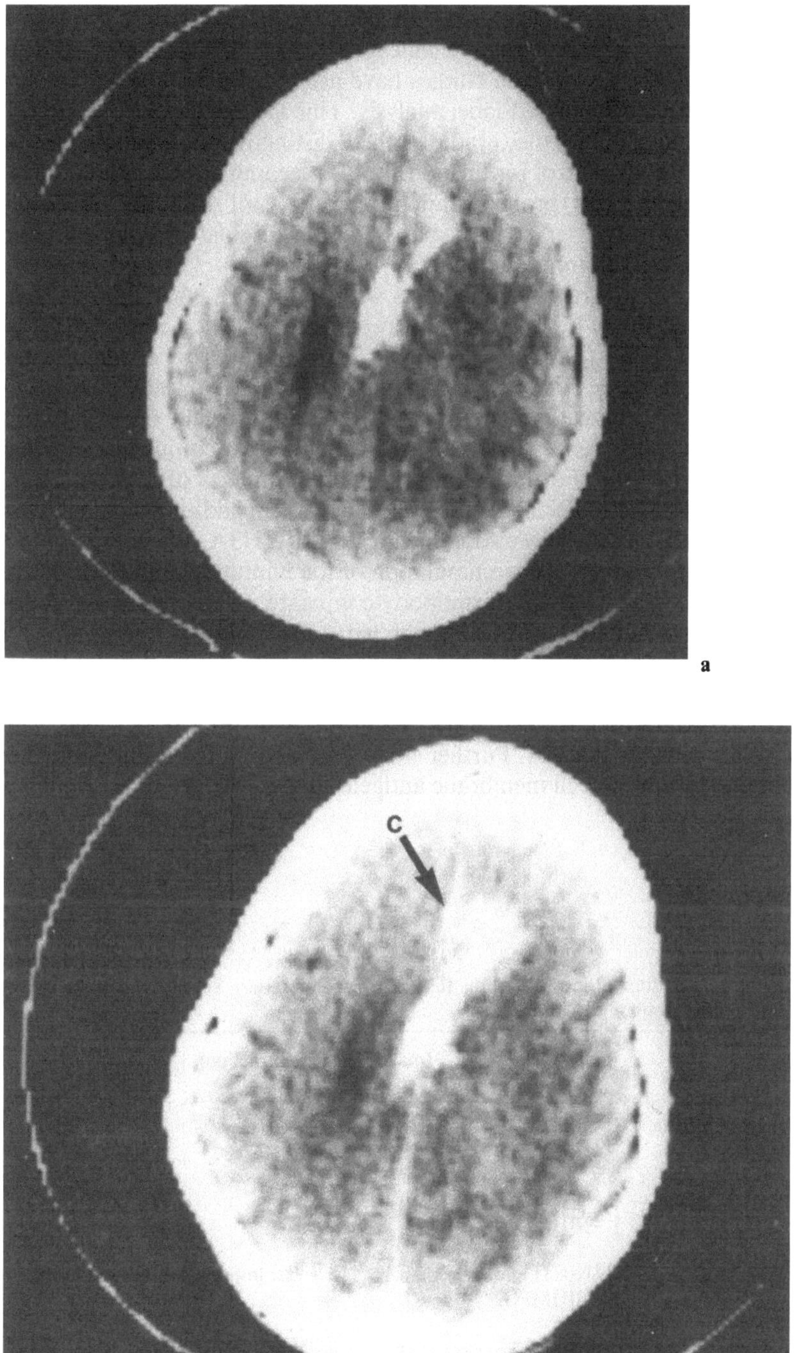

Fig. 6.3. a Computerised tomographic scan of patient no. 5 with a large oligoastrocytoma diagnosed 16 years previously by parietal burr hole biopsy. The tumour occupies much of the right cerebral hemisphere. Calcification is present antero-medially. **b** In the same patient, following Conray injection, a small, but definite area of enhancement is seen anteriorly (arrowed).

Specificity of Brain Tumour Radioimmunolocalisation

The original experiments of Pressman and colleagues (1957) were exemplary and set a standard to which very few human studies have aspired. These workers emphasised the importance of using paired-label analysis. This means the use of appropriate specific and control antibodies, radiolabelled distinctively and administered synchronously, in order to control for the non-specific accumulation of immunoglobulin within a tumour. This protein trapping property of tumours, especially gliomas, is well known and served as a basis for the original imaging of brain tumours with ^{131}I-labelled albumin (Chou et al. 1951).

We therefore studied a further five patients with the paired-label analysis technique using specific antibody UJ13A and non-specific HMFG2 as a control (Taylor-Papadimitriou et al. 1981) (Table 6.6). ^{131}I and ^{125}I were used to distinguish the antibodies in resected tissue analysis. Using this method it was not possible to demonstrate specificity, as measurement of the isotopes in surgically resected tissues showed no significant differences in uptake between the two conjugates in either normal brain or in tumour. Furthermore, scintigraphic images of a glioma were produced using [^{131}I]HMFG2 (Plate 5) and, conversely, in an additional patient with a carcinoma metastasis, an image was obtained with [^{131}I]UJ13A. We interpret these results as being due to non-specific accumulation of the immunoglobulin within the tumour tissue. The increased levels of antibody-conjugate within necrosis and cyst fluid which occur as a function of time may be part of this passive "sump effect". The avid binding of UJ13A to gliomas in vitro suggests that this antibody which is present in a tumour in vivo is likely to be bound to cell surfaces whereas the non-specific HMFG2 would be assumed to be free in the interstitial fluid space. This hypothesis is illustrated in Fig. 6.4. Further studies are needed to establish whether UJ13A is binding to tumour cell membrane antigens in vivo. A further possibility is

Table 6.6. Immunolocalisation of intra-vertebral tumours. Second series: Specific antibody UJ13A and control antibody HMFG2

Patient no.	Tumour	Radiolabels	Image	Subtraction
6	Malignant glioma	[^{131}I]UJ13A [^{125}I]HMFG2	Good	No
7	Malignant glioma	[^{131}I]UJ13A [^{125}I]HMFG2	Fair	No
8	Malignant glioma	[^{131}I]UJ13A [^{125}I]HMFG2	Fair	Yes: improved localisation
9	Malignant glioma	[^{131}I]UJ13A [^{125}I]HMFG2	Fair	Yes: improved localisation
10	Gliosarcoma	[^{131}I]HMFG2 [^{125}I]UJ13A	Good	No

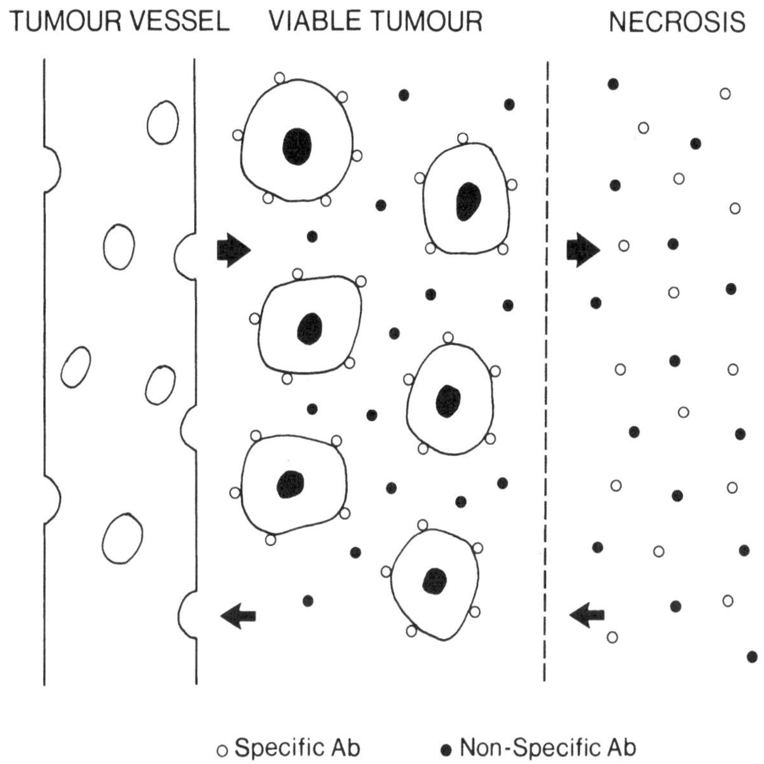

Fig. 6.4. Diagram indicating how the passive accumulation of a radiolabelled non-specific MCA in extracellular space and necrotic areas might mask the binding of the specific MCA (see text).

that the whole antibody used in this study is binding to Fc receptors of lymphoreticular cells within the tumours (Wood et al. 1980). However, these assumptions must await experimental verification.

Clearly these significant problems of dose delivery of antibody to tumour and of non-specific protein accumulation are impeding progress towards radioimmunodiagnosis or targeted radiation therapy for solid brain tumours. The use of antibody more specific for tumour, Fab or $F(ab')_2$ fragments, and BBB modification may all play a part in overcoming these problems. It is now becoming apparent that different murine and rat MCAs exhibit variability of behaviour in humans (Sikora et al. 1984). The idiosyncratic binding pattern seen with these reagents might also contribute to current difficulties in RIL of brain tumours. The use of human MCAs offers significant advantages in many respects. Unfortunately, instability of human hybridomas means these valuable reagents are at present in short supply. Sikora and Phillips (1981) produced hybridomas from the B lymphocytes harvested from a human glioma and infused the antibodies, radiolabelled, into the patient. Preferential uptake of the relevant antibody compared with a control was found by immunoscintigraphy and examination of tumour cyst fluid (Phillips et al. 1983).

Intrathecal Targeting for Leptomeningeal Malignancy

These problems of accessibility in targeting MCAs to tumours are not relevant in situations where natural barriers do not exist. Thus more favourable results would be expected by administering diagnostic or therapeutic conjugates directly into malignant effusions of the pleural, pericardial and peritoneal cavities (Courtenay-Luck et al. 1984).

We have recently obtained highly encouraging results in a case of widespread leptomeningeal infiltration by a recurrent pineocytoma following conventional therapy. The malignant cells obtained from the cerebrospinal fluid (CSF) were examined immunocytologically and found to express the UJ181.4 antigen not found on normal central nervous tissue. This provided the opportunity for in vivo targeting with direct access to tumour cells and with a tumour-specific reagent. In a study employing paired-label analysis, scintigraphy and external scintillation counting were carried out following the intrathecal administration of 0.5 mCi [^{131}I]UJ181.4 and 0.5 mCi [^{125}I]HMFG2 as a control (H. B. Coakham et al. unpubl. data).

Results from external scintillation counting and direct counting of radiation from CSF indicated that the ^{131}I-conjugate localised to the neuraxis. The non-specific ^{125}I-conjugate disappeared more rapidly from the CSF with retention of the specific label in the tumour cells. This led to very favourable ratios of up to 30 : 1 specific to non-specific activity, together with a persisting [^{131}I]UJ181.4 scintigraphic image of the spinal cord and base of brain. Subsequent myelography confirmed the presence of multiple nodules of neoplastic tissue involving the cord and nerve roots. Localisation of the specific ^{131}I activity in centrifuged CSF cell pellets exceeded that in the supernatant by 10 : 1. With this encouraging evidence of specific binding in vivo, the patient was given intrathecal therapy with 23 mCi[^{131}I]UJ181.4 and within a few weeks this produced a clinical improvement with reversion of CSF cell counts and chemistry to normal. The patient remains in remission at 10 months.

Conclusions

Mouse monoclonal antibody (MCA) will cross the blood–brain barrier (BBB) in the majority of human primary brain tumours, but the BBB may be impermeable to immunoglobulin in certain cases, particularly lower-grade gliomas. Accumulation of antibody-conjugate within a tumour compared with normal brain increases with time. Similarly, there is a time-related deposition of antibody in necrotic and cystic areas. Ratios in necrotic tissue relative to normal brain as high as 19:1 have been obtained. Despite these high ratios only a minute fraction of the intravenous radiation dose will ultimately localise in the tumour, making this at present a poor method of delivering radiation compared with interstitial brachytherapy.

The demonstration of specific localisation of an antineuroectodermal MCA to solid brain tumours is not yet possible since identical results are obtained by scintigraphy and direct scintillation counting of resected tissues when paired-label analysis is performed using a control antibody.

In other human solid tumours studied by radioimmunolocalisation, claims for in vivo specificity of antibodies have been less impressive when paired-label analysis has been employed (Mach et al. 1981, Larson et al. 1983, Baldwin et al. 1984). However, the high specificity index (relevant:control antibody) that can be obtained when radiolabelled antibody is administered intrathecally suggests that specific binding does occur with solid brain tumours; this awaits experimental verification.

The accessibility of antibody to tumour in targeting against malignancy in the cerebrospinal fluid (CSF) means that high doses of radiation can be appropriately delivered with relatively less radiation to other organs. Preliminary data suggest that this form of therapy may be extremely valuable in patients with neuroectodermal or lymphoid malignancy to whom neuraxis irradiation has already been given and who relapse with CSF malignancy. If appropriate human MCAs were available then such cases could receive multiple treatments in the hope of achieving long remissions.

We thank the staff of the Nuclear Medicine Department, Mrs G. Wenczek and Mrs A. White for preparing the manuscript, and the staff of medical illustration and library, Frenchay Hospital, Bristol. This work was supported by the Brain Cancer Research Fund and the Imperial Cancer Research Fund. A.G.D. is a Thorne Research Fellow and S.P.B. is supported by the Newman Foundation.

References

Allan PM, Garson JA, Harper EI, Asser U, Coakham HB, Brownell B, Kemshead JT (1983) Biological characterisation and clinical applications of a monoclonal antibody recognising an antigen restricted to neuro-ectodermal tissues. Int J Cancer 31: 591–598

Baldwin RW, Pimm MV, Embleton MJ, Armitage NM, Farrands PA, Hardcastle JD, Perkins A (1984) Monoclonal antibody 791T/36 for tumour detection and therapy for metastases. In: Nicholson GL, Milas L (eds) Cancer invasion and metastasis: Biologic and therapeutic aspects. Raven Press, New York, pp 437–455

Begent RHJ, Stanway G, Jones BE, Bagshawe KD, Searle F, Jewkes RF, Vernon P (1980) Radioimmunolocalisation of tumours by external scintigraphy after administration of ^{131}I antibody to human chorionic gonadotrophin: Preliminary communication. J R Soc Med 73: 624–630

Belitsky P, Ghose T, Aquino J, Norvell ST, Blair AH (1978) Radionuclide imaging of metastases from renal-cell carcinoma by ^{131}I-labelled antitumour antibody. Radiology 126: 515-517

Berche C, Mach J-P, Lumbroso J-D, Langlais C, Aubrey F, Buchegger F, Carrel S, Rougier P, Parmentier C, Tubina M (1982) Tomoscintigraphy for detecting gastrointestinal and medullary thyroid cancers: First clinical results using radiolabelled monoclonal antibodies against carcinoembryonic antigen. Br Med J 285: 1447–1451

Beverley PC, Callard RE (1981) Distinctive functional characteristics of human "T"-lymphocytes defined by E rosetting or a monoclonal anti-T cell antibody. Eur J Immunol 11: 329–334

Bourdon MA, Wikstrand CJ, Furthmayr H, Matthews TJ, Bigner DD (1983) Human glioma-mesenchymal extracellular matrix antigen defined by monoclonal antibody. Cancer Res 43: 2796–2805

Bourdon MA, Coleman RE, Bigner DD (1984) The potential of monoclonal antibodies as carriers of radiation and drugs for immunodetection and therapy of brain tumours. Prog Exp Tumor Res 28: 79–101

Chou SN, Aust JB, Moore GE, Peyton WT (1951) Radioactive iodinated human serum albumin as tracer agent for diagnosing and localising intracranial lesions. Proc Soc Exp Biol Med 77: 193–195

Coakham HB, Garson JA, Brownell B, Kemshead JT (1984) Monoclonal antibodies as reagents for brain tumour diagnosis: A review. J R Soc Med 77: 780–787

Courtenay-Luck N, Epenetos AA, Halnan KE, Hooker G, Hughes JMB, Krausz T, Lambert J, Lavender P, MacGregor WG, McKenzie CJ, Munro A, Myers J, Orr JS, Pearse EE, Snook D, Webb B, Burchell J, Durbin H, Kemshead JT, Taylor-Papadimitriou J (1984) Antibody-guided irradiation of malignant lesions: three cases illustrating a new method of treatment. Lancet I: 1441–1443

Day ED, Lassiter S, Woodhall B, Mahaley JL, Mahaley MS (1965) The localisation of radioantibodies in human brain tumours. I. Preliminary exploration. Cancer Res 25: 773–778
Deane BR, Papp MI, Lantos PL (1984) The vasculature of experimental brain tumours. III. Permeability studies. J Neurol Sci 65: 47–58
DeLand FH, Kim EE, Simmons G, Goldenberg DM (1980) Imaging approach in radioimmunodetection. Cancer Res 40: 3046–3049
Edwards PAW, Smith CM, Neville AM, O'Hare MJ (1982) A human-human hybridoma system based on a fast growing mutant of the ARH-77 plasma cell leukaemia-derived line. Eur J Immunol 12: 641–648
Epenetos AA, Mather S, Granowska M, Nimmon CC, Hawkins IR, Britton KE, Shepherd J, Taylor-Papadimitriou J, Durbin H, Malpas JS, Bodmer WF (1982) Targeting of iodine-123-labelled tumour-associated monoclonal antibodies to ovarian, breast, and gastrointestinal tumours. Lancet II: 999–1004
Farrands PA, Perkins AC, Pimm MV, Hardy JD, Embleton MJ, Baldwin RW, Hardcastle JD (1982) Radioimmunodetection of human colorectal cancers by an anti-tumour monoclonal antibody. Lancet II: 397–400
Feizi T (1985) Demonstration by monoclonal antibodies that carbohydrate structures of glycoproteins and glycolipids are onco-developmental antigens. Nature (Lond) 314: 53–57
Garson JA (1982) The development and characterisation of monoclonal antibodies for use in neuropathology. MD thesis, Department of Immunology, University of Birmingham
Garson JA, Beverley PCL, Coakham HB, Harper EI (1982) Monoclonal antibodies against human T lymphocytes label Purkinje neurones of many species. Nature (Lond) 298: 375–377
Ghose T, Blair AH, Martin RH, Norvell ST, Ramakrishman S, Belitsky P, Imai K, Ferrone S (1982) Tumour imaging by antitumour antibody-linked radionuclides: Experimental models and clinical applications. In: Burchiel SW, Rhodes BA, Friedman B (eds) Tumour imaging. Masson, New York, pp 167–178
Giacomelli F, Wiener J, Spiro D (1979) The cellular pathology of experimental hypertension. V. Increased permeability of cerebral arterial vessels. Am J Pathol 59: 133–160
Gold P, Freedman SO (1965) Demonstration of tumour specific antigens in human colonic carcinoma by immunological tolerance and absorption techniques. J Exp Med 121: 439–462
Goldenberg DM, Deland F, Kim E, Bennett S, Primus FJ, van Nagell JR, Estes N, DeSimone P, Rayburn P (1978) Use of radiolabelled antibodies to carcinoembryonic antigen for the detection and localisation of diverse cancers by external photoscanning. N Engl J Med 298: 1384–1388
Goldenberg DM, Kim EE, DeLand FH, van Nagell JR, Javadpour N (1980) Clinical radioimmunodetection of cancer using radioactive antibodies to human chorionic gonadotropin. Science 208: 1284–1286
Goldenberg DM, Kim EE, DeLand FH (1981) Human chorionic gonadotropin radioantibodies in the radioimmunodetection of cancer and for disclosure of occult metastases. Proc Natl Acad Sci USA 78: 7784–7758
Goldenberg DM, Deland FH, Bennet SJ, Primus FJ, Nelson O, Flanigan RC, McRoberts JW, Bruce A, Mahan DE (1983) Radioimmunodetection of prostatic cancer. J Am Med Assoc 250: 630–635
Goldman A, Vivian G, Gordon I, Pritchard J, Kemshead J (1984)) Immunolocalisation of neuroblastoma using radiolabelled monoclonal antibody UJ13A. J Pediatr 105: 252–256
Groothius DR, Fischer JM, Lapin G, Bigner DD, Vick NA (1982) Permeability of different experimental brain tumour models to horseradish peroxidase. J Neuropathol Exp Neurol 41: 164–185
Haisma H, Goedmans W, De Jong M, Hikens J, Hilgers J, Dullens H, Den Otter W (1984) Specific localisation of In-111-labelled monoclonal antibody versus 67-Ga-labelled immunoglobulin in mice bearing human breast carcinoma xenografts. Cancer Immunol Immunother 17: 62–65
Halsall AK, Fairweather DS, Bradwell AR, Blackburn JC, Dykes PW, Howell A, Reeder A, Hine KR (1981) Localisation of malignant germ cell tumours by external scanning after injection of radiolabelled anti-alpha-fetoprotein. Br Med J 283: 942–944
Kemshead JT, Fritschy J, Garson JA, Allan P, Coakham HB, Brown S, Asser U (1983) Monoclonal antibody UJ127:11 detects a 220 000–240 000 kdal glycoprotein present on a sub-set of neuroectodermally derived cells. Int J Cancer 31: 187–195
Kemshead JT, Jones DH, Goldman A, Richardson RB, Coakham HB (1984) Is there a role for radioimmunolocalisation in diagnosis of intracranial malignancies? Discussion paper. J R Soc Med 77: 847–854
Kohler G, Milstein C (1975) Continuous cultures of fused cells secreting antibody of predefined specificity. Nature (Lond) 256: 495–497
Lane D, Koprowski H (1982) Molecular recognition and the future of monoclonal antibodies. Nature (Lond) 296: 200–202
Larson SM, Carrasquillo JA, Krohn KA, Brown JP, McGuffin RW, Ferens JM, Graham MM, Hill LD,

Beaumier PL, Hellstrom KE, Hellstrom I (1983) Localisation of ^{131}I-labelled p97-specific Fab fragments in human melanoma as a basis for radiotherapy. J Clin Invest 72: 2101–2114
Mach J-P, Buchegger F, Forni M, Ritschard J, Berche C, Lumbroso J-D, Schreyer M, Girardet C, Accolla RS, Carrel S (1981) Use of radiolabelled monoclonal anti-CEA antibodies for the detection of human carcinomas by external photoscanning and tomoscintigraphy. Immunol Today 2: 239–249
Mach J-P, Chatal J-F, Lumbroso J-D, Buchegger F, Forni M, Ritschard J, Berche C, Douillard J-Y, Carrel S, Herlyn M, Steplewski Z, Koprowski H (1983) Tumour localisation in patients by radiolabelled monoclonal antibodies against colon carcinoma. Cancer Res 43: 5593–5600
Miller RA, Maloney DG, Warnke R, Levy R (1982) Treatment of B-cell lymphoma with monoclonal anti-idiotype antibody. N Engl J Med 306: 517–522
Neuwelt EA, Frenkel EP, Diehl J, Vu LH, Rapoport S, Hill S (1980) Reversible osmotic blood-brain barrier disruption in humans: Implications for the chemotherapy of malignant brain tumours. Neurosurgery 7: 44–52
Ott RJ, Grey LJ, Zivanovic MA, Flower MA, Trott NG, Moshakis V, Coombes RC, Neville AM, Ormerod MG, Westwood JH, McCready VR (1983) The limitation of the dual radionuclide subtraction technique for the external detection of tumours by radioiodine-labelled antibodies. Br J Radiol 56: 101–108
Phillips J, Alderson T, Sikora K, Watson J (1983) Localisation of malignant glioma by a radiolabelled human monoclonal antibody. J Neurol Neurosurg Psychiatr 46: 388–392
Pressman D, Keighley G (1948) The zone of activity of antibodies as determined by the use of radioactive tracers: The zone of activity of nephritoxic antikidney serum. J Immunol 59: 141–146
Pressman D, Day ED, Blau M (1957) The use of paired labelling in the determination of tumour-localising antibodies. Cancer Res 17: 845–850
Reese TS, Karnovsky MJ (1967) Fine structure localisation of a blood-brain barrier to exogenous peroxidase. J Cell Biol 34: 207–217
Richarsdon RB, Davies AG, Bourne S, Staddon GE, Kemshead JT, Coakham HB (1985) Radioimmunolocalisation of brain tumours. I. Scintigraphic studies. J Neuro-oncol (in press)
Ritz J, Best RC, Clavell LA, Hercend T, Sallan SE, Lipton JM, Feeney M, Nathan DG, Schlossman SF (1982) Autologous bone-marrow transplantation in CALLA-positive acute lymphoblastic leukaemia after in-vitro treatment with J5 monoclonal antibody and complement. Lancet II: 60–63
Schnegg JF, Diserens AC, Carrel S, Accolla RS, de Tribolet N (1981) Human glioma-associated antigens detected by monoclonal antibodies. Cancer Res 41: 1209–1213
Sikora K, Phillips J (1981) Human monoclonal antibodies to glioma cells. Br J Cancer 43: 105–107
Sikora K, Alderson T, Finan P, Lennox E, Markham N, Ritson A, Smedley H (1984) The selection of monoclonal antibodies for tumour localisation in patients with colorectal carcinoma. Med Oncol Tum Pharmacother 1: 63–71
Stevenson G, Stevenson F (1975) Antibody to a molecularly defined antigen confined to a tumour cell surface. Nature (Lond) 254: 714–716
Taylor-Papadimitriou J, Peterson JA, Arklie J, Burchell J, Ceriani RL, Bodmer W (1982) Monoclonal antibodies to epithelium-specific components of the human milk fat globule membrane: Production and reaction with cells in culture. Int J Cancer 28: 17–21
Treleaven JG, Ugelstad J, Philip T, Gibson FM, Rembaum A, Caine GD, Kemshead JT (1984) Removal of neuroblastoma cells from bone marrow with monoclonal antibodies conjugated to magnetic microspheres. Lancet I: 70–73
Wood GW, Morantz RA, Tilzer SA, Gollahon KA (1980) Immunoglobulin bound in vivo to Fc receptor-positive cells in human central nervous system tumours. J Natl Cancer Inst 64: 411–418

7 Surgery for Primary Brain Tumours

J. R. W. Gleave

Introduction

The term primary brain tumour may be defined as either an intracranial tumour that is not a metastasis, or a tumour arising from the substance of the brain itself. It is those tumours covered by the second definition which provide the greatest problem because they are not only the most numerous, but also the least amenable to treatment.

It is just a century since the first operations were carried out both for a tumour arising from the substance of the brain itself and for an extracerebral tumour not presenting as a calvarial mass, though there had been earlier operations for hyperostosing meningiomas (Pecchioli 1838, Macewan 1879). The diagnosis of these tumours and their intracranial localisation was made entirely on clinical grounds. The surgeons concerned were Rickman Godlee (Bennett and Godlee 1885) and Francesco Durante (1886). Godlee's patient survived the operation but succumbed from meningitis on the twenty-eighth post-operative day and would thus in most modern series be counted as a post-operative death. Durante's patient was alive and well 4 years later. Although it seems likely that Durante carried out his operation before Godlee, his work never received as much publicity as Godlee's because he did not publish it until later and the general press seem not to have been involved as they were in Godlee's case (*The Times*, 16 December 1884).

This was the beginning of neurosurgery as it is known today and the development of the art was for a long time based largely upon the treatment of tumours. This aspect of the work still occupies the centre of the neurosurgical stage with regard both to the volume of work and to the introduction of new techniques of diagnosis, surgery and other therapy. It would therefore seem appropriate to review in a global fashion the role of surgery in the management of the major groups of primary brain tumours.

In order to do this all the patients with tumours admitted to a Regional Neurosurgical Centre over the 20 year period 1963–1982 have been considered, the population served being approximately 2 million. During this time the aims of surgery have not changed, though there have been developments in diagnostic techniques, such as the introduction of computerised tomography (CT) in 1975, and refinements in surgical techniques including the availability of stereotaxy since 1964, the operating microscope since 1965, the carbon dioxide laser since 1978, and the Cavitron since 1981. For those tumours that are not surgically curable there have been developments in radiotherapy and chemotherapy, but these are beyond the scope of this discussion. The basic tumour statistics are set out in Table 7.1.

The aims of surgery may be summarised as follows:

1) to make a firm diagnosis,
2) to cure if possible,
3) to allow the best chance for other treatment to be effective if surgical cure is impossible or inappropriate,
4) to palliate symptoms.

Two principles have also guided the approach. The first is that if a tumour is surgically curable and there is no alternative effective treatment, some additional disability may be acceptable if the patient agrees, viz. the infliction of a facial palsy on a patient with an acoustic neurinoma. The second principle is that the infliction of global aphasia or the prolongation of life in the presence of global aphasia is not tolerable.

The remainder of this chapter presents the results of treatment for the individual tumour types from the Cambridge Regional Neurosurgical Centre.

Table 7.1. Brain tumour surgery in Cambridge (1963–1982)

Tumour type	No. of patients
Meningioma	377
Acoustic neurinoma	125
Haemangioblastoma	50
Craniopharyngioma	20
Astrocytoma including glioblastoma	1107[a]
Cerebral	1046
Optic chiasma/hypothalamic	9
Cerebellar	39
Brain stem	13
Oligodendroglioma	42
Ependymoma	43
Cerebral	10
Cerebellar	28
Brain stem	5
Microglioma	11
Medulloblastoma	48
Neuroblastoma	6
Ganglioneuroma	1
Germinoma	17
Brain stem (presumed glioma)	11

[a] Nine tumours associated with von Recklinghausen's disease.

Tumours of Extracerebral Origin

The major intracranial tumours of extracerebral origin are the meningiomas, acoustic neurinomas, haemangioblastomas and craniopharyngiomas. In these tumours surgery has the primary role in treatment and the results in the first three groups are reasonably satisfactory, as shown in Table 7.2.

Table 7.2. Results of surgery in intracranial tumours of extracerebral origin (Cambridge 1962–1981)

Type of tumour	No. of patients	Surgical removal		Further surgery (recurrence or new tumour)	Mortality	
		Total	Subtotal		Operative	From tumour
Meningioma	377	330 (87%)	47 (13%)	27 (7%)	26 (7%) (13 pulmonary emboli)	9 (2%)
Acoustic neurinoma	125					
Suboccipital	73	44 (60%)	29 (40%)	0	15 (20%)	4 (5%)
Trans-labyrinthine	52	51 (98%)	1 (2%)	0	2 (4%)	1 (2%)
Haemangioblastoma (including 4 medullary)	50	50 (100%)	0	9 (18%)	2 (4%) (both pulmonary emboli)	1 (2%)
Craniopharyngioma	20	8	12	8 (2 total resection)	1	3

The following individual comments may, however, be made.

Meningiomas

The results for meningiomas are very similar to those published from the Mayo Clinic by McCartey and Taylor (1979) except that re-operation in our patients did not carry the increased post-operative mortality that they described. Detailed results are presented in Tables 7.3 and 7.4.

There are a few meningiomas that appear to be surgically incurable though symptoms resulting from their bulk may be alleviated by surgery (Fig. 7.1). However, this number is becoming smaller as operations such as extended petrusectomy become more feasible. There were 10 patients over and above those included in the surgical series in whom operation was not advised as their symptoms did not warrant it and they were aged 80 or more. A careful watch was kept on them and in one patient a ventriculo-atrial shunt provided relief of her symptoms until she died from other causes. Radiotherapy has a place where there is doubt about the total removal of a tumour which histologically shows malignant characteristics.

Table 7.3. Results of surgical treatment for meningiomas

Location		Primary resection		Subsequent surgery		Operative mortality		% overall mortality	Death from tumour
		Total	Subtotal	After total resection	After subtotal resection	Total resection	Subtotal resection		
Parasagittal	92	79	13	4	5	2	1	3%	4
Cerebral convexity	84	83	1	2	1	1	0	2%	2
Sphenoid wing	58	50	8	1	3	3	4	10%	1
Olfactory groove	31	31	0	1	0	6	0	20%	1
Tentorial	29	23	6	0	3	1	1	7%	-
Suprasellar	28	25	3	0	0	2	1	11%	-
Middle fossa	18	14	4	1	3	1	0	5%	-
Cerebello-pontine angle	9	6	3	0	1	0	1	11%	-
Multiple	7	4	3	0	0	0	0		-
Petrous ridge	6	4	2	1	0	0	0		1
Clivus	5	1	4	0	1	0	0		-
Intraventricular	4	4	0	0	0	0	0		-
Foramen magnum	3	3	0	0	0	0	2	66%	-
Cerebellar convexity	2	2	0	0	0	0	0		-
Optic nerve	1	1	0	0	0	0	0		-
Totals	377	330	47	10	17	16	10		9
(2.4%)									
				(27 = 7%)		(26 = 7%)			

Table 7.4. Meningioma: Timing of subsequent surgery

Location	After total resection	After subtotal resection
Parasagittal	1(S), 2(S), 13(M), 29(M)	1(S), 2(S), 3(M), 9, 17
Cerebral convexity	1(S), 2, 4, 6	1(S)
Sphenoid wing	6	2, 10, 11(S)
Olfactory groove	2(S)	
Middle fossa	7	1, 7, 10
Cerebello-pontine angle		2
Petrous ridge	5(S) (met)	
Clivus		5

Figures indicate time in years from primary resection. Abbreviations: met, metastasis to liver; M, multiple; S, sarcoma.

Acoustic Neurinoma

The figures for the suboccipital approach in acoustic neurinomas are derived from the first 15 years of the series. Patients were not usually referred until in serious

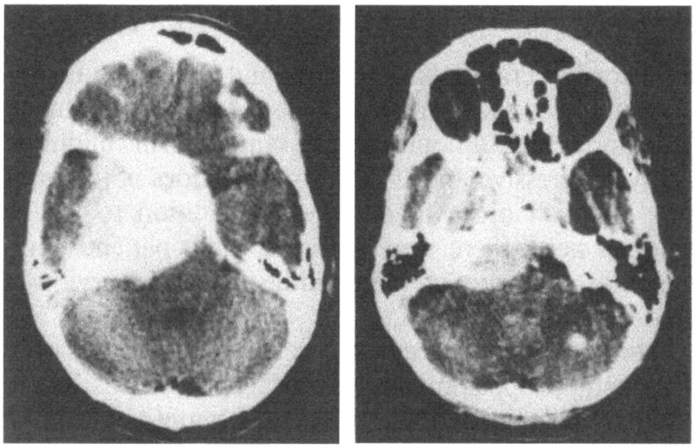

Fig. 7.1 Ineradicable meningioma of base of skull, biopsied trans-sphenoidally.

trouble from raised intracranial pressure or brain stem compression. Eighty-eight per cent of these tumours were graded as large, and 12% as intermediate. There were no small tumours.

In the last 5 years of the series a more enlightened attitude to unilateral deafness was adopted by ENT surgeons and CT scanning became available. This resulted in a team approach by ENT surgeons and neurosurgeons which has led to earlier diagnosis and treatment of these tumours. The results, with regard to both mortality and function, are correspondingly better.

However, surgery is not always essential for acoustic neurinomas and two patients have been followed up for 20 and 22 years respectively with probable acoustic neurinomas graded as large who presented with trigeminal neuralgia. An alcohol injection cured the neuralgia and, as they had no further symptoms nor any other disability, they declined surgery as under no circumstances did they wish for a facial palsy.

Leksell (1982) gave a very favourable report on a small series of tumours measuring up to 25 mm in diameter that were treated with stereotactic radiosurgery. The maximum follow-up was 11 years and only one patient had to be re-irradiated. There was sometimes preservation of useful hearing and no other cranial nerve loss.

Haemangioblastoma

The mortality from haemangioblastoma in our series is a great improvement on the previously reported studies in which it was 8%–15% (Mondkar et al. 1967, Palmer 1972, Jeffreys 1975). This improvement reflects the fact that all the patients in the series have had the advantage of modern neuroanaesthetic techniques and surgical instrumentation whereas the previous large series date back to a period before these benefits were available.

It is possible that Leksell's stereotactic radiosurgical treatment unit would be of value in cases of a small lesion in the mid-brain or pons, though a tumour in one of these sites did not occur in our series. Certainly this form of treatment has proved very useful in a patient with a small pontine arteriovenous malformation.

Craniopharyngioma

The variability in the natural history of craniopharyngiomas and the small number of patients with such tumours coming to each centre make assessment of treatment very difficult. There seems little doubt that tumours causing symptoms in childhood or adolescence are more rapidly progressive and that if a patient does not present until later in life the outlook is much more favourable. In addition to the 20 surgically treated cases mentioned here, there were a further eight patients, presumed to have craniopharyngiomas, who presented in middle age or older without symptoms and were discovered incidentally.

Extirpation at the first operation is probably the best procedure and the Cavitron has made this a much more realistic proposition. Indeed it has proved possible to remove totally two tumours that had given rise to recurrent symptoms after a previous partial removal.

Radiotherapy, the injection of radionuclides into the cystic component and the Leksell stereotactic radiosurgery apparatus may all have a part to play in the treatment of craniopharyngiomas, but insufficient experience has so far been obtained.

Primary Cerebral Tumours

If a primary brain tumour is defined as a tumour arising in the substance of the brain and derived from cells from which the brain itself is formed, a very different picture emerges. It is only in some small subgroups of these tumours that surgery, or indeed any form of treatment, has made any impact.

There is still debate about the precise classification of brain tumours (Butler et al. 1982). Kernohan's modification of the Bailey-Cushing scheme seems the most practical, steering as it does a middle course between too many and too few categories. However, in this series an attempt has been made to divide ependymomas into high-grade and low-grade malignancy tumours. Doubts must also be expressed whether glioblastoma multiforme is invariably a grade 4 astrocytoma; it is possible that it may be the final common path of all the glial tumours. In spite of this reservation glioblastoma multiforme has in fact been included with the grade 3–4 astrocytomas because its behaviour is similar.

Each tumour was graded according to its most malignant portion, and in addition to the cytology such features as vascularity and above all necrosis were taken into account. Zülch's concept of total malignancy (Zülch and Woolf 1965) is excellent but hard to apply, because even with CT scanning the deep extent of the tumour may be hard to establish.

Accordingly for the purposes of this analysis the tumours have been grouped according to the embryonic cell type and subdivided by cytological and histological criteria into low-grade (1–2) and high-grade (3–4) malignancy where applicable. It is well recognised that tumours may contain more than one cell type but it is convenient to name the tumour by its prevalent cell type (Rubinstein 1964). Using this classification the ultimate outcome for the patient seems to be reasonably well correlated with grade, though there are inevitable exceptions.

Astrocytoma Including Glioblastoma

Astrocytomas formed 86% of the whole Cambridge series; 94% of them were situated in the cerebral hemispheres and basal ganglia. Eighty-one per cent of the tumours were of high-grade malignancy and 19% of low-grade malignancy. The high-grade tumours are predominantly a disease of late middle life (fifth and sixth decades) and there is a 1.5:1 predominance of males over females. The low-grade tumours have a wider spread and a less marked but earlier peak; there is a 1.7:1 male predominance.

It has become apparent over the course of the 100 years since operations were first carried out for brain tumours that surgery cannot cure these tumours even if a hemispherectomy is carried out as it was by Dandy. Nonetheless it is also generally accepted that the greater the bulk of tumour that can be resected, the better is the prognosis (Hitchcock and Sato 1964, Davidoff 1966).

The surgical management of these patients is guided by several factors:

1) The need to make a firm diagnosis, not only with regard to prognosis but also as a guide to treatment.
2) The condition and the physiological age of the patient.
3) The neurological deficit present.
4) The position and extent of the tumour.
5) The deficit likely to be perpetuated or inflicted by surgical intervention on the tumour itself.
6) The possibility of relieving symptoms by means other than a direct attack, such as a shunt or an external decompression.
7) The possible advantage to the oncologists concerned of having less bulk of tumour to treat.

For example, the attempt to remove in whole or in part deep-seated tumour situated in the basal ganglia or thalamus, or centred on the white centrum semi-ovale, would cause unacceptable disability for the patient. The diagnosis of the tumour type in such cases must therefore be made by a biopsy. The knowledge of the type of tumour, in conjunction with the patient's general neurological state and his wishes (if they are known) or those of his relatives would determine whether to proceed to an external decompression, a shunt if hydrocephalus was present, or directly to radiotherapy under the protective cover of dexamethasone.

Similar considerations apply to more superficial tumours in the Rolandic region, particularly tumours of the dominant hemisphere, and invariably those in Wernicke's area. Broca's area is not functionally so important and six tumours have been excised from this part of the brain with improvement in previously dysphasic patients.

If the tumour is largely confined to frontal, occipital or temporal lobes, extirpation by lobectomy may be carried out. Occipital or frontal lobectomy seems of greater benefit than temporal lobectomy because a temporal lobe tumour will more frequently have extended deeply than occipital or frontal lobe tumours will have involved the forceps major or forceps minor of the corpus callosum.

Surgery may therefore consist of:

1) Biopsy, guided either by intuition if the target is large enough or by a stereotactic technique.
2) External decompression to alleviate symptoms and allow further treatment.
3) Subtotal removal of the tumour to give more prolonged relief from its bulk effects and to allow further treatment to be more effective.

4) Apparent surgical extirpation.
The results for tumours classified as having a high grade of malignancy (grades 3–4 or glioblastoma multiforme) are shown in Figs. 7.2 to 7.5. Biopsy or external decompression were the only procedures that were feasible in 56% of these patients. The operative mortality, defined as a death occurring within a month of the operation, was 67% for a burr hole biopsy and 22% for external decompression and biopsy. The mortality fell slightly after the introduction of dexamethasone in 1970 and was also lower when stereotactic methods were used. The operative mortality for subtotal removal was 25% and that for macroscopic extirpation 3%.

The factors of most relevance to operative mortality were the site of the tumour and the general and neurological condition of the patient. It may be inferred from the results in this series that with favourably sited tumours in a conscious, albeit obtunded and drowsy patient, the operative mortality for major surgery is low. It would not be right to conclude that a carefully conducted burr hole biopsy under dexamethasone cover is necessarily dangerous.

With regard to the long-term outlook, the benefits of surgery cannot be considered in isolation because of the effects of succeeding radiotherapy or chemotherapy. With regard to disability, surgery was so planned that few of the surviving patients had their condition made significantly worse by the operation and the

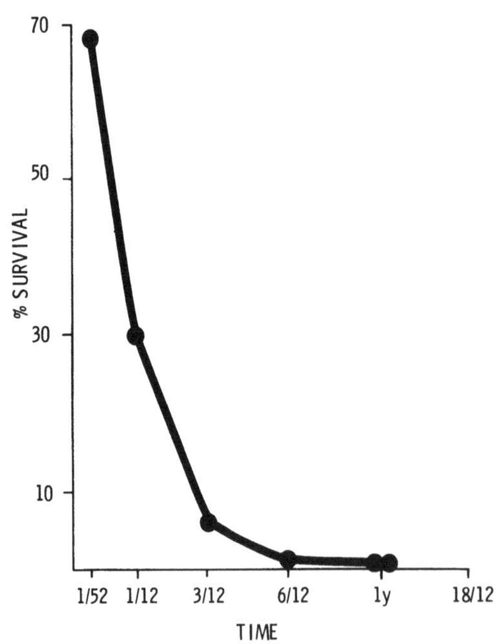

Fig. 7.2. Cerebral astrocytoma, high-grade malignancy: Survival following burr hole biopsy ($n = 348$, i.e. 41% of 848 high-grade astrocytomas treated).

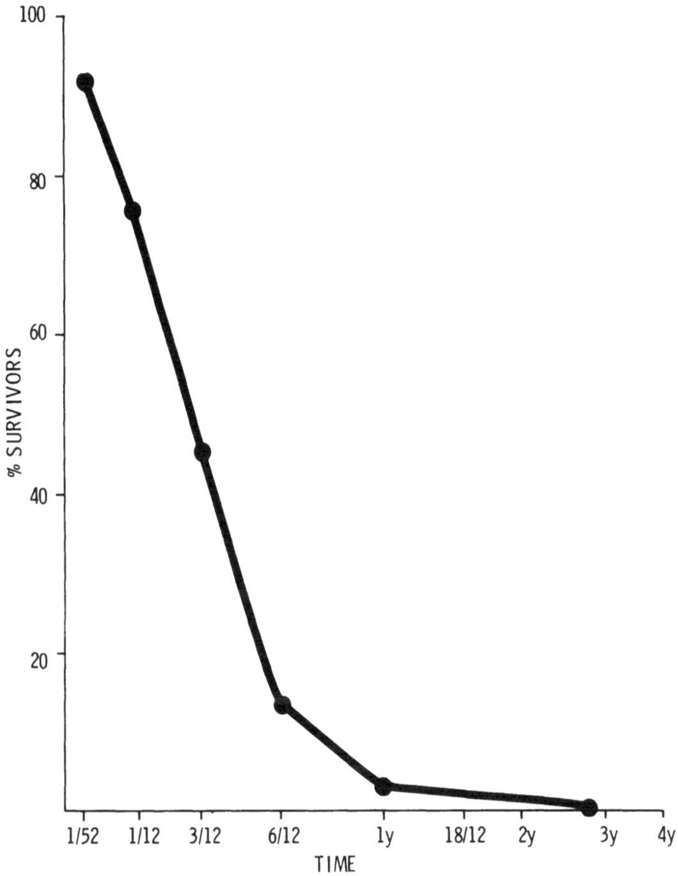

Fig. 7.3. Cerebral astrocytoma, high-grade malignancy: Survival following external decompression and biopsy ($n = 127$, i.e. 15% of 848 high-grade astrocytomas treated).

majority were significantly improved, with regard to both their level of consciousness and intellectual functioning, and their focal deficits. However, in commonsense terms it seems that survival for less than 6 months can hardly be called worthwhile except in very special circumstances, because the surgery and radiotherapy would occupy the best part of 3 months and final deterioration would have begun before convalescence was completed. Survival for 6 months to a year may be considered just worthwhile, for over a year worthwhile and for over 3 years very worthwhile. On these criteria the surgery and subsequent treatment were just worthwhile for 25% of the patients, worthwhile for 10% and very worthwhile for 2%. Of this last 2% six survived for more than 5 years, two more than 10 years, but none beyond 15 years.

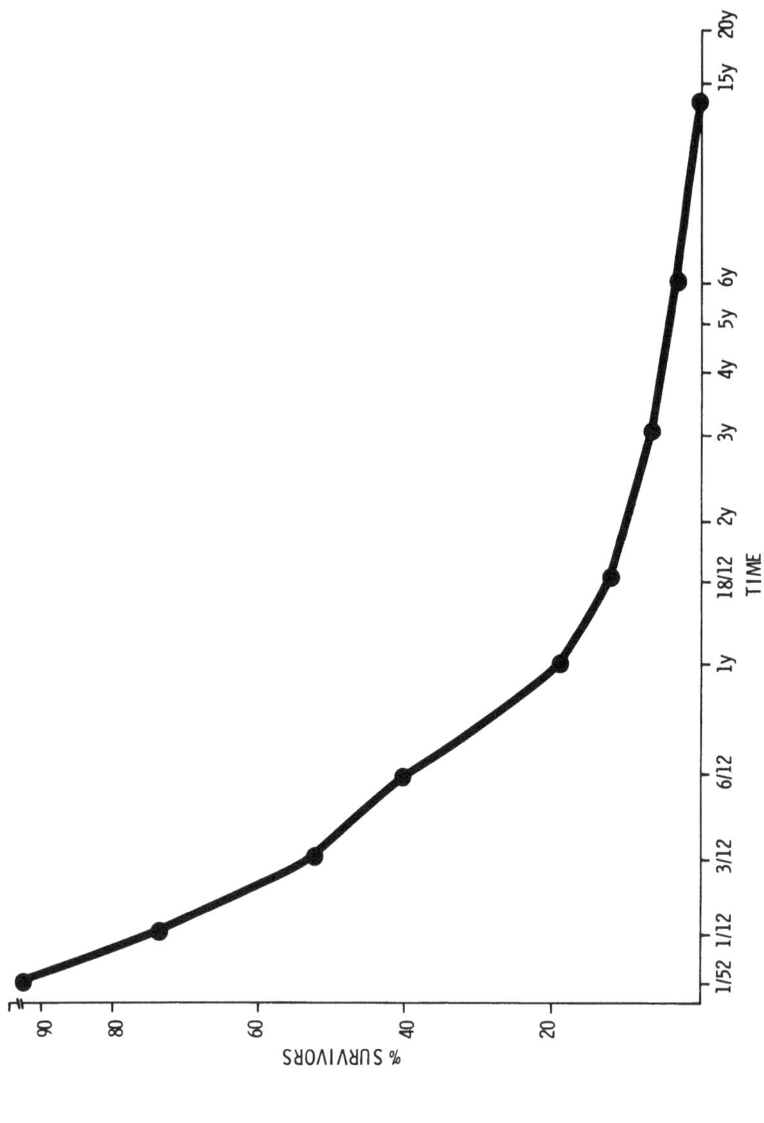

Fig. 7.4. Cerebral astrocytoma, high-grade malignancy: Survival following subtotal removal ($n = 178$, i.e. 21% of 848 high-grade astrocytomas treated).

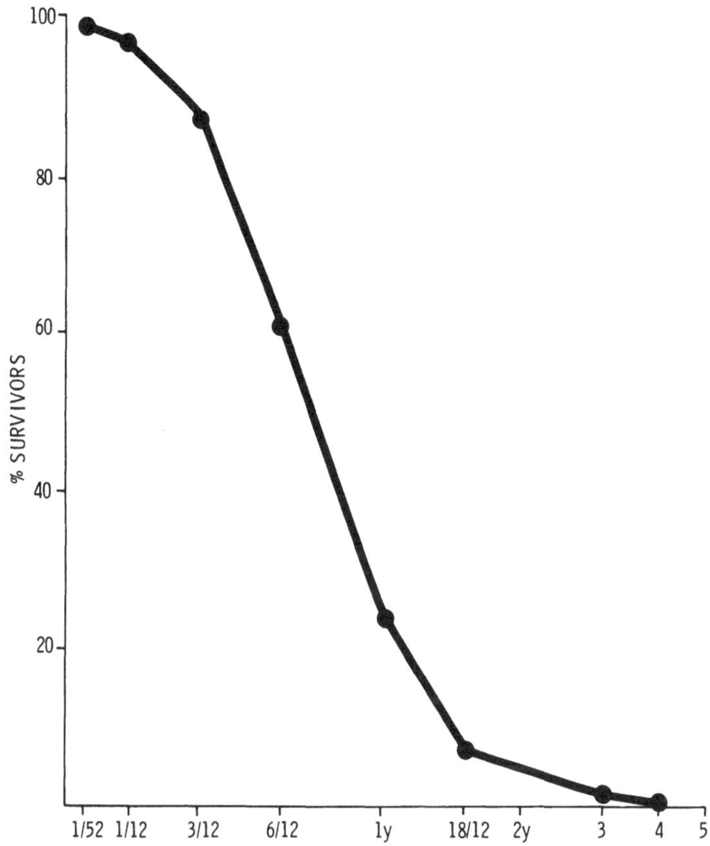

Fig. 7.5. Cerebral astrocytoma, high-grade malignancy: Survival following macroscopic total removal ($n = 195$, i.e. 23% of 848 high-grade astrocytomas treated).

The results for low-grade astrocytomas are much better, as shown in Figs. 7.6 to 7.9. Unfortunately, there are far fewer of these tumours. Biopsy with or without external decompression was the only feasible treatment in 50% of patients but the operative mortality was far lower, being 15% for a burr hole biopsy and nil when an external decompression was also carried out. For subtotal removal the operative mortality was 15% but for extirpation it was nil. Extirpation was carried out in somewhat over a quarter of the cases. Just worthwhile survivals amounted to 62%, worthwhile survivals to 50% and very worthwhile survivals to 30%. Of the long-term survivors, 15% lived more than 5 years, 8% more than 10 years, 2% have lived more than 15 years and 1% more than 20 years. Seven per cent of this group are still alive and well more than 5 years after the operation.

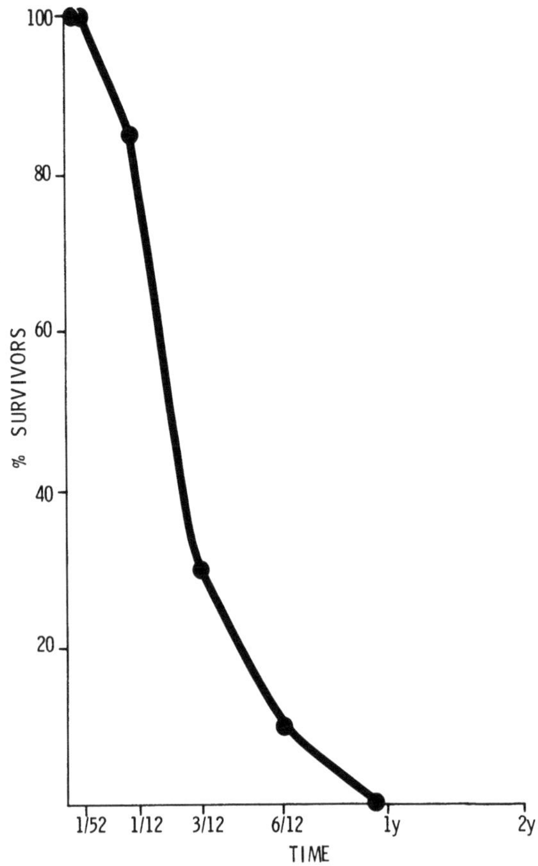

Fig. 7.6. Cerebral astrocytoma, low-grade malignancy: Survival following burr hole biopsy ($n = 44$, i.e. 22% of 198 low-grade astrocytomas treated).

Cerebellar Astrocytomas. The cerebellar astrocytomas form a special group. Seventy per cent of them occur in childhood and adolescence and these are dealt with by Bloom in another chapter of this book. Nearly 90% are low-grade tumours and the results are accordingly very good (Table 7.5). The operative mortality in our series of 39 patients was nil and total removal was carried out in 33 of them. Twenty-six were then subjected to radiotherapy (22 of those with low-grade tumours and the four patients with high-grade tumours). All four of the patients with high-grade tumours were dead by the end of the year and three of them had undergone what was thought to be a complete removal. Of those with low-grade tumours, three had died by the end of 3 years and all of them had undergone X-ray treatment. In two it was thought that a complete removal had been achieved. Two of the patients survived more than 20 years, ten more than 15 years, 20 more than 10 years, 28 more than 5 years and 32 more than 3 years.

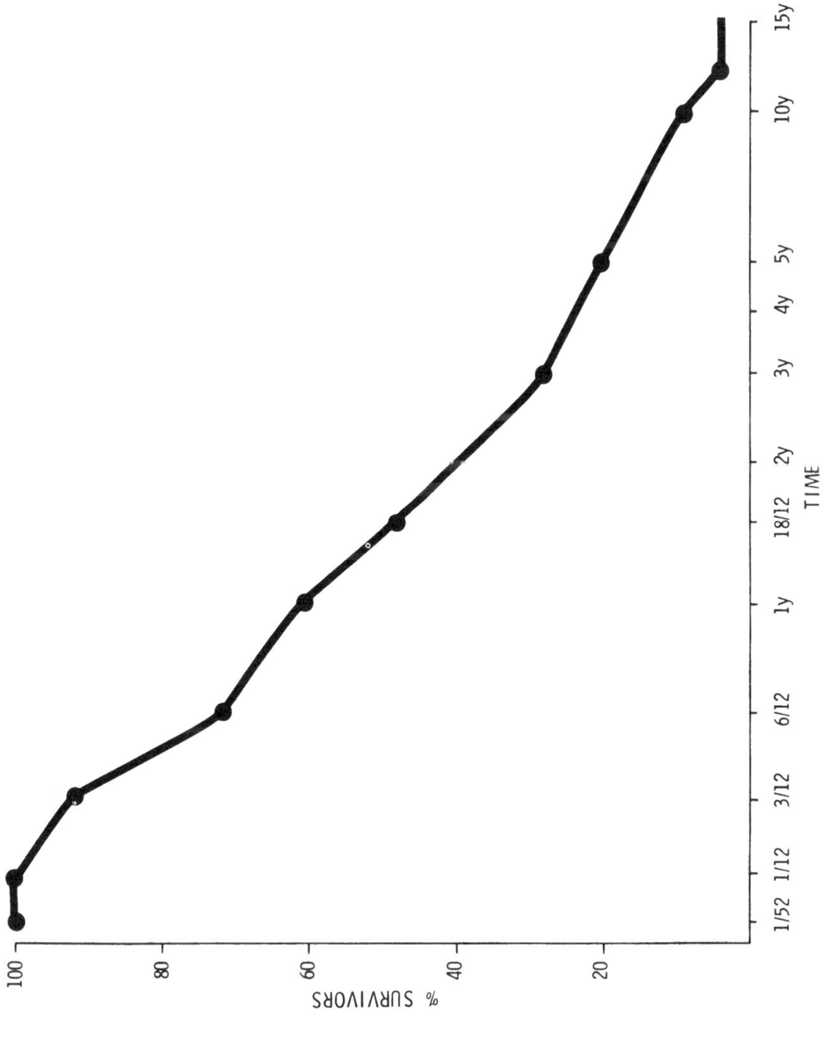

Fig. 7.7. Cerebral astrocytoma, low-grade malignancy: Survival following external decompression and biopsy ($n = 55$, i.e. 28% of 198 low-grade astrocytomas treated).

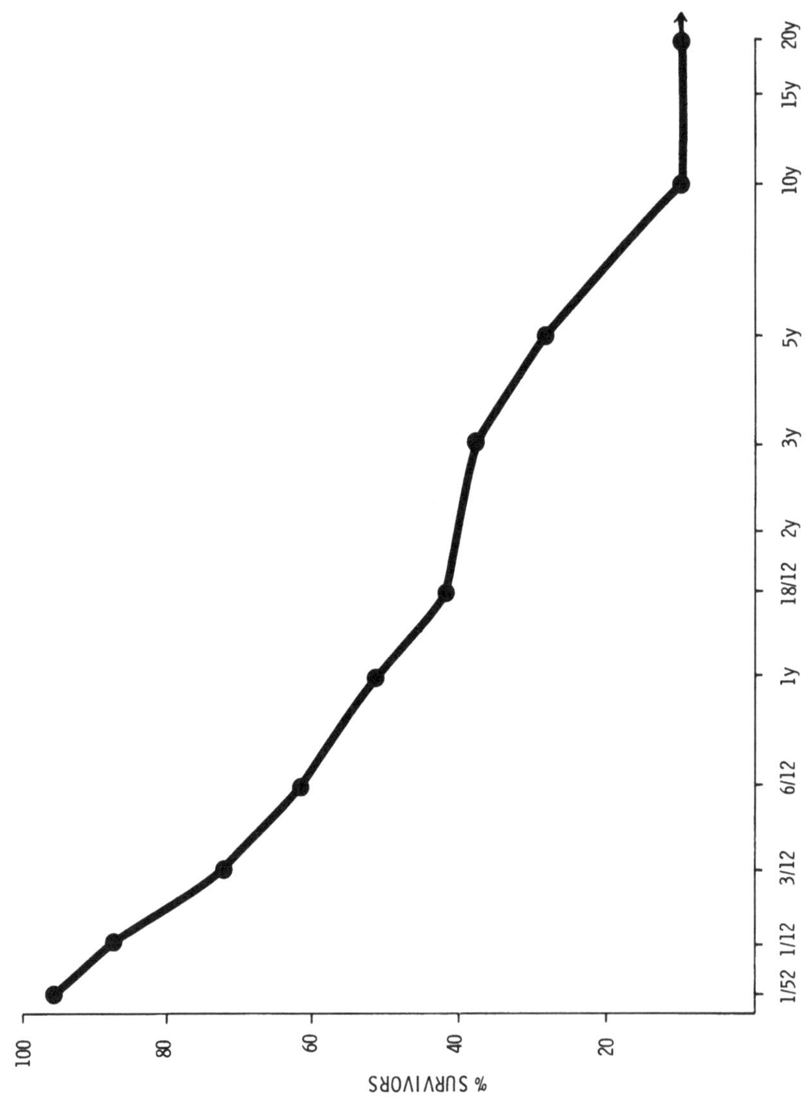

Fig. 7.8 Cerebral astrocytoma, low-grade malignancy: Survival following subtotal removal ($n = 46$, i.e. 23% of 198 low-grade astrocytomas treated).

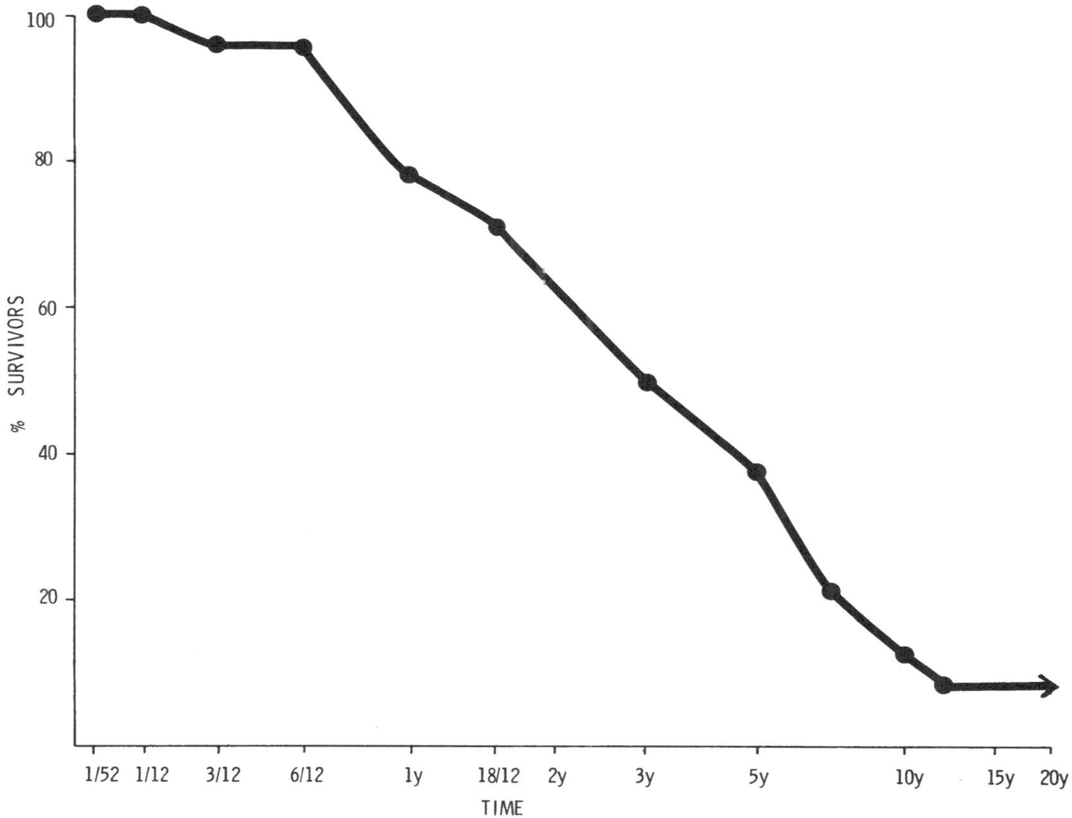

Fig. 7.9. Cerebral astrocytoma, low-grade malignancy: Survival following macroscopic total removal ($n = 53$, i.e. 27% of 198 low grade astrocytomas treated).

Table 7.5. Results of treatment of 39 patients with cerebellar astrocytoma

(*a*) *Patient details*

	Total no.	Age	No.	Removal		Operative mortality	Radiotherapy
				Total	Subtotal		
Low-grade (1–2)	35	0–9	12	11	1	Nil	8
		10–19	17	16	1		9
		20–29	3	1	2		2
		30–39	2	2	0		2
		40–49	1	0	1		1
High-grade (3–4)	4	0–9	2	2	0	Nil	2
		40–49	1	1	0		1
		50–59	1	0	1		1

(*b*) *Survival data*

	Deaths from tumour	Length of survival
Low-grade	3	6 months (subtotal; RT)[a]
		1 year (total)
		3 years (total; RT)
High-grade	4	6 months (subtotal; RT)
		9 months (total; RT)
		12 months (total; RT)
		12 months (total; RT)

Survivors	Length of follow-up (years)
2	20+
8	15+
10	10+
8	5+
4	1+
32	

[a]RT, radiotherapy.

Hypothalamic and Chiasmatic Astrocytomas. With only nine tumours in the series situated in the hypothalamic and chiasmatic regions it is impossible to see any definite pattern of the results of treatment. Surgical extirpation is out of the question and biopsy (either by open operation or stereotactically), shunting and radiotherapy are the procedures that have been undertaken. Seven of the patients have had tumours of low-grade malignancy and two have had tumours of high malignancy. One patient died from the tumour before biopsy could be undertaken, one died after 3 years, one after 7 years, one after 18 years and one after 20 years. One patient is still alive at 9 years, two at 10 years and one at 17 years.

Brain Stem Astrocytomas. Brain stem astrocytomas have a less favourable outlook than other types of astrocytoma. Even stereotactic biopsy of the medulla, pons and lower mid-brain is out of the question though it is technically possible. It has been carried out at the junction of the upper mid-brain and the subthalamus. Diagnosis is made either at autopsy or because the tumour has erupted beyond the confines of the brain stem so as to allow access via a posterior fossa exploration. A shunt may be necessary and treatment is by radiotherapy. The operative mortality in our series is 23%. The survival beyond a year is 61% and beyond 3 years 30%. One patient has lived 10 years and one 20 years.

Astrocytomas confined to an optic nerve have not been included in this group but the results of excision of the affected nerve have been excellent in four cases.

Irradiation of two cases where the tumour had spread into the chiasm seems to have been followed by a prolonged halt in the progression of the tumour.

Astrocytomas Associated with von Recklinghausen's Disease. The astrocytomas associated with von Recklinghausen's disease are of low grade in over half of the cases and of correspondingly good prognosis wherever they may be situated. In the high-grade malignancies the prognosis is appropriately gloomy.

Oligodendroglioma

Oligodendroglioma carries a better prognosis overall than astrocytoma because only about a quarter of the tumours show a high grade of malignancy (Zülch 1964). Furthermore in our series they were anatomically better suited to extirpation, 40% lying in the frontal lobe and 30% in the occipital lobe. Thus it was possible to carry out macroscopic removal in 33% of cases and subtotal removal in 42%. Subsequently all patients received post-operative radiotherapy. An additional beneficial prognostic factor is that the maximum age incidence was in the fourth decade. There was a male predominance of 1.5:1. Overall the operative mortality was 2%. Using the same criteria as for the astrocytomas, we may judge that just worthwhile survival occurred in 76% of patients, worthwhile survival in 64% and very worthwhile survival in 38%.

It will be seen that these figures are in fact superior to those for the low-grade astrocytomas. This reflects the polar situation of the majority of the tumours and the fact that surgical extirpation could be carried out in 33% of cases compared with 27% for the astrocytomas. Fourteen per cent of patients lived more than 5 years and 2% are living beyond 15 years.

Ependymoma

The cerebral ependymomas are rare. They occur in the first four decades of life and there is a female preponderance of 1.5:1. In our small series there were seven of high-grade and three of low-grade malignancy. Extirpation was possible in four patients and radiotherapy was given to all. There was no operative mortality. There was worthwhile survival in seven cases and very worthwhile survival in five. Three patients are still living at 4, 6 and 20 years respectively.

The cerebellar ependymomas, on the other hand, do not carry as favourable an outlook as the cerebellar astrocytomas because there is a higher proportion of high-grade malignant tumours (46%). Furthermore only 76% could be extirpated as compared with 84% for the astrocytomas, and even in the patients assessed to have had a complete extirpation there was in fact some doubt about the attachment in the region of the obex in 45%. The operative mortality was 15% (compared with nil for the astrocytomas) because of the attachment of these tumours to the medulla. Radiotherapy was given to all. There was worthwhile survival in 69% of cases and very worthwhile survival in 50%. Thirty-eight per cent of patients survived more than 5 years, 15% more than 10 years and 8% more than 15 years.

Of the patients with brain stem ependymomas one survived 6 years but four had died by 18 months.

Brain Stem Glioma

Of the patients with brain stem gliomas where the histological diagnosis was unknown all had died by 18 months, with the exception of one who survived for 18 years.

Microglioma

There was only a small number of microgliomas. None of these was diagnosed pre-operatively. There was one operative death and one patient survived 3 years, at which point he died of a myocardial infarction. The remainder died between 6 and 18 months after the operation in spite of radiotherapy.

Medulloblastoma

The treatment of medulloblastomas is dealt with in the chapter by Bloom, but there are three points of interest arising from our series:

1) Of the 25% of patients who were adult there was no post-operative mortality and following radiotherapy there was a 50% 5-year survival.
2) In the children there was one post-operative death giving a mortality rate of nearly 3%.
3) One patient had a recurrence of the disease which did not manifest itself for 20 years.

Neuroblastoma

Of the patients with neuroblastoma five died within 6 months but one survived and is still alive at 18 years, following external decompression and radiotherapy.

Ganglioneuroma

A subtotal removal of the one ganglioneuroma in our series was undertaken and the patient is well 11 years later.

Germinoma

There were seven proven cases of germinoma in our series (three suprasellar and four pineal). These all showed an excellent response to radiotherapy, though one patient died later from an unrecognised retroperitoneal germinoma and a second from the development of a choriocarcinoma. The other patients have remained well for between 5 and 12 years. In addition there were ten patients with pineal tumours who have remained symptom free for between 8 and 20 years following shunting and radiotherapy. One of these had a pineocytoma and one possibly a pineocytoma.

The remainder of the tumours were not biopsied but it seems likely that they were germinomas. In contrast, ten patients with pineal tumours who were treated in the same way and died between 5 months and 3 years after treatment were all shown to have gliomas.

Discussion

A hundred years ago a writer to *The Times* expressed the hope that, as the result of what the paper 50 years later described as "the new brain surgery", "many men and women will henceforth be safe from prolonged torture and death". To some extent this hope has been fulfilled. As the result of continuous improvement in diagnostic, anaesthetic and surgical techniques, the operative mortality and morbidity have been reduced to low levels though not to the absolute zero which would be the ultimate desideratum. Survival for patients with some types of tumours has improved. However, with regard to the great body of intrinsic brain tumours, the results remain extremely disappointing and at the moment there seems no way forward. While many are working to improve results, the surgeons must do their best to minimise the suffering of the patients. Where low-grade tumours are in accessible positions, the results of surgery approach the standards seen with extrinsic tumours. Patients would be spared much pointless surgery if the nature of the tumours could be identified by investigative means with as much precision as their position and extent now are. However, the CT scan can still be misleading. In some cases it is obvious that a tumour is inoperable whatever may be its nature, but in other cases it is impossible to differentiate between a high-grade astrocytoma and an oligodendroglioma. Again, what appears to be a low-grade astrocytoma with a relatively good prognosis may in fact turn out to be highly malignant (Fig. 7.10).

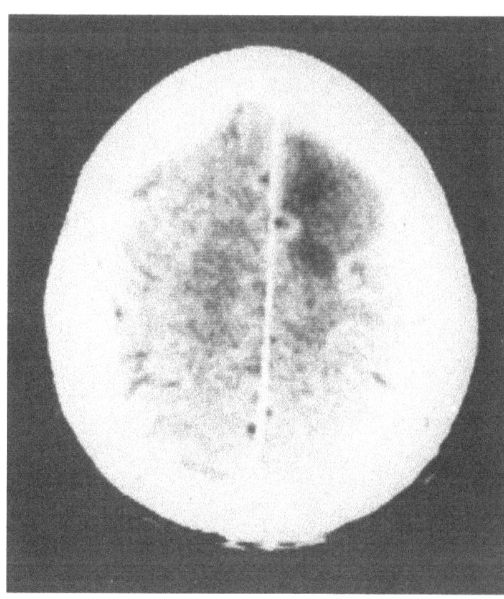

Fig. 7.10. Left frontal glioma diagnosed as low-grade astrocytoma, found at surgery to be glioblastoma multiforme.

Possibly magnetic resonance imaging or some new radionuclide technique may help. Be that as it may, from our present standpoint it would seem that surgery can never provide the answer to these problems and that with these tumours the future must lie with the oncologist.

I am grateful to Mr D. G. Hardy for the information on acoustic neurinomas; to Mr A. E. Holmes for the information on oligodendrogliomas; and to Mr L. Pobereskin for help in retrieving the data on meningiomas.

References

Bennett AH, Godlee LJ (1885) Case of cerebral tumour. The surgical treatment. Br Med J i: 988-989

Butler AB, Brookes WH, Netsky MG (1982) Classification and biology of brain tumours. In: Youmans neurological surgery, vol 5. WB Saunders, Philadelphia, pp 2659-2701

Davidoff LM (1966) Some random thoughts on the astrocytomas. Bull NY Acad Med 42: 85-99

Durante F (1886) Estirpazione di un tumore endocranico. Arch Atti Soc Ital Chir (Roma) 2: 252-255

Hitchcock E, Sato F (1964) Treatment of malignant gliomata. J Neurosurg 21: 497-505

Jeffreys R (1975) Clinical and surgical aspects of posterior fossa haemangioblastoma. J Neurol Neurosurg Psychiatr 38: 105-111

Leksell L (1982) Cairns Memorial Lecture (unpublished)

MacCarty CS, Taylor WF (1979) Intracranial meningiomas. Experiences at the Mayo Clinic. Neurol Med Chir (Tokyo) 19: 569-574

Macewan W (1879) Tumour of the dura mater; convulsions; removal of tumour by trephining; recovery. Glasgow Med J 12: 210-213

Mondkar VP, McKissock W, Russell RWR (1967) Cerebellar haemangioblastomas. Br J Surg 54: 45-49

Palmer JJ (1972) Haemangioblastomas: A review of eighty one cases. Acta Neurochir (Wien) 27: 125-148

Pecchioli Z (1838) Soria di un fungo della dura madre operato coll'estirpazione del Professor Zanobi Pecchioli. Nuovo Giornale de'Letterati-Scienze 36: 39-44

Rubinstein LJ (1964) Morphological problems of brain tumours with mixed cell population. Acta Neurochir Suppl 10: 141-165

Zülch KJ (1964) On the definition of the polymorphous oligodendroglioma. Acta Neurochir Suppl 10: 166-172

Zülch KJ, Woolf AL (eds) (1965) Classification of brain tumours. Acta Neurochir Suppl: 10

8 Treatment of Brain Gliomas in Children

H. J. G. Bloom

Introduction

Some neurologists and paediatricians regard the great majority of children with brain tumours as being incurable and suspect that in any long-term survivors the quality of remaining life following treatment will inevitably be greatly impaired. This general pessimism is not supported by the current results of modern treatment and past opinions may need to be revised. In fact, the survival outlook for children with intracranial gliomas is considerably better than that for adults, and this applies to tumours of both low-grade and high-grade malignancy.

At the Royal Marsden Hospital (RMH) between 1952 and 1976 a total of 461 children under age 16 years with primary intracranial tumours were referred for radiotherapy. The actuarial survival rate for all cases at 5 years was 48%, at 10 years 41% and at 20 years 38% (Fig. 8.1). Of the 415 children who completed a radical course of irradiation, given either post-operatively or as the sole treatment, 53% were still alive at 5 years, 45% at 10 years and 41% at 20 years (Fig. 8.1). Overall survival was influenced by age, the best results being seen in children aged 10–15 years and the worst in children under 3 years (Fig. 8.2).

Tumours of the Cerebral Hemispheres

About 25% of intracranial tumours in children are located in the cerebral hemispheres, the majority being astrocytomas of low- or intermediate-grade malignancy. If surgery is feasible, as much of the tumour as possible is removed and this should be followed by large-volume radiotherapy. By virtue of their size and position many

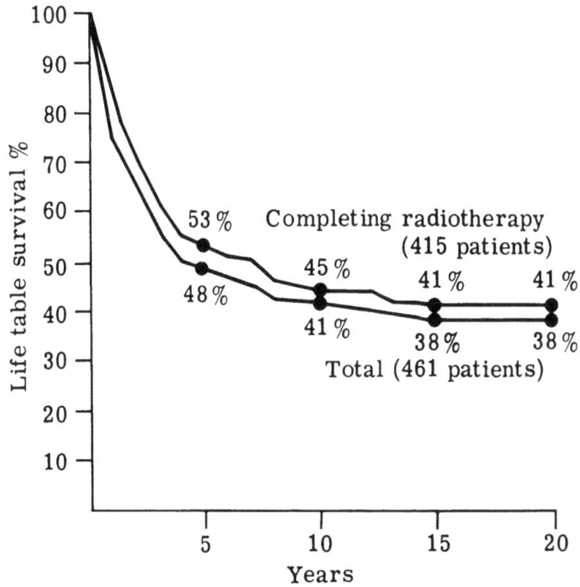

Fig. 8.1. Actuarial survival of all patients under 16 years of age with primary intracranial tumours seen at the RMH (1952–1976).

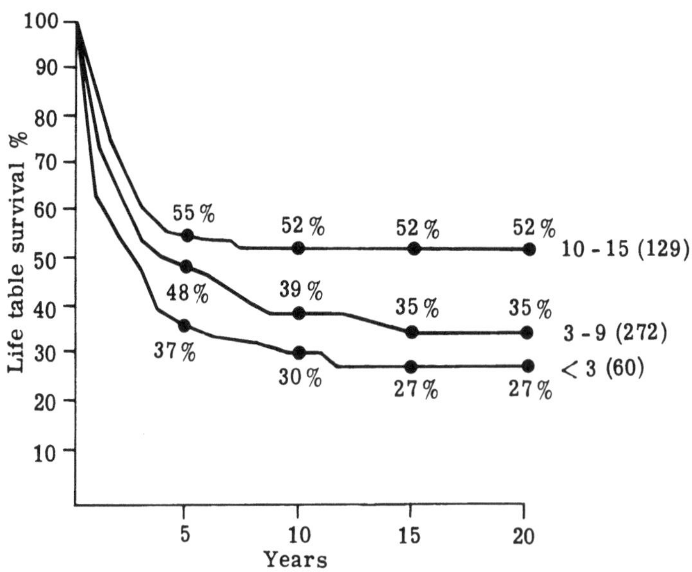

Fig. 8.2. Influence of age on survival for 461 children with intracranial tumours seen at the RMH (1952–1976).

deep-seated lesions, such as may occur in the thalamus and hypothalamus, are inoperable because of the high surgical risks to life and function. Such patients are best treated by radiotherapy alone, with or without a preliminary cerebrospinal fluid (CSF) shunt.

Because of their well-differentiated histology and slow growth, low-grade astrocytomas are widely regarded as being radioresistant. The available evidence, however, suggests that this is not the case. Such tumours may respond to irradiation and postoperative survival is greater following adjuvant radiotherapy than after surgery alone (Bouchard 1966, Bloom and Walsh 1975, Liebel et al. 1975, Fazekas 1977, Wara 1981).

In the RMH series, the 5-year survival rate for 88 children with cerebral hemisphere gliomas (excluding verified ependymomas) was 45% at 5 years and 38% at 10 years (Bloom 1982). Of 43 children in whom histological grading was available, 62% of grade 1 and 2 cases were alive at 5 years, compared with 28% of grade 3 and 4 cases (Fig. 8.3). The 5-year survival of 79 children completing radical radiotherapy was 43% in those with gliomas of the cerebral lobes and lateral ventricles, 71% in patients with tumours of the third ventricle and hypothalamus, and 28% in those with tumours of the thalamus.

High-Grade Cerebral Astrocytomas

Fortunately, high-grade cerebral astrocytomas are uncommon in children, constituting only about 5% of all intracranial tumours under the age of 15. Prognosis is profoundly influenced by age, children having a better prognosis than patients in middle age who in turn survive longer than the elderly (Penman and Smith 1954, Stage and Stein 1974). For example, at the RMH the 5-year survival rate for 141 adult patients with high-grade cerebral hemisphere astrocytomas was 6% (Bloom 1982), compared with 28% for 26 children under age 16 with tumours of similar grade (Fig. 8.3).

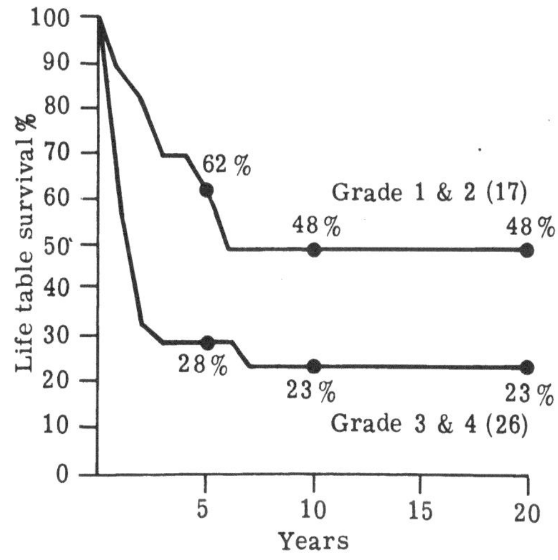

Fig. 8.3. Influence of tumour grade on survival for 43 children with cerebral astrocytoma seen at the RMH (1952–1976).

Thalamic and Other Deep-Seated Gliomas

Computerised tomographic (CT) scanning has assisted in the diagnosis of deep-seated hemisphere tumours and in assessing their extent, but histological verification still remains a problem because of the considerable surgical risk, even of biopsy of such lesions. CT-assisted or stereotactic CT-assisted needle biopsy carries far less risk than open operation, but failure to obtain adequate tissue for diagnosis by the needle is not uncommon.

Because the operative mortality for surgical approaches to thalamic tumours has been as high as 30%–40%, even in selected cases, radiotherapy with or without a preliminary CSF shunt has become the generally recommended treatment without a tissue diagnosis.

In neuro-oncological practice the radiotherapist is not infrequently called upon to treat patients with clinico-radiological evidence of an inoperable brain tumour and without a tissue diagnosis because surgery, even biopsy, is considered inadvisable. In these circumstances there is naturally reluctance to embark on radical radiotherapy or chemotherapy in a child with an unverified brain tumour. Nevertheless, the diagnosis of glioma is generally correct and the risk of such treatment is invariably less than the risk of leaving the lesion untreated, particularly if there is evidence of tumour progression. In our experience, the overall survival for children with unverified intracranial tumours treated by radiotherapy is virtually identical to that found in all children with histologically confirmed lesions treated by surgery and radiotherapy.

It is interesting that the prognosis for children with deep-seated inoperable tumours in the cerebral hemispheres may differ considerably according to the precise site of the lesion. Thus in a small group of children with gliomas involving the hypothalamus (6 cases) the 5-year survival rate was 83%, whereas only 20% of patients with thalamic tumours (18 cases) survived for this period. Difference in tumour histological grade is likely to be the explanation for this marked difference in prognosis (Bloom 1982).

Primitive Neuroectodermal Tumours of the Cerebrum

Anaplastic tumours composed of sheets of small primitive cells with ovoid hyperchromatic nuclei, similar in histological appearance to medulloblastomas, may occur in the cerebral hemispheres of children and young adults. These tumours are highly malignant and generally run a rapidly fatal course, even after radical treatment. Hart and Earle (1973) coined the term primitive neuroectodermal tumour (PNET) for tumours of this type and reported an average survival time of only 18 months in a series of 23 patients.

We have found 18 examples of PNET among 636 primary cerebral hemisphere tumours in the histopathological files of the RMH covering 1971 to 1980—an incidence of 2.8% (Gaffney et al. 1985). In 15 patients the undifferentiated component comprised more than 80% of the tumour seen in histological sections. Attempts at cellular differentiation occur along neuronal and glial lines. Tumours generally recur locally but may also spread via the CSF pathways and occasionally to extraneurogenic sites.

In the RMH series, 5 of 14 (36%) patients referred for radiotherapy were alive at 2 years and 3 of 12 (25%) at 5 years. Survival was influenced by the extent of

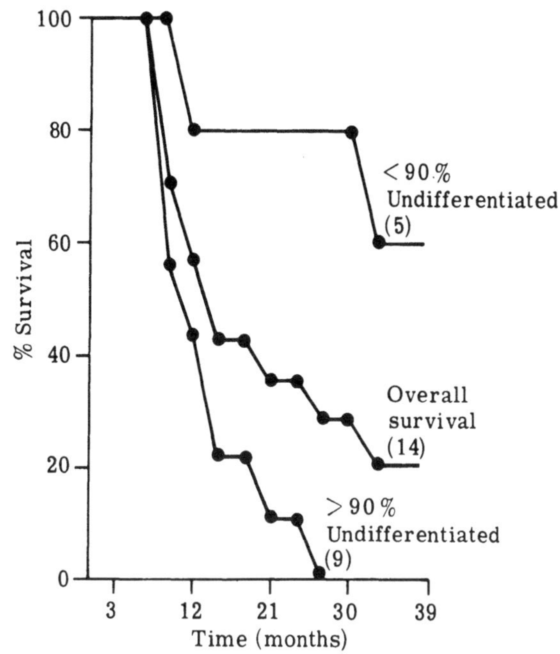

Fig. 8.4. Primitive neuroectodermal tumours of cerebral hemispheres: survival of 14 cases, overall and by extent of tumour differentiation. Note marked difference between when more than 90% and less than 90% of the tumour is undifferentiated.

undifferentiation. Thus, all 9 patients with more than 90% of the tumour undifferentiated were dead by 30 months, whereas 4 of 5 cases (80%) showing less than 90% undifferentiation were alive at this time (Fig. 8.4). We do not regard cerebral PNETs simply as supratentorial medulloblastomas. Apart from certain other differences, with regard to degree and type of differentiation, staining for glial fibrillary acidic protein and the mode of spread, the two tumours differ substantially in their response to treatment and in prognosis. Medulloblastomas are more responsive to irradiation and patients have a considerably greater survival rate. Whereas only between 20% and 25% of patients with PNETs survive 5 years (see review by Humphrey et al. 1981, Gaffney et al. 1985), 50%–70% of children with medulloblastoma are alive at this time (Bloom and Thornton-Jones 1983).

The three long-term survivors in our series (for 7, 9 and 11 years) all had adjuvant chemotherapy and two of these received whole cerebrospinal axis irradiation. A treatment policy similar to that used for medulloblastoma, involving radical surgery where feasible, whole central nervous system irradiation and adjuvant chemotherapy, may improve the survival of children with highly malignant PNETs.

Chemotherapy of Low-Grade Astrocytomas

Because of kinetic factors associated with low-grade gliomas, such as the long doubling times and the relatively few cells undergoing active division, such tumours may not be expected to respond effectively to cytotoxic agents. In our experience, however, recurrent low-grade gliomas in adults not only do respond to chemotherapy, but do so more frequently (8 of 15 grade 1–2 cases, 53%) than high-grade lesions (11 out of 121 grade 3–4 cases, 9%) (H. J. G. Bloom and D. Good, unpubl. obs.) There may be a role for chemotherapy alone in children with recurrent low-grade gliomas, or in combination with radiotherapy for the primary treatment of inoperable cerebral hemisphere tumours. However, further studies are required to assess the value of such treatment.

Medulloblastoma

Medulloblastoma is the most common brain tumour in children. Approximately 80% of all cases occur during the first 15 years of life, mainly during the first decade, with two incidence peaks at 3–4 years and 8–9 years. Boys are affected more often than girls (sex ratio 1.5–2:1) and tend to have a worse prognosis (Bloom 1971).

Medulloblastoma is not only the most frequent type of intracranial cancer found in children, but also the most malignant. The first treatment is the only one which carries any hope of cure. At present, all therapeutic efforts directed against recurrences can only achieve palliation.

Knowledge of the natural history of medulloblastoma and experience of the failure to control the disease by surgery alone and by radiotherapy when limited to the posterior fossa, have determined the current treatment policy. This now includes whole cerebrospinal axis irradiation together with the administration of greater doses, especially to the posterior cranial fossa. Nevertheless, surgery still remains the important initial attack. Its aim is to relieve intracranial hypertension and local pressure effects, to safeguard vision, to re-establish the normal CSF circulation, to obtain tissue for histology, to stage the tumour and to reduce the tumour mass as much as possible prior to adjuvant treatment. With improvement in surgical and anaesthetic techniques and with better pre- and post-operative care, the surgical mortality has been reduced from 30% or more to approximately 10% and now perhaps even to less than 10%.

Medical centres with experience in treating substantial numbers of children with medulloblastoma and whose series include 40–120 patients have, in recent times, reported 5-year survival rates in the region of 40%–55%, with up to 30%–40% still alive at 10 years (Harisiadis and Chang 1977, Hirsch et al. 1979, Schweisguth 1979, Berry et al. 1981, Silverman and Simpson 1982, Bloom 1983).

These figures, however, do not represent the general outlook for all children with medulloblastoma, since the operative deaths, the deaths prior to radiotherapy and those patients failing to complete the course of radiation are often excluded from the survival data reported from radiotherapy departments. To obtain the true picture concerning the fate of these children one must turn to national or regional statistics which report survival of *all* children with medulloblastoma occurring in a particular geographical region. In Britain, for example, the 5-year survival rate for 491 children under the age of 15 and registered with the diagnosis of medulloblastoma between 1962 to 1970 was 18% (Draper et al. 1982). An identical figure was reported for 117 patients from the state of Connecticut in the United States between 1935 and 1973 (Farwell et al. 1977).

A few authors have published unusually high survival rates for medulloblastoma: in the region of 60%-80% at 5 years. Such figures are generally based on small numbers of patients (8-15 cases) or on series containing a number of adults who have a better initial prognosis than children, or on selected small subgroups that have received what is considered to be the "optimum" treatment (Hope-Stone 1970, Sheline 1975, Tokars et al. 1979, Berry et al. 1981, Chin and Maruyama 1981, Deutsch 1984).

An overview of current results suggests that 5-year survival rates of 50%-55% would at present be a realistic goal to reach for children under age 16 with medulloblastoma treated by surgery and post-operative megavoltage radiotherapy. It would seem that higher rates, perhaps in the region of 60%-70%, may be attained in certain favourable subgroups such as older children with low-stage tumours which have been macroscopically totally excised and in whom high-dose radiotherapy has been completed.

There is evidence that the overall survival for children with medulloblastoma is increasing. Thus, in Britain the 5-year survival rate for 491 children treated between 1962 and 1970 was 18% (Draper et al. 1982), for 214 patients treated between 1971 and 1974 it was 27%, and for 154 patients between 1975 and 1977, 38% (Stiller and Lennox 1983).

Having taken surgery to its limits and having applied post-operative radiotherapy with the maximum possible effect and accuracy within the limits of reasonable safety to the child with medulloblastoma, it would seem that everything possible has been done to eradicate the tumour and that current results have now reached a plateau above which no further improvement can be expected with surgery and conventional megavoltage radiotherapy.

Adjuvant Chemotherapy

Because we cannot expect further improvement in treatment results due to the obvious limitations of radical surgical excision and of radiation dosage, attention must be directed to increasing tumour cell kill by enhancing or adding to the effects of irradiation. Since medulloblastoma is an embryonic tumour, it was only natural to consider cytotoxic agents as being of possible value in the treatment of this disease in view of the remarkable success of chemotherapy in other primitive tumours of childhood.

In developing cytotoxic drug regimes for children with medulloblastoma we need effective agents which must be able to pass the blood-brain barrier. Treatment with such drugs must also be haematologically feasible since marrow reserve in these patients is inevitably compromised by cerebrospinal axis irradiation. A combination of chemotherapy and radiotherapy needs to be reasonably safe since enhanced changes may occur, not only against the tumour but also in normal brain tissue. This would lead to an increase in possible late sequelae, especially in the very young children in whom the developing brain is particularly vulnerable to toxic injury. Finally, any potentially useful drug treatment must not jeopardise radiotherapy, which, for the present, remains the principal and most effective adjuvant treatment for this disease.

The RMH Chemotherapy Study (1970-1983). In 1970 a pilot study was started to assess the feasibility and possible value of adjuvant chemotherapy for medulloblastoma following radical surgery and megavoltage radiotherapy (Bloom 1975).

Between 1970 and 1983, 47 children were treated using mainly intravenous vincristine at weekly intervals during radiotherapy, followed by intermittent maintenance courses of vincristine and CCNU, cycled every 6 weeks over a period of approximately one year (Bloom 1982). The survival for this group is greater than that for an earlier historical series of 87 patients treated at the same centre between 1952 and 1970 in whom chemotherapy was not used (Fig. 8.5). The difference between the two groups at 5 years is highly significant ($P<0.001$).

In this study chemotherapy was reasonably well tolerated but, as expected in children undergoing prior craniospinal irradiation, marked myelosuppression occurred in some patients which made a reduction in the dose of CCNU or delays in drug administration inevitable. Serious neurotoxicity with vincristine was rarely encountered and full dosage of this agent throughout was generally achieved. There were no drug-related deaths.

Historical controls, of course, are highly unsatisfactory and in recent years advances in neurosurgery and improvements in megavoltage irradiation techniques have led to increased survival rates in children with medulloblastoma without the addition of chemotherapy. To assess the value of adjuvant chemotherapy for children with medulloblastoma a prospective controlled study was required.

Medulloblastoma Trial of the International Society of Paediatric Oncology (SIOP). In 1975 the Brain Tumour Committee of SIOP started a multicentre prospective randomised trial. Forty-four centres from 15 countries entered 286 children with medulloblastoma into the study, which was closed in September 1979. Details of the treatment protocol and of the statistical analysis have been given elsewhere (Bloom et al. 1982), but briefly the test arm involved post-operative radiotherapy with the administration of weekly intravenous vincristine during radiation and, commencing 1 month after completion of radiotherapy, a maintenance programme using a combination of CCNU (day 1) and vincristine (days 1, 8 and 15), cycled every 6 weeks for a total of eight courses. The control arm received post-operative radiotherapy alone.

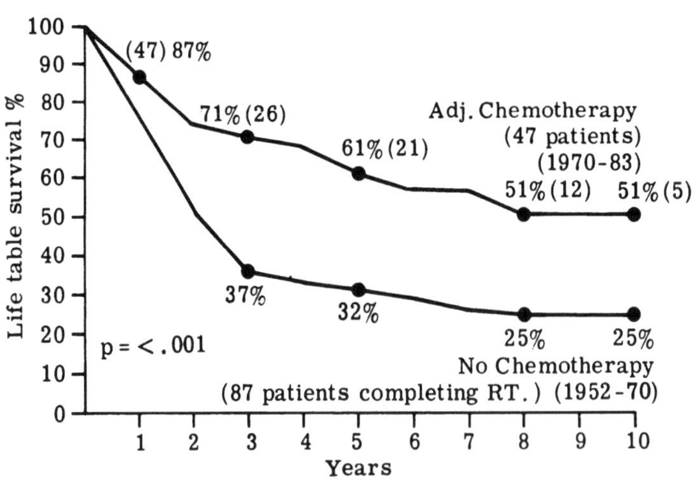

Fig. 8.5. Survival of 47 children with medulloblastoma treated between 1970 and 1983 who received adjuvant chemotherapy, compared with 87 cases treated previously without adjuvant chemotherapy.

The results, as reported to the SIOP Annual Conference in Barcelona in September 1984, revealed only a small difference in disease-free survival between the two principal arms of the trial in favour of adjuvant chemotherapy which, at that time, was not statistically significant ($P=0.06$). However, more striking results were obtained in favour of chemotherapy in certain high-risk subgroups, namely children aged less than 2 years ($P=0.08$) and 2–9 years ($P=0.04$); those having only partial or subtotal excision as opposed to total macroscopic removal ($P=0.05$); those with brain stem involvement ($P=0.002$) (Fig. 8.6a, b); and those with more locally advanced primary tumours as defined in categories T3 and T4 based on the system proposed by Harisiadis and Chang (1977) ($P=0.003$).

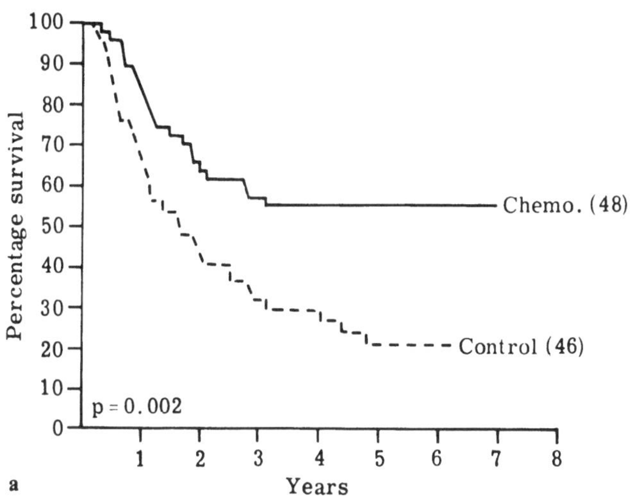

a

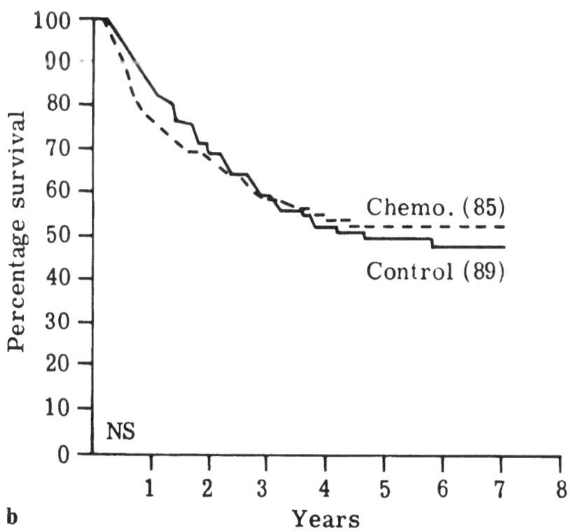

b

Fig. 8.6. Results of the SIOP Medulloblastoma Trial: note the significantly greater survival of patients with brain stem involvement by tumour who received adjuvant chemotherapy, compared with those who did not (**a**). No benefit was seen from chemotherapy when the brain stem was judged to be free from involvement (**b**).

The overall survival rate for the entire SIOP series at 3 years was 63% and at 5 years, 53%. Bearing in mind that 44 centres from many countries were involved in this study, these figures must be regarded as more than satisfactory and, indeed, they rank among the best reported from single large institutions in recent years.

On the basis of the present SIOP data it seems that adjuvant chemotherapy may improve the survival of children in certain high-risk groups and that further studies in this field are fully justified. A new SIOP Medulloblastoma Trial was launched in 1984 to evaluate post-operative and pre-irradiation chemotherapy using procarbazine, vincristine and high-dose methotrexate with citrovorum rescue. In high-risk cases (those with less than total or subtotal tumour removal, or with invasion of the brain stem or with evidence of metastatic disease within the central nervous system), post-irradiation maintenance chemotherapy is also given using CCNU and vincristine cycled every 6 weeks as in the first SIOP trial but for a total of six courses.

From the study at the RMH and the results of the SIOP trial there is hope that adjuvant chemotherapy will lead to greater survival rates, especially in children with high-risk factors. It is important to stress that the RMH study was not a controlled investigation and that in the SIOP trial the current difference in survival between the principal chemotherapy and control arms is not statistically significant ($P=0.06$). Nevertheless, these observations seem to be clinically important and the difference in favour of chemotherapy may be real, particularly in unfavourable cases. They should serve to encourage the search for more effective drugs and schedules.

Stiller and Lennox (1983) reviewed 368 children with medulloblastoma registered in Britain between 1971 and 1977. Of the 304 children completing radiotherapy, 90 received various types of adjuvant chemetherapy and 214 did not. The survival in the large series was better for the chemotherapy group, but the difference was not statistically significant (Fig. 8.7).

Intracranial Ependymoma

Ependymomas constitute about 10% of all intracranial tumours in children, with a peak incidence during the first decade. In about 40% of patients the tumour is found above and in 60% below the tentorium. Factors relating to tumour and host which may influence prognosis are, first and foremost, tumour grade and, to a lesser extent, tumour site, patient's age and perhaps sex. In our experience girls fare appreciably better than boys.

In the past, attempts to treat ependymomas by surgery alone were associated with a high operative mortality and poor results, the 5-year survival rate being in the region of only 15%–20%. The previous high operative mortality, in the region of 30%–40%, has decreased and, to improve results in survivors, post-operative radiotherapy involving high-dose, large-volume irradiation is mandatory. Following such treatment the overall 5-year survival rate has increased to 40%–50% (Salazar et al. 1975, 1983, Glanzmann et al. 1980, Bloom 1982, Marks and Adler 1982, Read 1984).

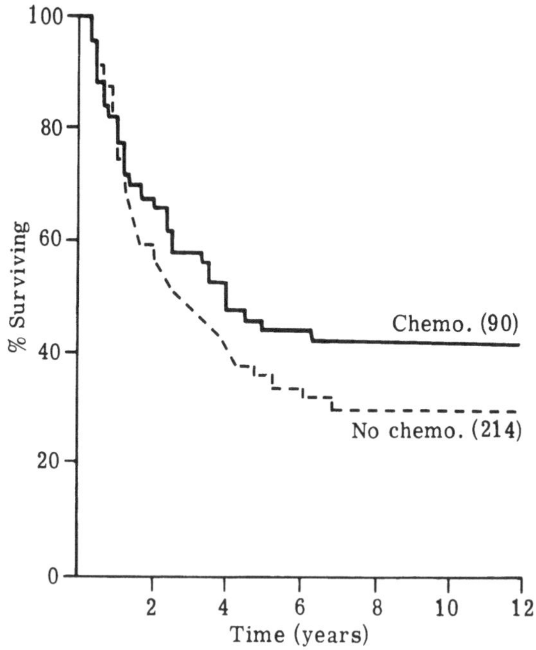

Fig. 8.7. Survival of 304 children with medulloblastoma in England, Wales and Scotland during 1971–1977: note the greater survival trend for those who received adjuvant chemotherapy (Stiller and Lennox 1983).

Ependymomas may seed along the CSF pathways forming widespread satellite nodules and this risk will influence radiotherapy policy. However, opinions vary regarding the frequency of this complication. The average incidence among some 600 cases collected from the literature was only 12% but with a range mainly from 0–33% (Bloom 1982). The incidence depends upon the primary tumour site, histological grade and, of course, whether the diagnosis of seeding is based on clinical, radiological, cytological or autopsy findings.

A rational approach to deciding on the volume to be irradiated in patients with intracranial ependymomas is based on the expected incidence of seeding according to tumour site and histological grade. Taking the collected experience of Kim and Fayos (1977), Bloom (1975) and also Pierre-Kahn et al. (1983), seeding of supratentorial tumours occurred rarely in low-grade lesions and in about 4% of high-grade cases. On the other hand, for ependymomas in the posterior fossa this complication was found in 16% of low-grade and in over 50% of high-grade cases (Table 8.1). For all patients with high-grade tumours and for those with tumours of any grade situated in the posterior fossa we recommend irradiation to the whole cerebrospinal axis. The risk of dissemination in supratentorial low-grade tumours seems to be quite small and for these lesions treatment may be limited to the primary site with a substantial margin of clearance but without the need to irradiate the whole brain and spinal cord.

Table 8.1. Spinal tumour seeding in patients (all ages) with intracranial ependymoma. Collected results from three series[a] according to tumour site and grade

Site	Grade	Cases	Seeding
Supratentorial	Low	22	0 (0%)
	High	27	1 (4%)
Infratentorial	Low	32	5 (16%)
	High	29	15 (52%)
Total		110	21 (19%)

[a]Bloom and Walsh (1975), Kim and Fayos (1977) and Pierre-Kahn et al. (1983).

The RMH Series

Of 47 children with histologically verified ependymoma referred for radiotherapy to the RMH between 1952 and 1976, 53% survived 5 years, 37% 10 years and 32% 20 years (Fig. 8.8). The 10-year survival rate for 28 children with infratentorial ependymoma was 43%, compared with 26% for 19 patients with supratentorial lesions. Prognosis for ependymoma is largely determined by histological grade: for grade 1–2 cases the 5-year survival rate was 63%, compared with 38% for those with grade 3–4 lesions (Fig. 8.9). The 5-year survival rate was 72% for patients aged 10–15 years, 53% for those aged 3–9, and 33% for children aged less than 3. Sixty-one per cent of girls were alive at 5 years, compared with 42% of boys.

The overall survival nationally for 226 children with intracranial ependymoma registered in Britain between 1962 and 1970 was 23% at 5 years and 18% at 10 years (Draper et al. 1982).

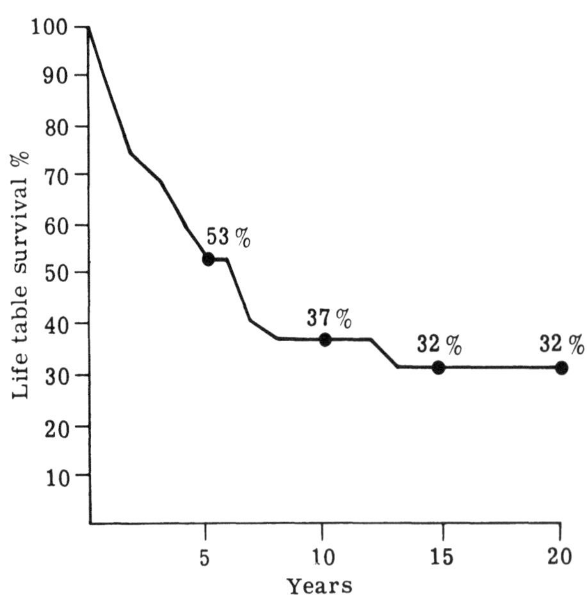

Fig. 8.8. Survival of 47 children with ependymoma treated by radiotherapy at the RMH (1952–1976).

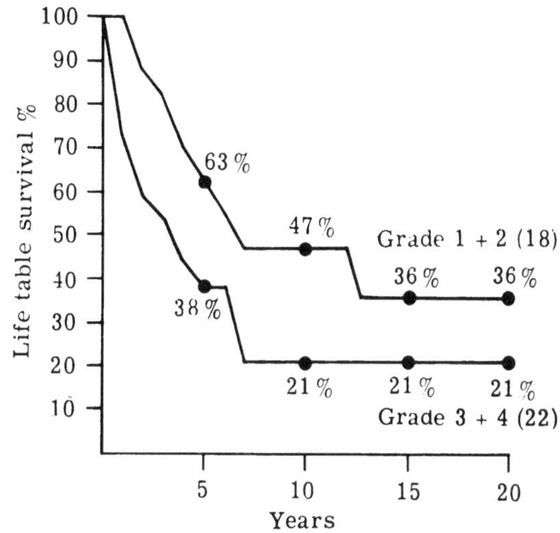

Fig. 8.9. Survival of 40 children with ependymoma according to histological grade (RMH 1952–1976).

Adjuvant Chemotherapy

Because of the ultimate poor results in children with high-grade ependymoma following surgery and radiotherapy, a pilot adjuvant chemotherapy study was initiated at the RMH. This was designed to assess the value of adjuvant chemotherapy in such patients using the same drug schedule as for children with medulloblastoma. Although the early results were encouraging, with 71% alive at 5 years compared with 48% in historical controls not receiving chemotherapy, improvement with adjuvant cytotoxic agents was not maintained beyond 6 years. Thus, life appeared to have been prolonged without an increase in cure rate (Bloom 1982).

Tumours of the Brain Stem

Gliomas of the medulla and pons make up about 10% of all intracranial tumours in childhood. They cause considerable disability from involvement of closely packed neurogenic components in a small vital anatomical structure which forms the highway for information between body and brain. Surgical intervention, even biopsy, is fraught with danger and hence, in most cases, no tissue diagnosis is available. Apart from a possible CSF shunt, radiotherapy is the only feasible treatment.

Most of these tumours respond to irradiation with gratifying reduction of distressing symptoms and signs. In 223 collected cases from the literature 68% responded to this treatment (Bloom 1983). However, such treatment is usually only palliative since in most cases the tumour recurs, resulting in progressive disability and death within 24 months. The 5-year survival rate following treatment is generally only 15%–20% (Bloom 1982). A mere 6% of all children with "pontine" tumours registered in Britain between 1961 and 1968 were still alive at 5 years (Stewart et al. 1973).

The RMH Series

Of 57 children with tumours of the brain stem, treated at the RMH between 1952 and 1976, 17% were still alive at 5 years and this same figure was projected to 20 years (Fig. 8.10). Ten children failed to complete treatment and 60% of the children were dead within the first year. Age appears to influence prognosis, with 27% of the older children (aged 10–15) surviving 5 years.

Gliomas of the brain stem represent a great challenge to the radiotherapist since the tumour burden is often small, there is a good initial response to irradiation but there is a high recurrence rate without dissemination. As little further progress can be expected from megavoltage radiotherapy alone, attention has been given to the use of cytotoxic drugs and chemical radiosensitisers to increase the degree and duration of the radiation response. Although chemotherapy using CCNU, procarbazine, methotrexate and vincristine as single agents or in combination may induce a response and increase survival in patients with recurrent brain stem tumours, there is no evidence that such treatment administered as an adjuvant with radiation is of benefit (Fulton et al. 1981). At the RMH we have found chemotherapy of little value in recurrent cases of brain stem glioma (all ages), with only 1 partial response being seen in 12 patients treated with CCNU, with or without procarbazine and vincristine.

The situation regarding brain stem tumours seems to be ideal for exploring the value of chemical radiosensitisers in the hope of rendering residual hypoxic tumour tissue, following the initial good response to irradiation, more vulnerable to treatment. However, a pilot study at the RMH in which misonidazole was used as a radiosensitiser in the primary treatment of children with brain stem tumours (Bloom and Bugden 1982) has, so far, failed to improve survival.

Of all children with intracranial tumours those suffering from intrinsic brain stem gliomas have the worst prognosis, with a fatality rate of 60% within the first year of treatment. At present, therapeutic endeavours are hampered by the dangers of operation, and the vulnerability of the normal brain stem structures to irradiation as well as the tumour's resistance to current cytotoxic drugs. Hope must lie in finding more effective adjuvant cytotoxic agents and chemical radiosensitisers.

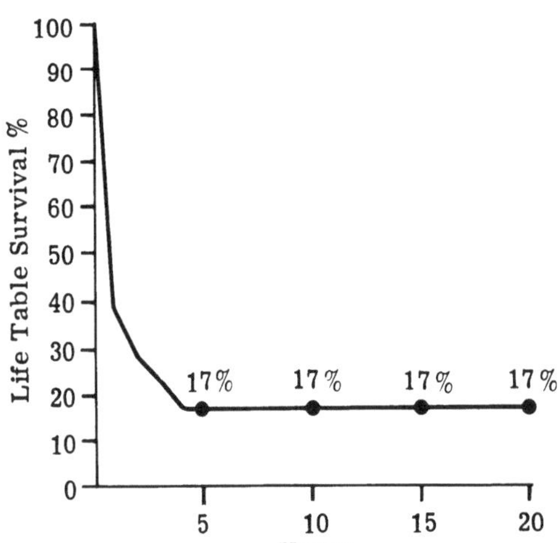

Fig. 8.10. Survival of 57 children with brain stem tumours (RMH 1952–1976).

Cerebellar Astrocytomas

The low-grade astrocytoma of the cerebellum is one of the most important tumours seen in children, with a peak incidence between 6 and 9 years of age. It is among the most frequent intracranial neoplasms and is also one of the most curable. The majority are slow-growing, well-circumscribed, often cystic lesions with a mural nodule, and are frequently amenable to total excision. In such circumstances a 100% cure rate is expected. However, in about 30% of children total removal may be extremely difficult or not possible.

There appear to be two distinct histological types of cerebellar astrocytoma in children. First, there is the more common juvenile piloid grade 1 lesion characterised by elongated unipolar and bipolar cells, rare mitosis, prominent fibrillary processes and Rösenthal fibres. Tumours of this type are associated with a 25-year survival rate exceeding 90%. Second, there is a less common, diffuse type of lesion, often histologically grade 2. Only some 30%–40% of patients with such tumours remain alive at 25 years (Gjerris and Klinken 1978).

Post-operative adjuvant treatment is unnecessary in children with the juvenile type of astrocytoma when total macroscopic excision has been performed. However, for children with the more diffuse type of lesion or grade 2 tumours, and for those in whom total excision of more circumscribed tumours was grossly incomplete, post-operative radiotherapy is recommended.

Many neurosurgeons believe that radiotherapy has no place in the treatment of low-grade cerebellar astrocytomas because of their indolent nature and assumed radioresistance. However, from our experience in children with low-grade astrocytomas in the cerebellum, in the cerebral hemispheres, particularly the hypothalamic region (Bloom and Walsh 1975, Bloom 1982), and in the optic pathways (Horwich and Bloom 1985), it is evident that such tumours may, in fact, respond remarkably well to irradiation. Several other authors have published results which suggest that post-operative radiotherapy in patients with low-grade astrocytomas improves survival, compared with surgery alone (Bouchard 1966, Stage and Stein 1974, Fazekas 1977, Griffen et al. 1979, Wara 1981).

The RMH Series

Of the 30 children with unfavourable cerebellar astrocytomas referred to the RMH for post-operative radiotherapy, 70% were alive at 5 years and 58% from 10 to 20 years (Bloom 1983) (Fig. 8.11). Once again, the prognosis was found to be more favourable for older children: some 70% of those aged 10–15 and 5–9 years survived 10 years or more, compared with only 44% of children under the age of 5.

Optic Glioma

The majority of optic gliomas (80%) occur in childhood, mostly within the first 5 years of life, and constitute some 4% of all intracranial tumours in children. In the

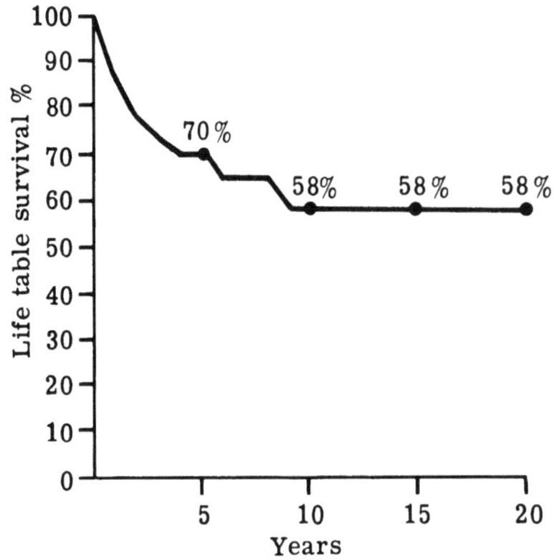

Fig. 8.11. Survival of 30 children with cerebellar astrocytomas (RMH 1952–1976).

United States Hoyte and Baghdassarian (1969) regard optic gliomas as being congenital, non-neoplastic, self-limiting lesions akin to hamartomas. The generally held view, however, is that these lesions are slow-growing, low-grade astrocytomas, and their true neoplastic nature is supported by the diffuse invasion of optic pathways, by the presence of direct infiltration of the subarachnoid space or hypothalamus and by the rare occurrence of higher-grade astrocytomas. The natural history of optic gliomas is in keeping with that of other low-grade midline astrocytic tumours of the cerebrum and cerebellum in childhood.

Death in this disease is usually due to untreated hydrocephalus, involvement of the hypothalamus by posterior-placed tumours, operative intervention especially in chiasmal lesions and occasional transformation into more malignant tumours. The latter event is more likely to occur in older patients.

For gliomas of the diffuse type or for those involving the chiasm, attempts at excision are contra-indicated and radiotherapy is the treatment of choice. Some authors have questioned the value of irradiation for low-grade gliomas in general. Histologically mature glial tumours may, in fact, respond well to irradiation.

Our experience with optic gliomas (all ages) has been limited to advanced cases. Of 29 such patients treated by radiotherapy, 27 (93%) were alive 1–30 years after treatment. Good or useful vision was present in 85% of 27 surviving traced patients (Horwich and Bloom 1985).

In spite of the emphasis by various authors on the benign nature and slow development of optic gliomas, progressive growth resulting in blindness and death is not infrequent, especially in patients with chiasmal lesions. Radiotherapy may result in marked reduction in size and prolonged control of these tumours with prevention of death and with retention of or improvement in vision.

Late Effects Following Treatment

Associated with the improving survival rates of children treated for intracranial tumours is an increasing awareness and concern over possible late sequelae affecting mental function and somatic development. This may be especially significant in the very young, where a high percentage of those treated survive to adult life (Fig. 8.12).

Several authors have reported favourably on the overall functional results in children treated for brain tumours by irradiation: some 70%–80% of surviving patients were leading apparently normal or active useful lives (Bouchard 1966, Bloom et al. 1969, Jenkin 1969, Onoyama et al. 1975, Bloom 1979). The criteria for making these assessments were crude, though, and based principally on general clinical observation and social enquiry. Clearly there is a need for a more detailed and precise investigation of intellectual capabilities and socio-economic status by specially trained personnel. What at first may appear to be an active useful life with little or no neurological deficit may, in fact, turn out to be one that is significantly altered by changes in intellect and behaviour which may not be obvious on general examination.

The frequency and the degree of late changes in intellectual, academic and emotional function seen in children receiving brain irradiation for intracranial tumours, or prophylactically for acute leukaemia, seem to vary in different reports. There is also a considerable range in the individual educational and employment attainments in different series and also between individuals having similar treatment in the same series.

Host, tumour and treatment factors which may influence the presence and the degree of subsequent psychological sequelae and the level of education and job attainment are:

(i) Age of patient at time of treatment. Serious changes are more likely to occur in children less than 3 years of age.

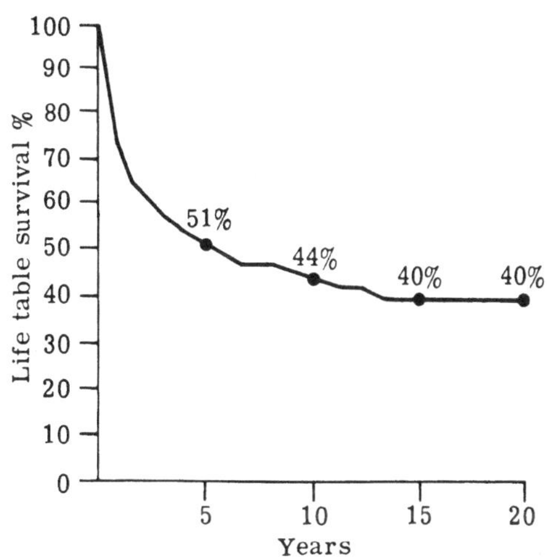

Fig. 8.12. Survival of 136 children under 6 years of age treated for intracranial tumour (all types, by radiotherapy, with or without prior surgery) (RMH 1952–1976).

(ii) The site and extent of the brain tumour. Tumour involvement of lower neurogenic centres may be related to higher centre disturbance. Invasion of the hypothalamus (Danoff et al. 1982) or of the brain stem (Hirsch et al. 1979) seems to be associated with a far greater incidence of mental impairment than occurs in patients in whom these structures are not affected.
(iii) The presence, degree and duration of hydrocephalus.
(iv) The extent of surgery.
(v) Endocrine disturbance induced by tumour or by treatment.
(vi) The volume and dose-time factors used in radiotherapy, especially dose per fraction.
(vii) Combined treatment using chemotherapy or radiosensitisers and irradiation.
(viii) Special sensory defects such as impaired vision or hearing which may interfere with education.
(ix) The opportunities available for rehabilitation and catch-up education.

It is clear from a number of reports that a significant number of young children treated successfully for brain tumours subsequently show deficient or borderline intelligence function, particularly with regard to learning ability, memory and power of concentration, and that these changes are more likely to be present in those who have received brain irradiation (Bamford et al. 1976, Hirsch et al. 1979, Danoff et al. 1982, Kun et al. 1983). Until we have found more efficient and more selective treatments for brain tumours we may have to accept some morbidity. This may include a possible reduction in mental capacity, perhaps some emotional disability and neurogenic and endocrine dysfunction as the price for an otherwise healthy and active child who is capable of some education and training and will eventually be able to earn his or her own living, although probably at a reduced level. It would seem that radiotherapy should not be withheld from the treatment of young children with intracranial tumours, unless the degree of disability already existing due to tumour or operation is unacceptable. This is a conclusion also reached by Deutsch (1982), who reported on children under the age of 5 with brain tumours, and by Spunberg et al. (1981), who studied the effect of treatment on children under the age of 2 years.

When all treatment has been completed, continued regular follow-up and supervision is necessary to deal with general rehabilitation and with any problems relating to lost schooling, reduced vision or hearing, impaired physical and mental function, behaviour changes and endocrine disturbance. It requires considerable teamwork to provide adequate and comprehensive care for children who have been treated for an intracranial tumour. The future for such children is by no means lost and to help manage these problems at the RMH we have set up a Brain Tumour Board and also an Endocrine and Growth Clinic, each body consisting of medical and paramedical staff representing the relevant issues of treatment, rehabilitation, education and employment.

References

Bamford FN, Jones PM, Pearson D, Ribeiro GG, Shalet M, Beardwell CG (1976) Residual disabilities in children treated for intracranial space-occupying lesions. Cancer 37: 1149–1151

Berry MP, Jenkin RDT. Keen CW, Nair BD, Simpson WJ (1981) Radiation treatment for medulloblastoma: A 21 year review. J Neurosurg 55: 43–51

Bloom HJG (1971) Concepts in the natural history and treatment of medulloblastoma in children: Increasing survival rates and possible risks with current therapy techniques. CRC Crit Rev Radiol Sci 2: 89–143

Bloom HJG (1975) Combined modality therapy for intracranial tumours. Cancer 35: 111–120

Bloom HJG (1979) Recent concepts in the conservative treatment of intracranial tumours in children. Acta Neurochir 50: 103–116

Bloom HJG (1982) Intracranial tumours: Response and resistance to therapeutic endeavors, 1970–1980. Int J Radiat Oncol Biol Phys 8: 1083–1113

Bloom HJG (1983) Tumours of the posterior fossa in childhood: Role of radiotherapy and chemotherapy. In: Jensen H-P, Brock M, Klinger M (eds) Advances in neurosurgery vol 11. Springer-Verlag, Berlin, pp 209–227

Bloom HJG, Bugden RD (1982) Radiation and misonidazole in children with brain stem gliomas and supratentorial glioblastoma. In: Kärcher KH, Kogelnik HD, Reinartz G (eds) Progress in radio-oncology vol 2. Raven Press, New York, pp 203–211

Bloom HJG, Thornton-Jones H (1983) Adjuvant chemotherapy for medulloblastoma: The multicentre controlled trial of the International Society of Paediatric Oncology (SIOP). In: Proceedings of the 13th International Congress of Chemotherapy, Vienna, 28 August–2 September 1983, vol 10. Egermann, Vienna, p 208/19–25

Bloom HJG, Walsh L (1975) Tumours of the central nervous system. In: Bloom HJG, Lemerle J, Neidhardt MK, Voûte PA (eds) Cancer in children: Clinical management. Springer-Verlag, Berlin, pp 93–119

Bloom HJG, Wallace ENK, Henk JM (1969) The treatment and prognosis of medulloblastoma in children: A study of 82 verified cases. Am J Roentgenol 105: 43–62

Bloom HJG, Thornton H, Schweisguth O (1982) SIOP medulloblastoma and high grade ependymoma therapeutic clinical trial: Preliminary results (1975–1981). In: Raybaud C, Clement R, Lebreuil G, Bernard JL (eds) Paediatric oncology. Proceedings of the 13th meeting of the International Society of Paediatric Oncology, Marseilles, 15–19 September 1981. Excerpta Medica, Amsterdam, pp 309–322

Bouchard J (1966) Radiation therapy of tumours and diseases of the nervous system. H. Kimpton, London

Chin HW, Maruyama Y (1981) Results of radiation treatment of cerebellar medulloblastoma. Int J Radiat Oncol Biol Phys 7: 737–742

Danoff BF, Cowchock FS, Marquette C, Mulgrew L, Kramer S (1982) Assessment of the long-term effects of primary radiation therapy for brain tumours in children. Cancer 49: 1580–1586

Deutsch M (1982) Radiotherapy for primary brain tumours in very young children. Cancer 50: 2785–2789

Deutsch M (1984) The impact of myelography on the treatment results for medulloblastoma. Int J Radiat Oncol Biol Phys 10: 999–1003

Draper GJ, Birch JM, Bithell JF et al. (1982) Childhood cancer in Britain: Incidence, survival and mortality. Her Majesty's Stationery Office, London (Studies on medical and population subjects no. 37)

Farwell JR, Dohrmann GJ, Flannery JT (1977) Central nervous system tumours in children. Cancer 40: 3123–3132

Fazekas JT (1977) Treatment of grades I and II brain astrocytomas: The role of radiotherapy. Int J Radiat Oncol Biol Phys 2: 661–666

Fulton DS, Levin VA, Wara WM, Edwards MS, Wilson CB (1981) Chemotherapy of paediatric brain stem tumours. J Neurosurg 54: 721–725

Gaffney CC, Sloane JP, Bradley NJ, Bloom HJG (1985) Primitive neuroectodermal tumours of the cerebrum: Pathology and treatment. J Neuro-Oncol 3: 23–33

Gjerris F, Klinken L (1978) Long term prognosis in children with benign cerebellar astrocytoma. J Neurosurg 49: 179–184

Glanzmann CH, Horst W, Scheiss K, Friede R (1980) Considerations in the radiation treatment of intracranial ependymoma. Strahlentherapie 156: 97–101

Griffin TW, Beaufait D, Blasko JC (1979) Cystic cerebellar astrocytoma in childhood. Cancer 44: 276–280

Harisiadis L, Chang CH (1977) Medulloblastoma in children: A correlation between staging and results of treatment. Int J Radiat Oncol Biol Phys 2: 833–841

Hart MN, Earle KM (1973) Primitive neuroectodermal tumours of the brain in children. Cancer 32: 890–897

Hirsch JF, Renier D, Czernichow P, Benveniste L, Pierre-Kahn A (1979) Medulloblastoma in childhood: Survival and functional results. Acta Neurochir 48: 1–15

Hope-Stone H (1970) Results of treatment of medulloblastomas. J Neurosurg 32: 83–88

Horwich A, Bloom HJG (1985) Optic gliomas: Radiation therapy and prognosis. Int J Radiat Oncol Biol Phys 11: 1067–1079
Hoyte WF, Baghdassarian SA (1969) Optic glioma of childhood. Br J Ophhalmol 53: 793–798
Humphrey GB, Dehner LP, Kaplan RJ, Waters KD, Jenkin RDT, Wara WM (1981) Overview on the management of primitive neuroectodermal tumours. In: Humphrey GB, Dehner LP, Grindey GB, Acton RT (eds) Paediatric oncology vol 1. Martinus Nijhoff, The Hague, pp 289–294
Jenkin RDT (1969) Medulloblastoma in children: Radiation therapy. Can Med Assoc J 100: 51–53
Kim YH, Fayos JV (1977) Intracranial ependymomas. Radiology 124: 805–808
Kun LE, Mulhern RK, Crisco J (1983) Quality of life in children treated for brain tumours. J Neurosurg 58: 1–6
Leibel SA, Sheline GE, Wara WM, Boldrey EB, Neilsen SL (1975) The role of radiation therapy in the treatment of astrocytoma. Cancer 35: 1551–1557
Marks JE, Adler SJ (1982) A comparative study of ependymomas by site of origin. Int J Radiat Oncol Biol Phys 8: 37–43
Onoyama Y, Abe M, Takahashi M, Yabumoto E, Sakamoto T (1975) Radiation therapy of brain tumours in children. Radiology 115: 687–693
Penman J, Smith MC (1954) Intracranial gliomata: Some clinical, radiological and therapeutic aspects of 298 cases. Her Majesty's Stationery Office, London (Medical Research Council Special Report no. 284)
Pierre-Kahn A, Hirsch JF, Roux FX, Renier D, Saint-Rose C (1983) Intracranial ependymomas in childhood. Survival and functional results of 47 cases. Childs Brain 10: 145–156
Read G (1984) The treatment of ependymoma of the brain or spinal canal by radiotherapy: A report of 79 cases. Clin Radiol 35: 163–166
Salazar OM, Rubin P, Bassano D, Marcial VA (1975) Improved survival of patients with intracranial ependymomas by irradiation: Dose selection and field extension. Cancer 35: 1563–1574
Salazar OM, Castro-Vita H, Van Houtte P, Rubin P, Aygun C (1983) Improved survival in cases of intracranial ependymoma after radiation therapy. J Neurosurg 59: 652–659
Schweisguth O (1979) Tumeurs solides de l'enfant. Flammarion Médicine-Sciences, Paris
Sheline GE (1975) Radiation therapy of tumours of the central nervous system in childhood. Cancer 35: 957–964
Silverman CL, Simpson JR (1982) Cerebellar medulloblastoma: The importance of posterior fossa dose to survival and patterns of failure. Int J Radiat Oncol Biol Phys 8: 1869–1876
Spunberg JJ, Chang CH, Goldman M, Auricchio E, Bell JJ (1981) Quality of long-term survival following irradiation for intracranial tumours in children under the age of 2. Int J Radiat Oncol Biol Phys 7: 727–736
Stage WS, Stein JJ (1974) Treatment of malignant astrocytomas. Am J Roentgenol 120: 7–18
Stewart AM, Lennox EL, Sanders BM (1973) Group characteristics of children with cerebral and spinal cord tumours. Br J Cancer 28: 568–574
Stiller CA, Lennox EL (1983) Childhood medulloblastoma in Britain 1971–1977: Analysis of treatment and survival. Br J Cancer 48: 835–841
Tokars RP, Sutton HG, Griem ML (1979) Cerebellar medulloblastoma: Results of new method of radiation treatment. Cancer 43: 129–136
Wara WM (1981) Advantages and disadvantages of adjuvant chemotherapy in the treatment of primary CNS tumours. In: Humphrey GB, Dehner LP, Grindey GB, Acton RT (eds) Paediatric oncology vol 1. Martinus Nijhoff, The Hague, pp 199–211

9 Normal Tissue Tolerance and Radiation Therapy of Gliomas of the Adult Brain

Glenn E. Sheline

Introduction

Over 95% of gliomas of the adult brain are unifocal, hence, effective local therapy should be curative. Results of therapy, however, have been dismal. Restrictions imposed by the necessity of preserving function limit the extent of resection and the radiation dose that may be delivered. Because of the limitations placed by radiation tolerance, this chapter will begin with a consideration of radiation effects on the normal brain. Subsequently it will review data from a number of clinical studies dealing with the treatment of gliomas in the adult. While emphasis will be on prospective randomised clinical trials, data from retrospective analyses will be included even though the latter are difficult to interpret.

Brain Tolerance to Therapeutic Irradiation

Most of the older literature on effects of ionising radiation on the central nervous system (CNS) of experimental animals is of little use to the clinician. Usually, the radiation doses were below those of clinical interest, large single doses were utilised, or the animal models were less than optimal for extrapolation to the human. Caveness and his group (1977), however, conducted primate investigations designed to give information pertinent to the clinical situation. Using macaque monkeys (*Macaca mulatto*) they first studied the effect of single megavoltage whole-brain radiation exposures on neurological function, visual evoked responses (VER), electroencephalograms (EEG) and histology. With a dose of 10 Gy no lesion was found. Exposure to 15 Gy produced small focal areas of necrosis in white matter by 6 months which, by 12 months, had developed into confluent areas of necrosis that included both grey and white matter. After 52 weeks loss of brain tissue led to ventricular dilatation. Animals given 20 Gy failed to survive beyond 6 months. Subsequently, Caveness studied the effects of fractionated radiation using daily doses of 2.0 Gy for 5 days per week for total doses of either 40, 60 or 80 Gy. Radiation effects after 40 Gy were negligible. Doses of 60 Gy produced widely scattered small necrotic lesions largely, but not exclusively, in white matter. These lesions appeared after latent intervals of weeks or months and tended to mineralise with time. By one year mineralisation, telangiectasia and minute breaks in the blood–brain barrier led to both oedema and papilloedema. Furthermore, altered VER and EEG occured in two of the three monkeys. A dose of 80 Gy gave similar microscopic lesions which, by 12 months, had become extensive, coalescent, and productive of gross brain destruction. Of the three monkeys studied at 12 months, all had abnormal VER, EEG and motor function; two had severe ataxia and were blind.

In another large-animal study Fike et al. (1984), at the University of California, San Francisco, have begun an investigation of the effects of radiation on the brain of adult beagle dogs. In the preliminary phase of this study the four dogs that received 30 Gy to a single hemisphere died in 6 months but only two of the eight that received 15 Gy died. It appears that the dose to produce necrosis in the dog, as well as the monkey, brain is similar to that for the human brain. Fike developed a quantitative computerised tomography (CT) technique in which serial determinations of pre- and post-contrast CT numbers allow for the observation of development and progression of CNS damage without sacrifice of the dogs. This technique is now being used to study the effects of fractionated radiation exposures using total dose-fractionation combinations thought equivalent to single doses of 13.5–17 Gy.

Although in the past the human brain was considered relatively radioresistant, it has become evident that dose-fractionation schemes within the usual clinical range can cause functional changes, and even necrosis. When considering such CNS reactions to irradiation it is prognostically useful to view them according to time of appearance. For present purposes they will be divided into acute, early delayed and late delayed reactions.

Acute Reactions

Acute reactions are those that occur during or shortly after the course of radiotherapy. Generally they are of little consequence. When they occur they may be associated with increased intracranial pressure or an exacerbation of the symptoms or signs of the lesion being treated. Probably these reactions are due to oedema and they usually respond to corticosteroid therapy.

With conventional fractionation and prophylactic dexamethasone, Salazar et al. (1976, 1979) carried total doses as high as 80 Gy without encountering significant acute radiation complications.

The United States Radiation Therapy Oncology Group (RTOG) (Kramer et al. 1977) conducted a randomised trial which compared various dose-fractionation schemes in more than 1000 patients with brain metastases. Corticosteroid therapy was permitted. The schemes included 15 daily fractions of 2.67 Gy (total 40 Gy) in 3 weeks and 10 of 3 Gy (total 30 Gy) in 2 weeks. Both regimens were well tolerated.

Patients given steroids responded more promptly than did those without steroid therapy but after 4 weeks the result was the same whether or not steroids were used. Another RTOG study used five fractions of 6 Gy given twice-weekly, with misonidazole, to a total of 30 Gy. This regimen also was well tolerated (Phillips et al. 1984).

Young et al. (1974) used two increments of 7.5 Gy to the whole brain and had a complication rate of 49% compared with 15% in patients treated with 15 increments of 2 Gy. The complications included headache, nausea, vomiting, temperature elevation and cerebral herniation. With a single dose of 10 Gy to the whole brain Hindo et al. (1970) reported four deaths in 54 patients within 48 hours and a fifth within 7 days. There was no beneficial effect of concomitant corticosteroid therapy. The severe and fatal complications found by both Young and Hindo occurred in patients who had major pre-treatment neurological deficits and the precise role of irradiation is not entirely clear.

In summary, with daily fractions of 2 Gy, total doses up to 60 or even 80 Gy are usually well tolerated. With commensurate reduction of the total dose, fractions as high as 6 Gy are tolerated, but larger fractions should be given with caution. Corticosteroid therapy may prevent or ameliorate symptoms but appears to have little long-term benefit.

Early Delayed Reactions

Early delayed reactions appear a few weeks to months post-radiation and, like the Lhermitte's syndrome of the spinal cord, are usually transient. Although the spinal cord syndrome is widely recognised as a clinical entity, the brain syndrome is less well known. As early as 1929 Druckman (1929) reported that 3% of children irradiated for ringworm of the scalp developed a marked but transient somnolence 6–8 weeks after treatment. Rider (1963) reported two adult patients who had received about 55 Gy, in 16 or 27 fractions, for extracranial lesions and 10 weeks later developed nausea, vomiting, dysarthria, dysphagia, cerebellar ataxia, nystagmus and a positive Romberg's sign. Recovery began after 4 weeks and was complete in 6–8 weeks. Both patients were alive and well 6 years later. Boldrey and Sheline (1967) described transient adverse signs and symptoms which appeared about 2 months after partial brain irradiation for low-grade gliomas, meningiomas and pituitary adenomas.

The above observations were largely ignored until 1973 when Freeman et al. (1973) reported transient somnolence and lethargy in 80% of children given prophylactic CNS irradiation for acute lymphoblastic leukaemia. The children had received 24 Gy to the whole brain in 20 fractions over 4 weeks in conjunction with either spinal irradiation or intrathecal methotrexate.

Hoffman et al. (1979) reported on adult patients with malignant gliomas treated with daily fractions of 1.8 Gy to a total of 60 Gy. Within 18 weeks 49% had deteriorated sufficiently to suggest tumour progression; however, nearly 30% improved spontaneously without change of therapy. Since the latent interval corresponded with myelin turnover time, it is postulated that transient demyelination might have occurred.

The importance of recognising the early delayed brain syndrome resides in the fact that generally it is transient and that the appearance of new or exacerbated signs and symptoms shortly after radiotherapy does not necessarily indicate treatment failure nor the need to alter therapy. Occasionally, however, the brain syndrome is progressive and fatal (Lampert et al. 1959, Lampert and Davis 1964).

Late Delayed Reactions

Late delayed reactions appear from several months to years after radiotherapy and constitute the major hazard of brain irradiation. The lesion may present as necrosis with volume loss or as a glial reaction masquerading as an intracranial tumour. White matter tends to be more radiosensitive than grey matter. While the evidence suggests a role for demyelination in the early delayed reactions, vasculopathies and direct effects on neurons appear to be more important with the passage of time.

The effect of radiotherapy on intellectual functions of the adult has received relatively little attention. Hochberg and Slotnick (1980) described difficulties in problem-solving and failure to resume active lives in 12 patients who had had surgery, radiotherapy and chemotherapy for astrocytomas that, presumably, were under control. It is unclear whether the tumour or a component of the therapy was responsible. Although we have not studied the problem systematically, it is our impression that, with radiation doses in the order of 60 Gy given in daily increments of 1.8–2 Gy, some patients experience a decrease in memory and the more cognitive functions, and that the loss is more marked in those who have also received chemotherapy. In this regard it should be noted that methotrexate and BCNU have produced encephalopathies even without irradiation (Shapiro et al. 1980, Burger et al. 1981).

Nearly all studies on radiation necrosis of the brain have failed to relate number of cases to the population at risk, hence, it is possible only to provide an estimate of the relation between necrosis and dose, number of fractions and treatment time. Lindgren (1958) constructed a log–log plot of dose versus duration of treatment for radiation necrosis. Two lines were drawn: one joined the lowest doses reported to produce necrosis and the other was a regression line representing the dose associated with a "great risk" of cerebral necrosis. The slope of each line was 0.26. Lindgren's diagram was based on only 17 patients. Furthermore, some had had an interruption of therapy with extension of treatment time. If dose had been plotted against number of fractions, the slope would have been greater.

Kramer (1968) reviewed the literature and found 57 cases acceptable as radiation necrosis. He concluded that the normal brain will "tolerate a tissue dose of 65 to 70 Gy in 6.5 to 8 weeks delivered by 5 daily fractions per week using supervoltage techniques" but that such doses occasionally produce necrosis. DiLorenzo et al. (1978) also reviewed the literature on cerebral radionecrosis.

Sheline et al. (1980) analysed the realtionship between dose, time, number of fractions and injury of the human brain. This analysis was based on 80 patients in the literature of whom 28 had been treated for an extracranial tumour, 20 for a pituitary tumour or craniopharyngioma, and 32 for a primary brain tumour. In 68 the diagnosis of necrosis had been confirmed by tissue analysis. Of the other 12 patients, 4 had been irradiated for extracranial lesions and in 8 the injury was sufficiently removed from the tumour site that it could not be explained by a recurrence of the tumour. Reported doses were converted to megavoltage rad equivalents (MRE) and log–log diagrams were constructed in which MRE was plotted against either time or number of fractions. Lines were drawn such that most of the points were either on or above them. These lines represent the thresholds at which brain necrosis had been reported: namely, approximately 35 Gy for 10 fractions, 60 Gy for 35 fractions, and 70 Gy for 60 fractions.

In this plot of dose versus fraction number the slope of the line was 0.44. To the extent that an isoeffect formula of the Ellis (1969) type (dose = equivalent dose $\times N^a T^b$) is appropriate the slope should equal the sum of the exponents for N (number of fractions) and T (total time in days). Numerous animal and human studies have indicated that for the CNS the exponent for N is at least 0.4 while that for time is very small (Reinhold et al. 1984). In a review of radiation tolerance of the spinal cord van der Kogel (1979) concluded that in the human the log-log plot of tolerance dose versus number of fractions has a slope of 0.4 and that, at least up to 6 weeks, the time exponent is negligible. Pezner and Archambeau (1981) derived a formula for human brain tolerance in which the N exponent was 0.45 and the T exponent 0.03. If the T exponent is in the order of 0.0 to 0.04, then our analysis suggests an exponent of about 0.42 for N. This gives much greater emphasis to the number of fractions and less to time than does the Ellis formula. The extent to which the equation or these exponents are applicable to very small or large numbers of fractions or very short or long overall times is questionable. Recent experimental results on the rat cervical spinal cord failed to show a further increase in tolerance dose as fraction sizes were decreased below 2 Gy (Reinhold et al. 1984), suggesting that caution should be used in extrapolating to a large number of small doses as used in hyperfractionation studies.

Marks et al. (1981) reported nine instances of radiation necrosis in 139 patients who had received at least 45 Gy at 1.8–2.0 Gy per day 5 days per week. They used the formula ED $= DN^{-0.377}\, T^{-0.058}$ to convert various total dose (D)/time(T)/fraction number (N) combinations to equivalent doses (ED). With an ED $\leqslant 1250$ ($1250 \equiv 60$ Gy/34 fractions) there was no necrosis in 51 patients. Between ED 1251 and 1330 ($1330 \equiv 60$ Gy/31 fractions or 66 Gy/38 fractions) necrosis occurred in 4 of 60 (7%) patients. Between ED 1331 and 1460 ($1460 \equiv 60$ Gy/25 fractions or 70 Gy/75 fractions) 5 of 28 (18%) developed necrosis. No necrosis occurred below a dose equivalent to 54 Gy in 30 fractions.

The extent to which chemotherapeutic agents influence the production of radiation necrosis is poorly documented. There is, however, evidence suggesting that certain of these agents do play a role. For example, children with acute lymphoblastic leukaemia treated with aggressive chemotherapy, both intravenous and intrathecal, plus prophylactic brain irradiation have developed brain damage following doses as low as 24 Gy in 1.2–2.0 Gy fractions. These doses, without chemotherapy, would be considered well within safe limits. Burger et al. (1979) reported radiation necrosis of brain or brain stem in 5 adults after 60 Gy in 1.8–2.0 Gy fractions. Four of these patients had received seven to 10 courses of BCNU, procarbazine or dibromodulcitol. Pratt et al. (1977) documented a case of fatal cerebral necrosis after 30 Gy in 10 fractions plus multi-agent chemotherapy —again, a radiation dose that should have been tolerated.

Glioma Classification

In the initial United States Armed Forces Institute of Pathology (AFIP) fascicle on tumours of the CNS Kernohan and Sayre (1952) stated that "prior to 1926 there was great confusion in the classification and nomenclature of gliomas". Unfortunately, the confusion remains. Bailey and Cushing (1926) had proposed a classification system based on presumed histogenesis. They used terms such as astrocytoma, astroblastoma, spongioblastoma polare and glioblastoma multiforme. In 1949 Kernohan et al. (1949) proposed a classification based on the assumption that gliomas are derived from astrocytes, ependymal cells or oligodendrogliocytes and that behavioural differences within each cell type are a function of the degree of anaplasia. For example, it was assumed that astrocytomas and glioblastoma multiforme simply represent different degrees of dedifferentiation of astrocytes. For the astrocytic series it was proposed that they be classified as astrocytoma grade 1, 2, 3 or 4, depending on the degree of anaplasia. Evaluation of anaplasia was to be based on pleomorphism, hyperchromatism and number of mitotic figures. In the Kernohan system the older term astrocytoma was replaced by astrocytoma grade 1; astroblastoma became astrocytoma grade 2; and glioblastoma multiforme became astrocytoma of grade either 3 or 4. In 1952 this grading system was introduced into the first AFIP fascicle on CNS tumours (Kernohan and Sayre 1952). The second AFIP fascicle on CNS tumours, written by Rubinstein (1972), reverted to a modification of the Bailey and Cushing system and referred to these tumours as astrocytoma, which included malignant astrocytoma as a subtype, polar spongioblastoma and glioblastoma multiforme. Thus, different classification systems are in use. Furthermore, some authors have assumed that glioblastoma multiforme is synonymous with the Kernohan astrocytoma grade 4, while others have lumped grades 3 and 4 together under this term.

As will be seen, when comparing data from different centres it is essential to know the classification system used. At the University of California, San Francisco, (UCSF) we have tended to separate these gliomas into three main groups: astrocytoma, anaplastic or malignant astrocytoma and glioblastoma multiforme. At present we are investigating the prognostic and therapeutic value of subdividing the anaplastic astrocytomas.

Astrocytoma

There has been no randomised clinical trial evaluating radiation therapy for treatment of astrocytomas. Furthermore, most authors (Bouchard 1973, Bouchard and Pierce 1960, Scanlon and Taylor 1979) have reported survival rates for either irradiated or non-irradiated patients without either a control group or a clear description of the selection factors employed. At UCSF (Leibel et al. 1975) the records of 122 consecutive patients with astrocytoma were reviewed. In 14, predominantly with cystic cerebellar astrocytoma in childhood, the tumours were thought to have been completely excised. At the time of review there was no recurrence among this group with completely resected lesions. Of the 108 patients with incompletely resected tumours, 71 received post-operative radiotherapy whereas 37 did not; there was no discernible difference in patient population or extent of resection between the two groups. Twenty-two per cent of the surgery only group and 30% of the surgery plus radiotherapy group were children. The usual tumour dose was around 50–55 Gy given in 1.8 Gy daily fractions, five times a week. The overall 5-year recurrence-free survival rate for incomplete resection alone was 19% (7/37) as compared with 46% (33/71) when radiotherapy was added. The 10-year survival rates were 11% (4/37) and 35% (19/54), respectively. The survival curve for the irradiated group appeared to be flattening out after about 15 years. For adults, the 5-year survival rates were 10% (3/29) for surgery alone versus 32% (16/50) when radiotherapy was added. One histological subgroup, namely the gemistocytic astrocytomas, had a particularly poor prognosis: only one in seven irradiated patients and none of the four non-irradiated patients survived 5 years.

Although, normally, we do not use the Kernohan grading system, an attempt was made to subclassify our astrocytomas into grade 1 and grade 2. While Kernohan found grade 1 to be less frequent than grade 2 (46% versus 54%), our review resulted in a grade 1 to 2 ratio of approximately 3 to 1 (76% versus 24%). Either we had a different mix of astrocytomas than at the Mayo Clinic or we applied the grading criteria differently. At UCSF the 5-year survival rates for grade 1 with and without irradiation were 58% and 25%, respectively. For grade 2 they were 25% and 0%. The original Mayo Clinic paper (Svien et al. 1949) reported a 63% 3-year survival rate for grade 1 versus 16% for grade 2; however, a more recent Mayo paper (Scanlon and Taylor 1979) reported similar survival data for patients with grades 1 and 2 astrocytoma. Apparently both the application of the grading system and its prognostic usefulness vary with the criteria used by individual pathologists.

Marsa et al. (1975) had a 41% actuarial 5-year survival for a group of 40 patients, mostly adults, with irradiated hemispheric astrocytomas. Fazekas (1977) compared 32 patients who had had incomplete excision plus adjuvant irradiation with 15 who had had incomplete excision alone. The actuarial 5-year survival was 41% with radiation therapy versus 13% without. Bloom (1982) reported 5-year survival rates of 33% for grade 1 and 21% for grade 2 astrocytomas in 120 adults with irradiated supratentorial tumours. Survival decreased to 16% and 6%, respectively, at 10 years. Neither Marsa nor Bloom reported survival data for patients with non-irradiated astrocytomas.

In summary, the data available from retrospective reviews suggest that for incompletely resected astrocytomas, post-operative radiotherapy improves 5-year and 10-year survival rates. Even with radiation therapy, however, the survival rates, especially in adults, leave much to be desired. Nevertheless, with these often slowly progressing lesions, increasing the dose and volume probably is not the solution as it could lead to incapacitating brain injury before tumour recurrence would otherwise have occurred (Bloom 1982).

Anaplastic Astrocytoma and Glioblastoma Multiforme

A retrospective review at UCSF showed a 5-year recurrence-free survival of 7/31 for patients with post-operatively irradiated anaplastic astrocytoma (malignant astrocytoma) versus 0/40 for those with glioblastoma multiforme (Sheline 1975). No non-irradiated patient with either diagnosis survived 5 years. Marsa et al. (1975) reported a similar experience for irradiated tumours: the mean survival time was 20 months for malignant astrocytoma versus 9 months for glioblastoma multiforme, and the

5-year actuarial survival rates were 19% and 0%, respectively. Kramer (1973) had a 22% 5-year survival rate for patients with anaplastic astrocytoma. These lesions were reported as astrocytoma grade 3. However, Kramer believes the reason his results are similar to those at UCSF, at Stanford, and those to be described for the RTOG trial is that the pathologists at his institution actually applied the histological criteria of anaplastic astrocytoma rather than those enumerated by Kernohan for the grading system (Kramer pers. comm. 1983).

In 1969 the US Brain Tumor Study Group (BTSG) (Walker et al. 1978) initiated a post-operative prospective randomised multi-institutional clinical trial for adult patients with "anaplastic gliomas". The four arms of the study were: (1) supportive therapy only; (2) BCNU 80 mg/m^2 intravenously on three successive days repeated every 6–8 weeks; (3) whole-brain radiotherapy with 1.7–2.0 Gy per day, 5 days per week, to a total of 50–60 Gy; and (4) BCNU plus radiotherapy. Two hundred and twenty-two patients were entered into the study; on central review of the pathology 90% of the tumours were classified as glioblastoma multiforme (GBM) and 9% anaplastic astrocytoma (AA). The median survival times for the valid study groups were: supportive care, 14; BCNU, 19; radiotherapy, 36; and BCNU plus radiotherapy, 35 weeks. The survival difference between radiotherapy with or without BCNU and either supportive care alone or BCNU alone was significant with a P value of 0.001. Thus, for the first time, it was shown by a randomised trial that radiotherapy significantly increased median survival time. At 18 months, four patients treated by radiotherapy alone and 19 by radiotherapy plus BCNU were alive but there was no survivor among those who had received either supportive care alone or BCNU alone.

The next BTSG randomised trial (72-01: Walker et al. 1980) compared oral semustine (MeCCNU) (220 mg/m^2 repeated every 6–8 weeks), radiotherapy (60 Gy in 30–35 daily fractions), radiotherapy plus BCNU and radiotherapy plus MeCCNU in 358 patients (84% GBM, 11% AA). Median survival times were 24, 36, 51 and 42 weeks, respectively. Using the Cox model with adjustment for predictive variables such as age, symptom duration, pathology and performance status, the P value for difference between radiotherapy alone (36 weeks) and radiotherapy plus BCNU (51 weeks) was 0.11, suggesting a modest but non-significant gain accrued by the addition of BCNU.

BTSG study 75-01 randomised 527 adults (87% GBM, 11% AA) to receive post-operative radiotherapy plus either BCNU, procarbazine (orally, 150 mg/m^2 per day in three or four divided doses for 28 consecutive days repeated every 8 weeks), high-dose methylprednisolone (orally, 400 mg/m^2 per day in three divided doses for 7 consecutive days repeated every fourth week) or BCNU plus methylprednisolone (Green et al. 1983). The radiotherapy plus BCNU and radiotherapy plus procarbazine survival curves were virtually identical; the median survival was 50 weeks for radiotherapy plus BCNU versus 47 weeks for radiotherapy plus procarbazine. Addition of prednisolone did not improve the results of radiotherapy plus BCNU.

BTSG study 77-02 randomised 603 adult patients (86% GBM, 11% AA) to receive either radiotherapy plus BCNU, radiotherapy plus misonidazole and BCNU, radiotherapy plus streptozotocin, or hyperfractionated radiotherapy plus BCNU. The misonidazole dose was 1.5 g/m^2 twice a week for 6 weeks. The hyperfractionated radiotherapy was approximately 1.1 Gy twice a day, 5 days a week, to a total of 66 Gy. The results of this study have not yet been fully reported, but an abstract (Green et al. 1984) states that, after adjustment for the prognostic variables of age, performance status and histopathology, neither hyperfractionation nor misonidazole conferred a survival advantage and that streptozotocin appeared to be as effective as BCNU. Possibly the hyperfractionated radiotherapy was too conservative: in retrospect, larger fractions or a greater total dose might have been tolerated and have been more effective.

Between 1974 and 1979 the RTOG and the Eastern Cooperative Oncology Group (ECOG) (Chang et al. 1983) randomised 554 adult patients with malignant gliomas to receive either: (1) 60 Gy over 6–7 weeks to the whole brain; (2) 60 Gy to the whole brain plus a boost of 10 Gy in 1 week to the tumour volume; (3) 60 Gy plus BCNU (80 mg/m^2 per day for 3 days repeated every 8 weeks); or (4) 60 Gy to the whole brain plus MeCCNU (125 mg/m^2 repeated every 8 weeks) and DTIC (150 mg/m^2 per day for 5 days repeated every 4 weeks). The 70 Gy dose yielded essentially the same survival curve as did 60 Gy. Although the median survival times for patients receiving radiotherapy and BCNU (10.0 months), radiotherapy plus DTIC and MeCCNU (9.8 months), and radiation alone (9.9 months) were the same, the survival curves were slightly better with adjuvant chemotherapy. However, the only significant difference occurred in the 40–60 year age range where patients receiving radiotherapy plus BCNU ($P = 0.01$) or radiotherapy plus MeCCNU and DTIC ($P = 0.04$) had a significantly increased survival rate compared with patients who received radiation alone. In patients younger than 40 or older than 60 years neither chemotherapy regimen influenced survival. Severe thrombocytopaenia, the major acute toxicity, occurred in 6% of those receiving BCNU versus 23% for the MeCCNU plus DTIC combination. Thus, on the basis of toxicity, BCNU appeared preferable to MeCCNU plus DTIC.

Levin et al. (1979) reported a randomised clinical trial of the Northern Californian Oncology Group (NCOG) in which radiation therapy plus BCNU was compared with radiation therapy plus BCNU and hydroxyurea (HU) for glioblastoma multiforme. Both groups of patients received BCNU (80 mg/m^2 per day for 3 days) and whole-brain irradiation (50 Gy) with a boost of 10 Gy to the tumour volume. The radiation therapy was conventionally fractionated (1.7–2.0 Gy per day). HU (275 mg/m^2 every 6 hours) was given on alternate days until either completion of the radiotherapy or myelotoxicity forced dose reduction or its discontinuance. The median time to tumour progression was 41 weeks for those receiving HU versus 31 weeks for those without; the difference was statistically significant ($P = 0.03$).

These randomised trials have disclosed several prognostic criteria which should be noted before proceeding to review other clinical trials many of which were not randomised and/or failed to account for these criteria. The RTOG/ECOG study identified age as an important prognostic factor. Patients less than 40, 40–60 or older than 60 years of age had 18-month survival rates of 64%, 20% and 8%, respectively (Chang et al. 1983). The BTSG studies (Byer et al. 1983) also identified a significant age effect which persisted after multivariate analysis with adjustment for other factors such as duration of symptoms, performance status and histological type. Compared with patients of less than 45, those 45–54, 55–64, or older than 65 years of age had death rates of 1.75, 2.5 and 3.5 respectively.

A second important variable is initial performance status. In the RTOG/ECOG study, patients with a Karnofsky performance scale of 70–100 had a median survival of 12 months and 34% survived 18 months; with a performance rating of 40–60 the median survival was only 6 months and 13% survived 18 months (Chang et al. 1983). In the BTSG trials the death rates for patients with Karnofsky ratings of 70–80, 50–60 and 10–40 were 1.4, 2.0 and 2.9 times greater than for those with ratings of 90–100.

Histology is also important. In the BTSG trials (Byer et al. 1983) the death rates for patients with glioblastoma multiforme were 1.5–2.0 times higher than for those with other malignant gliomas. J. S. Nelson et al. (1983) reviewed the pathology material from 503 patients in the RTOG/ECOG trial. When results were analysed according to the Kernohan grading system the median survival times for astrocytoma grade 3 and grade 4 were virtually identical, namely 10 versus 9 months, respectively. A recent review from the Mayo Clinic (Scanlon and Taylor 1979) also failed to find a difference in survival when malignant gliomas were classified as grade 3 or 4.

However, when the tumours were reclassified retrospectively as astrocytoma with anaplastic foci (AAF) or glioblastoma multiforme (GBM), marked differences in both median survival time and 18-month survival rate were found. In this review the essential feature used to distinguish these two categories was the presence in GBM of foci of unequivocal coagulation necrosis involving neoplastic astrocytes. The median survival time for AAF was 28 months versus 8 months for GBM. The survival at 18 months was 62% and 15%, respectively. It was evident that while the Kernohan grading was of little value in this study for assessing prognosis, histology was, nevertheless, a useful prognostic indicator.

Fulling and Garcia (1984) examined AAF tumours for the presence of histological features considered indicative of anaplasia. Vascular endothelial proliferation and number of mitoses were inversely correlated with median actuarial survival; however, there was no correlation between survival and nuclear pleomorphism, cell density or the presence of secondary structures. As mentioned above, we at UCSF also are attempting to subclassify anaplastic astrocytomas.

Thus, although other factors of such as seizures, duration of symptoms and the occurrence of certain neurological abnormalities may correlate with prognosis, it is clear that age, performance status and histological category are very strong prognostic variables. When comparing results within or between randomised trials it is important to ensure that either the patient groups are similar in composition with respect to these variables or that means have been used to adjust for the differences. This becomes even more critical when using data from non-randomised studies.

Radiosensitisers

It is generally thought that malignant gliomas contain areas of hypoxic but viable tumour cells. In support of this concept, Hoshino et al. (1972) found a low tritiated thymidine labelling index in cells adjacent to necrotic areas. If the low labelling is due to hypoxia and reoxygenation does not occur during fractionated radiotherapy, hypoxia may play a significant role in the failure of low linear energy transfer (LET) radiation to control malignant gliomas. Various methods to circumvent the presumed effects of hypoxia have been investigated. These include irradiation under hyperbaric oxygen conditions and the use of hypoxic cell radiosensitisers or high LET irradiation.

In a non-randomised pilot study, Chang (1977) found a median survival of 38 weeks for patients irradiated in oxygen at 3 atmospheres pressure compared with 31 weeks for patients irradiated in air. There were two long-term survivors in the hyperbaric oxygen group. This study suffers from lack of randomisation, small numbers and failure to consider the prognostic variables.

Certain electron affinic chemicals serve as substitutes for oxygen in fixing DNA damage caused by radiation. Theoretically these compounds, which have the advantage of not being metabolised while diffusing through tissue, should increase the radiosensitivity of hypoxic cells without corresponding sensitisation of euoxic cells. To date, results for two electron affinic radiosensitisers have been reported. Urtasun et al. (1976) used a 5-nitroimidazole derivative, metronidazole (Flagyl), in a randomised trial involving 36 patients with supratentorial "glioblastoma multiforme". They gave nine fractions of 3.33 Gy each in 19 days for a total of 30 Gy (1290 rets according to the Ellis formula). Comparing patients who did and did not recieve metronidazole showed that those receiving the drug experienced an additional 4 month delay before onset of disease progression. The control patients, however, did poorly compared with patients treated in other trials by higher-dose radiotherapy alone. The metronidazole appears to have offset the unfavourable results of inadequate radiotherapy, but lack of stratification by the variables and the small number of patients make any interpretation difficult.

There have been several clinical trials with misonidazole (1-(2-nitro-1-imidazole)-3-methoxy-2-propanol) (MISO). Oral administration of 1.5–2.5 g/m^2 of MISO yields serum concentrations of about 50–100 μg/ml which may be expected to give a radiation sensitising efficiency, or enhancement ratio, of approximately 1.5 to 1.7 (Dische et al. 1976, 1978). Toxicity studies have shown that single doses greater than around 5 g/m^2 produce severe nausea and vomiting. With divided doses, the total dose that can be given is in the order of 10 or 12 to 18 g/m^2, dependent on the size of the individual dose, overall time and possible other factors such as the administration of phenytoin or dexamethasone. Various study groups have utilised the total tolerable dose of MISO in different ways. Some have used multiple small doses with conventionally fractionated radiotherapy. However, since larger enhancement ratios are associated with larger doses of MISO, the majority of trials have used fewer but larger doses of MISO together with larger than conventional daily radiation doses.

The unsuccessful BTSG trial using 1.5 g/m^2 MISO twice weekly with conventional fractionation was described above.

Bleehen et al. (1981) conducted a clinical trial in which 55 patients with "grade 3 or 4 supratentorial astrocytoma" were randomly allocated to one of three treatment groups. Group A received 28 equal fractions of 2.02 Gy over 5½ weeks for a total dose of 56.6 Gy. Group B received 2.94 Gy on Monday and Wednesday and 5 Gy on Friday for a total of 43.6 Gy in 12 fractions over 4 weeks. Group C was given the same radiation schedule as group B but also received 3 g/m^2 MISO 4 hours before the Friday radiation dose. The three groups were stratified according to biopsy only versus resection and grade 3 versus grade 4, but not by performance status or other histological measures. The median survival times for groups A, B and C were 251, 220 and 270 days, respectively—not significantly different. The small number of patients and lack of stratification by the major prognostic variables, however, make interpretation uncertain.

Urtasun et al. (1982) randomly assigned 66 patients with supratentorial "high grade astrocytomas", stratified by functional level and tumour grade, to three treatment groups. Group I received 1.93 Gy per day, 5 days a week for 6 weeks (total 58 Gy). Group II received 4.33 Gy three times per week for 3 weeks (total 39 Gy) plus 6 g/m^2 metronidazole (METRO) 4 hours before each radiation fraction. Group III had the same radiation therapy as group II but received 1.25 g/m^2 MISO rather than METRO. The median survival times for groups I, II and III were 26, 19 and 27 weeks, respectively. Neither length of remission nor probability of survival was improved by METRO or MISO.

The Medical Research Council (MRC 1983) reported 384 adult patients with "grade 3 or 4" supratentorial astrocytoma treated with modest doses of radiation and small daily doses of MISO. Each patient received 45 Gy in 20 equal fractions 5 days per week for 4 weeks. Patients were randomised to receive either 0.6 g/m^2 MISO or a placebo 4–5 hours before each radiation fraction. Twelve-month survival rates were 25% for the MISO patients versus 28% for those receiving the placebo. The survival curves were virtually superimposable out to 36 months. This study was not stratified by the major prognostic variables. As in other clinical trials, performance status, age and history of seizures were identified as prognostic factors but tumour grade was not prognostic.

The RTOG conducted a MISO trial on 245 adult patients with supratentorial malignant astrocytic glioma (D. Nelson et al. 1983). This randomised study was stratified according to age, performance status and histology. The age range was 18–70 years. A Karnofsky status of at least 40 was required. The permitted histologies were astrocytoma with anaplastic foci (AAF) and glioblastoma multiforme (GBM) as defined by J. Nelson et al. (1983). Group A received 2 Gy to the whole brain, five times per week for 6 weeks. Group B received 4.0 Gy on Mondays, 4 hours after 2.5 g/m^2 of MISO, and 1.5 Gy on Tuesdays, Thursdays and Fridays for 6 weeks. In the seventh week Group B received a boost of 9.0 Gy in five equal daily fractions. Thus both groups had a total of 60 Gy: they also received BCNU (80 mg/m^2 on days three, four and five during radiation therapy and repeated every 8 weeks for 2 years). According to a preliminary analysis (D. Nelson et al. 1983) the median survival for the control group A was 12.6 and for the MISO group B 10.7 months—not significantly different. For a subgroup of 50 patients with anaplastic astrocytoma (Nelson et al. 1985) the median survival without MISO was 168 weeks versus 48 weeks with MISO. The significantly poorer result with MISO was thought due to the radiation fractionation scheme, brain injury from MISO, or a combination thereof. Interestingly, a similar poorer result with MISO was seen in the RTOG study of 849 patients with brain metastases (Phillips et al. 1984).

In summary, METRO and MISO, as used to date, have failed to improve the results of radiation therapy alone, and MISO may be harmful. If hypoxia is a significant clinical problem and the radiosensitisers are to be useful, a better scheme of utilisation or a more effective agent is necessary.

Unconventional Fractionation

A number of clinical trials have been conducted with unconventional radiation fractionation regimens. The unsuccessful BTSG trial with 1.1 Gy twice a day, 5 days per week to 66 Gy in 6 weeks, has already been described (Green et al. 1984). Simpson and Platts (1976) compared 8 hour versus 24 hour intervals between treatments for 134 patients with "glioblastoma multiforme" (grades 3 and 4). They found no difference in survival between those on the thrice versus once daily fractionation schedules. However, the number of patients in their nine subgroups ranged from 7 to 28, total doses were only 30–40 Gy, and prognostic variables were not considered. Douglas and Worth (1982) treated 30 patients with a mixture of astrocytoma grades 3 and 4 with three 1.0 Gy fractions per day. The 12-month survival for patients with hyperfractionated radiotherapy was significantly higher than that for historical controls (44% verus 27%). Use of historical controls, small numbers, the system of tumour grading plus a lack of attention to prognostic factors render this trial uninterpretable.

Payne et al. (1982) carried out a prospective randomised trial with 157 patients with "malignant astrocytoma" (grade 3 or 4). The patients were stratified according to sex, age, extent of surgery, tumour site and performance status. All patients received CCNU and hydroxyurea. Both radiation regimes provided rather low total doses. One group received 50 Gy in 25 fractions over 5 weeks. The second group received 36–40 Gy in 36–40 fractions of 1.0 Gy each given four times a day for 2 weeks. There was no significant difference in survival or toxicity between the two groups.

Shin et al. (1983) randomised 69 patients with grade 3 or 4 astrocytoma to receive CCNU plus 50 Gy in either 25 fractions in 5 weeks or 50 fractions in 4 weeks (40 Gy in 45 fractions in 3 weeks plus 10 Gy in five fractions in 1 week). The 1-year survival was 54% versus 32% and the median survival 13 months versus 9 months for the groups receiving hyperfractionated and conventionally fractionated radiation, respectively. The differences were not statistically significant and could be accounted for by the small numbers and an imbalance in prognostic factors as well as actual differences in the treatment accorded the two groups. Thus the group receiving conventionally fractionated radiation required more steroid therapy (18 versus 9 weeks) and recieved less CCNU (18 versus 26 patients) than did the group having hyperfractionated radiation.

Fulton et al. (1984) recently reported a randomised trial comparing conventional fractionation (CF) with multiple daily fraction (MDF) with or without MISO. The individual radiation doses were similar to those of Payne et al. but the total doses were greater. The study included 128 patients and was stratified according to functional status and histology (anaplastic actrocytoma versus glioblastoma multiforme). CF consisted of 58 Gy in 30 daily fractions (1.93 Gy) in 6 weeks and MDF 0.89 Gy thrice daily for totals of 69 fractions and 61.4 Gy over $4\frac{1}{2}$ weeks. The MISO dose was 1.25 g/m^2 given three times a week for 3 weeks. Patients receiving MDF, with or without MISO, did significantly better ($P=0.002$) than those treated by CF, but MISO did not improve the result of MDF. The median survival time in weeks was 29 for CF, 45 for MDF, and 50 for MDF + MISO.

The European Organisation for Research on Treatment of Cancer (EORTC) (Ang et al. 1982) performed a pilot study of split-course multiple daily fractionated radiotherapy plus MISO. In this trial the patients received 2.0 Gy three times a day for 5 days with 1.2 g/m^2 MISO 2 hours before the first daily fraction. The regimen was repeated after a rest period of 2–4 weeks. Tolerance to this regimen was acceptable and a randomised trial has been initiated.

Particle Therapy

High-LET radiations have theoretical advantages over low-LET photon irradiation. These include a lower oxygen enhancement ratio, less repair of non-lethal radiation damage, and less variation of radiosensitivity over the cell cycle. While a few patients have been treated with neon ions at the University of California, Berkeley, or with pion beams (Nelson et al. 1985), the major experience with high-LET radiations to date is with neutrons. Laramore et al. (1978) treated 36 patients with neutrons either alone or in combination with megavoltage photons. Neutron doses thought biologically equivalent to those used in photon therapy increased the local tumour control rate; however, survival was not improved. In 14 of the 15 patients who underwent post-mortem examination the tumour apparently was eradicated but diffuse gliosis and demyelination were present in areas distant from tumour. Damage to normal CNS tissues was thought to be the cause of death. Catterall et al. (1980) reported a similar experience. The 12-month survival rate in their series was 36% for patients treated with photons versus 30% for those treated with neutrons. However, 69% of cases examined at post-mortem or second craniotomy were found to have either no tumour or only microscopic foci. Current RTOG trials are attempting to find a lower neutron dose that will retain the tumour control but produce less damage to normal tissue.

Brachytherapy

During the last 5 years interstitial brachytherapy has been used at UCSF (Gutin et al. 1984, Leibel et al. 1984) for treatment of recurrent "malignant" brain tumours. CT scans have been used both to determine treatment volume and to develop coordinates for the stereotaxic placement of removable afterloaded catheters. The technique has evolved over the 5 years; currently it allows implantation of up to four catheters with one to five radionuclide sources per catheter. At present the sources are 30–50 mCi ^{125}I seeds. The majority of these patients with recurrent tumours received tumour doses, calculated at the periphery of the contrast enhancing volume, of 80–120 Gy. Twenty-three of the first 43 patients had favourable clinical or CT-documented responses lasting from 2 to 17 or more months. Stabilisation of the disease for 3 to 12 months occurred in eight others. Median survival following implantation of these recurrent tumours was 18 months. Interestingly, the initial patient, who had a recurrent glioblastoma multiforme, is presently alive and in good functional condition more than 4 years after implant and subsequent resection of a localised necrotic area.

Encouraged by these results, a prospective randomised trial has been initiated. Previously untreated patients with malignant gliomas suitable for interstitial brachytherapy are randomly assigned to either an ^{131}I implant or a 5-bromo-2-deoxyuridine (BUdR) protocol study. The implant patients receive 60 Gy (1.8–2 Gy per day) external radiation, in combination with hydroxyurea, followed by a ^{125}I implant designed to deliver an additional 60 Gy, in 4–6 days, to the periphery of the contrast enhancing volume. Subsequently these patients receive cyclic chemotherapy (procarbazine, cyclophosphamide and vincristine) and surgical debulking of necrotic tissue when indicated. The BUdR study is based on the fact that halogenated pyrimidine analogues are incorporated into dividing cells where they substitute for thymidine in DNA and increase radiation sensitivity. The BUdR (0.8 g/m^2 per day, 4 days a week) is given weekly during conventional radiotherapy, by a 96 hour intravenous infusion. As in the implant protocol, the radiotherapy is followed by cyclical chemotherapy.

Target Volume and Radiation Dose

Optimum Treatment Volume. Concannon et al. (1960) compared tumour volume, as identified at post-mortem examination, with the volume previously irradiated and found that the treatment volume included the gross tumour plus a 1 cm margin in only 10% of their patients. Kramer (1969) subsequently recommended that for malignant gliomas the entire intracranial content should be irradiated. Influenced by such recommendations and because of difficulties in defining tumour volume, the earlier BTSG, NCOG and RTOG/ECOG clinical trials used whole-brain irradiation. Although a large well-controlled comparison of limited-field versus whole-brain irradiation has not been conducted, the results of several studies suggest that limited-field (Ramsey and Brand 1973, Sheline 1975, Fossati et al. 1979, Bleehen et al. 1981, Payne et al. 1982, Urtasun et al. 1982, MRC 1983) radiotherapy is as good as whole-brain irradiation. Urtasun et al. (1982), who used partial-brain irradiation ("2/3 of the brain volume"), obtained necropsies in 30% of patients and found no instance of tumour extending beyond the irradiated volume. Hochberg and Pruitt (1980) compared data from CT scans performed within 2 months of death with post-mortem findings. The CT scan volume plus a 2 cm margin included both the gross and microscopic tumour in 29 of 35 (80%) patients; the major source of error was subependymal spread which occurred in four patients. In addition to subependymal spread one of the 35 autopsied patients had microscopic infiltration more than 2 cm beyond the CT scan margin. Multicentricity occurred in 4% of previously untreated patients and in each case was identified by the CT scan. Serial CT scans in 42 patients showed that recurrences were within a 2 cm margin of the primary site in 90% of patients. The current RTOG and NCOG protocols use less than whole-brain radiotherapy. At UCSF we are treating with generous margins, in the order of about 2–3 cm around the contrast enhancing volume as identified by CT scan. Limiting the irradiated volume is important if, without missing tumour, it permits avoidance of tissues which if damaged may give rise to significant loss of function or mortality.

Optimum Radiation Dose. Selection of the optimum radiation dose for malignant gliomas has been as controversial as selection of the appropriate volume. In a retrospective review of the Mayo Clinic data, Scanlon and Taylor (1979) found that patients receiving less that 1400 rets did as well as those receiving higher doses. In a small series treated at the Royal Marsden Hospital, London, the mean survival decreased from 14 to 8 months when the dose was changed from 50 Gy in 5 weeks to 55 Gy in 6 weeks (Catterall et al. 1980). On the other hand, Salazar et al. (1976, 1979) reported an increase in survival time as the total dose was increased from 50 to 60 or 75 Gy. The median survival times for the three dose groups were 30, 42 and 56 weeks for grade 4 and 43, 82 and 204 weeks for grade 3, respectively. These data, however, must be accepted with caution: (1) the number of patients in each group was small; (2) the groups were treated chronologically not concurrently; (3) there was no consideration of the distribution of prognostic variables among the three dose groups; and (4) approximately one-fifth of the patients did not complete radiotherapy and were excluded from the analysis. Furthermore, in the highest dose group the quality of life, as indicated by performance status, declined steadily after radiotherapy with general debilitation evident by 18–24 months.

In large prospective randomised clinical trials both the BTSG and the RTOG/ECOG examined the question of optimum dose. The BTSG analysed data from 621 patients treated between 1966 and 1975 (Walker et al. 1979). These patients were retrospectively divided into three groups with median total doses of 50, 55 or 60 Gy. The median survival times were 28, 36 and 42 weeks, respectively. The difference between 50 and 60 Gy was significant at the $P = 0.004$ level. Since nearly 90% of the patients in the BTSG study had glioblastoma multiforme this dose-response effect applies to glioblastoma multiforme but not necessarily to other malignant gliomas. As described earlier the RTOG compared the effects of 60 Gy to the whole brain with 60 Gy to the whole brain plus a booster dose of 10 Gy to the tumour volume (Chang et al. 1983). Survival after 70 Gy was not better than after 60 Gy. Combining the results of the large randomised BTSG and RTOG/ECOG trials indicates that with conventional fractionation, i.e. single daily fractions of 1.8–2.0 Gy, given 5 times per week, the optimum dose for glioblastoma multiforme is around 60 Gy.

Oligodendrogliomas

Earlier attempts by Kernohan and Sayre (1952) to correlate oligodendroglioma "grade" with survival were unsuccessful. Recently, Smith et al. (1983) reviewed the pathology material from 323 cases of oligodendroglioma looking for predictive histological features. They evaluated endothelial proliferation, necrosis, nuclear/cytoplasmic ratio, cell density and pleomorphism. When viewed as single variables, only pleomorphism correlated with survival ($P = 0.01$). However, when the lesions were graded A to D based on all five histological features, the median survival times were: grade A, 94 months; grade B, 51 months; grade C, 45 months; grade D, 17 months. The 5-year survivals for grades A, B, C and D were 71%, 45%, 43% and 0%, respectively. Since survival times for grades B and C are about equal it appears that three prognostic groups may be distinguished and that the distinction is useful to 5 years. By 12–13 years, however, the survival curves for grades A, B and C converged at about 20%.

There has been no randomised clinical trial evaluating radiotherapy for oligodendrogliomas. Available studies are retrospective, non-randomised and contradictory. We reported a review of 32 patients (Sheline et al. 1964) of whom 16 received post-operative irradiation and 16 did not. The clinical records disclosed no recognisable difference in selection factors for the two groups. Specifically, there was no correlation between the use of irradiation and location of the tumour, completeness of resection, histology, patient age, duration of symptoms, or presence of tumour calcification. The 5-year and 10-year survival rates were 85% (11/13) and 55% (6/11) with radiation therapy, and 31% (4/13) and 25% (2/8) without. The difference at 5 years was statistically significant ($P = 0.02$). In the absence of discernible bias in treatment selection, these survival differences led us to believe that radiation therapy at least extended survival.

Neumann et al. (1978) reviewed the experience with oligodendroglioma at the University of Bonn. Patients were grouped according to degree of malignancy. After deleting patients who died post-operatively the average survivals in their groups I and II were less for irradiated than for non-irradiated patients. The average survival for group I was 3.5 years with radiotherapy and 5 years without, for group II the averages were 2 and 4 years, respectively. It was concluded that radiotherapy was useless. This report, however, ignored the fact that the only survivors in group III were irradiated and it failed to specify radiation dose, technique or relative characteristics of the patients who did or did not receive radiotherapy. The fact that the irradiated patients in groups I and II actually did worse than those not irradiated suggests that the radiation therapy was faulty or that the patients with poorer prognoses were selected for irradiation.

A recent, and in my opinion biased, paper from the Cleveland Clinic (Reedy et al. 1983) also failed to find a difference in 5-year survival between patients who did (68% of 27) or did not (70% of 21) receive radiation therapy. Although the authors of this report indicated an awareness that certain factors may be of prognostic significance, no effort was made to evaluate patient characteristics or treatment selection factors for the two groups. For example, complete resection occurred twice as frequently in the non-irradiated group. Furthermore, total radiation doses were as low as 22 Gy.

Chin et al. (1980) reported the experience with cerebral oligodendrogliomas at McGill University Hospitals. Again, there was little consideration of patient selection factors excepting that the majority were referred due to "incomplete radical resection". The irradiated patients received 53–70 Gy over 7–9 weeks. The 5-year survival after surgery alone was 9 of 11 (82%); however, only 5 (45%) were recurrence free. For the irradiated group the 5-year survival was 24/24 (100%) and 19 (79%) were recurrence free. Chin et al. concluded that in most cases post-operative radiotherapy is indicated.

A prospective randomised trial examing the role of radiation therapy for oligodendrogliomas would be useful. In the meantime, based on the experience at UCSF fortified by that from the Montreal group, it is our practice to give post-operative irradiation to these patients. Our approach is moderately conservative, using generous but less than whole-brain target volumes giving approximately 1.8 Gy per day, treating all radiation fields at each treatment session, and going to a total dose of about 55 Gy in 6 weeks.

References

Ang KK et al. (1982) Split course multiple daily fractionated radiotherapy schedule combined with misonidazole for the management of grade III and IV gliomas: A pilot feasibility study of the Radiotherapy Group of the EORTC. Int J Radiat Oncol Biol Phys 8: 1657–1664

Bailey P, Cushing H (1926) A classification of tumours of the glioma group on a histogenic basis with a correlated study of prognosis. Lippincott, Philadelphia

Bleehen NM, Wiltshire CR et al. (1981) A randomized study of misonidazole and radiotherapy for Grade 3 and 4 cerebral astocytoma. Br J Cancer 43: 436–442

Bloom HJG (1982) Intracranial tumours: Response and resistance to therapeutic endeavors, 1970–1980. Int J Radiat Oncol Biol Phys 8: 1083–1113

Boldrey E, Sheline G (1967) Delayed transitory clinical manifestations after radiation treatment of intracranial tumors. Acta Radiol 5: 5–10

Bouchard J (1973) Central nervous system. In: Gletcher G (ed) Textbook of radiotherapy, 2nd edn. Lea and Febiger, Philadelphia, pp 366–418

Bouchard J, Pierce CB (1960) Radiation therapy in the management of neoplasms of the central nervous system, with a special note in regard to children: Twenty years' experience, 1939–1958. Am J Roentgenol 84: 610–628

Burger PC, Kamenar E, Schold SC et al. (1981) Encephalomyelopathy following high-dose BCNU therapy. Cancer 48: 1318–1327

Burger PC, Mahaley MS, Dudka L, Vogel FS (1979) The morphologic effects of radiation administered therapeutically for intracranial gliomas: A post-mortem study of 25 cases. Cancer 44: 1256–1272

Byer DP, Green SB, Striker TA (1983) Prognostic factors for malignant glioma. In: Walker MD (ed) Oncology of the nervous system. Martinus Nijhoff, The Hague, pp. 379–395

Catterall M, Bloom HJG, Ash DV et al. (1980) Fast neutrons compared with mega voltage X rays in the treatment of patients with supratentorial glioblastoma. Int J Radiat Oncol Biol Phys 6: 261–266

Caveness WF (1977) Pathology of radiation damage to the normal brain of the monkey. Natl Cancer Inst Monogr 46: 57–76

Chang CH (1977) Hyperbaric oxygen and radiation therapy in the management of glioblastoma. Natl Cancer Inst Monogr 46: 163–169
Chang CH, Horton J, Schoenfeld D et al. (1983) Comparison of postoperative radiotherapy and combined postoperative radiotherapy and chemotherapy in the multidisciplinary management of malignant gloimas: A joint Radiation Therapy Oncology and Eastern Cooperative Oncology Group Study. Cancer 52: 997–1007
Chin HW, Hazel JJ et al. (1980) Oligodendrogliomas. I. A study of cerebral oligodendrogliomas. Cancer 45: 1458–1466
Concannon JP, Kramer S, Berry R (1960) The extent of intracranial gliomata at autopsy and its relationship to techniques used in radiation therapy of brain tumours. Am J Roentgenol 84: 99–107
DiLorenzo N, Nolletti A, Palma L (1978) Late cerebral radionecrosis. Surg Neurol 10: 281–290
Dische S et al. (1976) Clinical testing on the radiosensitiser Ro-07-0582-II radiosensitisation of normal and hypoxic skin. Clin Radiol 27: 159–167
Dische S et al. (1978) Hypoxic cell sensitisers in radiotherapy. Int J Radiat Oncol Biol Phys 4: 157–160
Douglas BG, Worth AJ (1982) Superfractionation in glioblastoma multiforme: Results of a Phase II study. Int J Radiat Oncol Biol Phys 8: 1787–1794
Druckman A (1929) Schlafsucht als Folge der Roñtgenbestrahlung. Beitrag zur Strahlenempfindlichkeit des Gehirns. Strahlentherapie 33: 382–384
Ellis F (1969) Dose, time and fractionation: A clinical hypothesis. Clin Radiol 20: 1–7
Fazekas JT (1977) Treatment of grades I and II brain astrocytomas: The role of radiotherapy. Int J Radiat Oncol Biol Phys 2: 661–666
Fike JR, Sheline GE, Cann CE, Davis RL (1984) Radiation necrosis. Prog Exp Tumour Res 28: 136–151
Fossati F, Jacker C, Tosi G (1979) Effect of field size and unconventional dose fractionation in the radiotherapy of malignant cerebral gliomas. In: Paoletti P, Walker MD, Butti G, Knerich R (eds) Multidisciplinary aspects of brain tumor therapy. Elsevier, Amsterdam, pp 106–115
Freeman JE, Johnston PGB, Voke JM (1973) Somnolence after prophylactic cranial irradiation in children with acute lymphoblastic leukaemia. Br Med J iv: 523–525
Fulling KH, Garcia DM (1984) Anaplastic astrocytoma of the adult cerebrum: Prognostic value of histologic features. Cancer (in press)
Fulton DS et al. (1984) Misonidazole combined with hyperfractionation in the management of malignant glioma. Int J Radiat Oncol Biol Phys 10: 1709–1712
Green SB, Byar DP, Walker MD et al. (1983) Comparisons of carmustine, procarbazine and high-dose methylprednisolone as additions to surgery and radiotherapy for the treatment of malignant glioma. Cancer Treat Rep 67: 121–132
Green SB, Byar DP, Strike TA et al. (1984) Randomised comparisons of BCNU, streptozotocin, radiosensitiser, and fractionation in the post-operative treatment of malignant glioma (Study 7702) (abstr). Proc Am Soc Clin Oncol 3: 260
Gutin PH et al. (1984) Brachytherapy of recurrent malignant brain tumors with removable high-activity iodine-125 sources. J Neurosurg 60: 61–68
Hindo WA, DeTrana FA, Lee MS, Hendrickson FR (1970) Large dose increment irradiation in treatment of cerebral metastases. Cancer 26: 138–141
Hochberg FH, Pruitt A (1980) Assumptions in the radiotherapy of glioblastoma. Neurology 30: 907–911
Hochberg FH, Slotnick B (1980) Neurophysiologic impairment in astrocytoma survivors. Neurology 30: 172–177
Hoffman WF, Levin VA, Wilson CB (1979) Evaluation of malignant glioma patients during the postirradiation period. J Neurosurg 50: 624–628
Hoshino T, Barker M, Wilson CB, Boldrey EB, Fewer D (1972) Cell kinetics of human gliomas. J Neurosurg 37: 15–26
Kernohan JW, Sayre GP (1952) Tumours of the central nervous system. Armed Forces Institute of Pathology, Washington DC
Kernohan JW, Mabon RF, Svien HJ, Adson AW (1949) A simplified classification of the gliomas. Proc Staff Meet Mayo Clin 24: 71–75
Kramer S (1968) The hazards of therapeutic irradiation of the central nervous system. Clin Neurosurg 15: 301–318
Kramer S (1969) Tumour extent as a determining factor in radiotherapy of glioblastoma. Acta Radiol 8: 111–117
Kramer S (1973) Radiation therapy in the management of malignant gliomas. 7th National Cancer Conference Proc., American Cancer Society, pp 823–826
Kramer S, Hendrickson F, Zelen M, Schotz W (1977) Therapeutic trials in the management of metastatic brain tumors by different time/dose fractionation schemes of radiation therapy. Natl Cancer Inst Monogr 46: 213–221

Lampert PW, Davis RL (1964) Delayed effects of radiation on the human central nervous system. "Early" and "late" delayed reactions. Neurology 14: 912-917

Lampert PW, Tom MI, Rider WD (1959) Disseminated demyelination of the brain following Co-60 (gamma) radiation. Arch Pathol 68: 322-330

Laramore GE et al. (1978) Fast neutron and mixed (neutron/photon) beam teletherapy for Grades III and IV astrocytomas. Cancer 42: 96-103

Leibel SA, Sheline GE, Wara WM et al. (1975) The role of radiation therapy in the treatment of astrocytomas. Cancer 35: 1551-1557

Leibel SA, Gutin PH, Phillips TL, Wara WM, Weaver KW, Lamb S (1984) Interstitial implantation of high-activity iodine-125 sources for the treatment of recurrent malignant brain tumors (abstr.). Proc Int J Radiat Oncol Biol Phys 10 [Suppl 2] 144

Levin VA, Wilson CB et al. (1979) A phase III comparison of BCNU, hydroxyurea, and radiation therapy to BCNU and radiation therapy for treatment of primary malignant gliomas. J Neurosurg 51: 526-532

Lindgren M (1958) On tolerance of brain tissue and sensitivity of brain tumors to irradiation. Acta Radiol [Suppl] 170: 1-73

Marks JE, Baglan RJ, Prassad SC, Bland WF (1981) Cerebral radionecrosis: Incidence and risk in relation to dose, time, fractionation and volume. Int J Radiat Oncol Biol Phys 7: 243-252

Marsa GE, Goffinet DR, Rubinstein LJ, Bagshaw MA (1975) Megavoltage irradiation in the treatment of gliomas of the brain and spinal cord. Cancer 36: 1681-1689

MRC Working Party (1983) A study of the effect of misonidazole in conjunction with radiotherapy for the treatment of grades 3 and 4 astrocytomas: A report from the MRC Working Party on Misonidazole in gliomas. Br J Radiol 56: 673-682

Nelson DF, Schoenfeld D, Weinstein AS et al. (1983) A randomized comparison of misonidazole sensitized radiotherapy plus BCNU and radiotherapy plus BCNU for treatment of malignant glioma after surgery; preliminary results of an RTOG study. Int J Radiat Oncol Biol Phys 9: 1143-1151

Nelson DF et al. (1985) Recent and current investigations of radiation therapy of malignant gliomas. Semin Oncol (in press)

Nelson JS, Tsukada Y, Schoenfeld D, Fulling K et al. (1983) Necrosis as a prognostic criterion in malignant supratentorial, astrocytic glioma. Cancer 52: 550-554

Neumann J, Kimpel J, Gulotta F (1978) Das Oligodendrogliom: der klinische Verlauf in Bezug zum histologischen grading. Neurochirurgia 21: 35-42

Payne DG et al. (1982) Malignant astrocytoma: Hyperfractionated and standard radiotherapy with chemotherapy in a randomized prospective clinical trial. Cancer 50: 2301-2306

Pezner RD, Archambeau JO (1981) Brain tolerance unit: A method to estimate risk of radiation brain injury for various dose schedules. Int J Radiat Oncol Biol Phys 7: 397-402

Phillips TL, Diener MD, Wasserman TH, Asbell SO, Chang CH, Urtasun RC, Moylan DJ (1984) Hypofractionated radiotherapy with or without misonidazole for the treatment of brain metastases. Proc Int J Radiat Oncol Biol Phys 10 [Suppl 2]: 145

Pratt RA, Di Chiro G, Weed JC (1977) Cerebral necrosis following irradiation and chemotherapy for metastatic choriocarcinoma. Surg Neurol 7: 117-120

Ramsey RG, Brand WN (1973) Radiotherapy of glioblastoma multiforme. J Neurosurg 39: 197-202

Reedy DP, Bay JW, Hahn JF (1983) Role of radiation therapy in the treatment of cerebral oligodendroglioma: An analysis of 57 cases and a literature review. Neurosurg 13: 499-503

Reinhold HS, van Putten WLJ, Hopewell JW, van der Kogel AJ (1984) The latent period in clinical radiation myelopathy. Int J Radiat Oncol Biol Phys 10: 2385-2387

Rider WD (1963) Radiation damage to the brain: A new syndrome. J Can Assoc Radiol 14: 67-69

Rubinstein LJ (1972) Tumors of the central nervous system. Armed Forces Institute of Pathology, Washington, DC

Salazar OM, Rubin P, McDonald JV, Feldstein ML (1976) High dose radiation therapy in the treatment of glioblastoma multiforme. Int J Radiat Oncol Biol Phys 1: 717-727

Salazar OM, Rubin P, Feldstein ML, Pizzutiello R (1979) High dose radiation therapy in the treatment of malignant gliomas: Final report. Int J Radiat Oncol Biol Phys 5: 1733-1740

Scanlon PW, Taylor WF (1979) Radiotherapy of intracranial astrocytomas: Analysis of 417 cases treated from 1960 through 1969. Neurosurg 5: 301-308

Shapiro WR, Allen JC, Horton BC (1980) Chronic methotrexate toxicity to the central nervous system. Clin Bull 10: 49-52

Sheline GE (1975) Conventional radiation therapy of gliomas. In: Hekmatpanah J (ed) Current concepts in biology, diagnosis and therapy. Springer-Verlag, Berlin (Recent results in cancer research), pp 125-134

Sheline GE, Boldrey E, Karlsberg P, Phillips TL (1964) Therapeutic considerations in tumours affecting the central nervous systems: Oligodendrogliomas. Radiol 82: 84-89
Sheline GE, Wara WM, Smith V (1980) Therapeutic irradiation and brain injury. Int J Radiat Oncol Biol Phys 6: 1215-1228
Shin KH, Muller PJ, Geggie PHS (1983) Superfractionation radiation therapy in the treatment of malignant astrocytoma. Cancer 52: 2040-2043
Simpson WJ, Platts ME (1976) Fractionation study in the treatment of glioblastoma multiforme. Int J Radiat Oncol Biol Phys 1: 639-644
Smith MT et al. (1983) Grading of oligodendrogliomas. Cancer 52: 2107-2114
Svien HJ, Mabon RF, Kernohan JW, Adson AW (1949) Astrocytomas. Proc Staff Meet Mayo Clin 24: 54-64
Urtasun RC et al. (1976) Radiation and high-dose metronidazole in supratentorial glioblastoma. N Engl J Med 294: 1364-1367
Urtasun R, Feldstein ML, Partington J et al. (1982) Radiation and nitroimidazoles in supratentorial high grade gliomas: A second clinical trial. Br J Cancer 46: 101-108
van der Kogel AJ (1979) Late effects of radiation on the spinal cord. Radiobiological Institute, TNO Rijswijk, The Netherlands, pp 118-121
Walker MD, Alexander E, Hunt WE et al. (1978) Evaluation of BCNU and/or radiotherapy in the treatment of anaplastic gliomas: A cooperative clinical trial. J Neurosurg 49: 333-343
Walker MD, Strike TA, Sheline GE (1979) An analysis of dose-effect relationship in the radiotherapy of malignant gliomas. Int J Radiat Oncol Biol Phys 5: 1725-1731
Walker MD, Green SB, Byar DP et al. (1980) Randomized comparisons of radiotherapy and nitrosoureas for the treatment of malignant glioma after surgery. N Engl J Med 303: 1323-1329
Young DF, Posner JB, Chu F, Nisce L (1974) Rapid-course radiation therapy of cerebral metastases: Results and complications. Cancer 34: 1069-1076

10 Third Ventricular Tumours

R. Berman, P. N. Plowman and A. E. Jones

Introduction

From its embryonic development the third ventricle has greater potential for diversity of tumour types than any other part of the central nervous system (CNS). When tumours do develop, because of juxtaposition of "eloquent structures" their manifestations attract the attention of both neurologists and endocrinologists. At the anterior end of the ventricle attention is claimed by pituitary and parasellar lesions (including those of the hypothalamus), while at the posterior end interest has long been centred on the pineal gland. The fascination of the pineal for biologists and physicians has for generations been out of proportion to its known physiological importance and this is further reflected in the study of its tumours.

The pineal gland arises as an evagination in the back of the embryonic ectoderm of the forebrain; consequently it is not surprising that the pineal should reflect this origin in producing neuroectodermal tumours. The morphology of pineoblastoma resembles that of the medulloblastoma-neuroblastoma group (including Homer-Wright rosette formation). The paradox is that the common tumour at this site is in fact a germinal cell tumour formed of neoplastic germ cells and reactive lymphocytes, identical in this two-cell pattern to its gonadal counterparts and as such highly radiosensitive. Such tumours are not confined to the pineal region, but also occur in the suprasellar region and hypothalamus.

Tumours at both ends of the ventricle commonly occur in adolescence but the sex ratio is interesting. Those in the pineal area occur predominantly in young males while for tumours in the suprasellar region the male/female ratio is almost equal. The well-known increased prevalence of germinoma in Japan (where it accounts for between 4% and 10% of all intracranial tumours, and about 20% of those in young males) is yet another facet of this oncogenetic conundrum.

There have been major advances in the study of third ventricular tumours during the last 10 years. These have come from more precise characterisation of the tumours, both in lineage and in metastatic potential; from delineation by computerised axial tomography (CT) scanning; from the recognition of biochemical markers in tumours and cerebrospinal fluid (CSF); from stereotactic biopsy to provide tissue diagnosis; from the increasing use of microsurgical techniques as both primary and salvage procedures; from greater sophistication of radiotherapeutic techniques including craniospinal irradiation; from the reawakened interest in chemotherapy; and from the summation of all of these into the formulation of treatment policies designed to improve the already considerable cure rates from irradiation. Of the important studies which have recently contributed to our understanding of these tumours the following should be mentioned especially: that of Rubinstein (1981) on the cytogenesis and differentiation of pineal neoplasms; the monograph on pineal tumours by Schmidek (1977); the extensive surgical experience of Sano (1983) from Tokyo; and the admirable review of intracranial germ cell tumours by Bloom (1983). All of these provide valuable data on which we have drawn considerably in this review.

Our comments are based on a series of 25 patients referred to the Department of Radiotherapy at St Bartholomew's Hospital in the period 1962 to 1984. Their investigation and treatment have been considered in the light of such studies as those mentioned above.

Pathology

The tortuous history of tumours of the pineal region (Borit 1981) has, as its latest unfolding, a generally recognised separation of those neoplasms of germ cell origin (including various types of teratoma and of mixed forms) from pineal parenchymal cell tumours and others of neuroectodermal origin. Thus we have the simplified classification as shown in Table 10.1. In a compilation of 278 histologically verified pineal tumours collected from 12 published series Bloom (1983) calculated the incidence of the various types to be: germinoma 45%, glioma 17%, mature and anaplastic teratoma 16%, pineal parenchymal tumours 15%, and others 7%.

Table 10.1. Classification of pineal and related tumours

I Germ cell tumours	(a) Germinoma
	(b) Anaplastic germ cell tumour and teratoma
	Embryonal cell tumour
	Choriocarcinoma
	Endodermal sinus (yolk sac) tumour
	Malignant teratoma with differentiation
	(c) Mixed germ cell tumour
	(d) Mature teratoma/dermoid cyst
II Pineal parenchymal tumours	(a) Pineocytoma
	(b) Pineoblastoma
III Glioma	Astrocytoma and ependymoma
IV Other	Meningioma, angioma, metastases, cysts, etc.

Germinoma

The commonest type of pineal tumour is a highly malignant tumour which infiltrates widely (Fig. 10.1) and gives rise to both ventricular and cerebrospinal subarachnoid deposits. Of its two component cell types—the large polygonal cells with central spherical nuclei, and the small darkly staining cells—only the former are neoplastic, the latter being lymphocytes whose presence may have an immunological significance. Certainly there is sometimes a paradoxically long history for such a malignant tumour. An overt admixture of teratomatous tissue may sometimes be apparent.

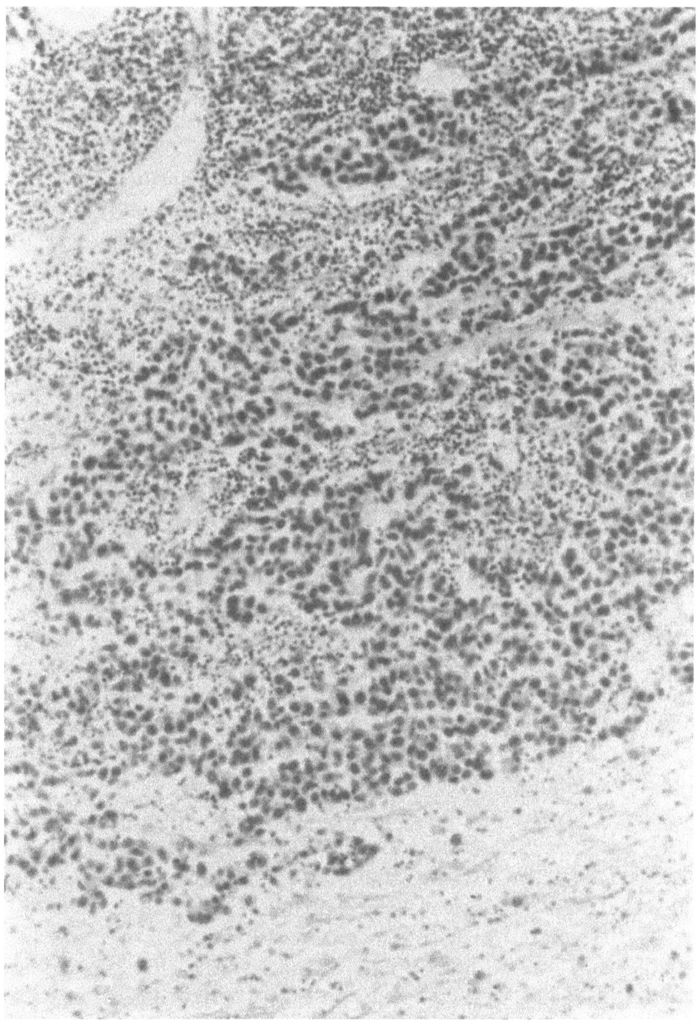

Fig. 10.1. Typical histological appearance of primary pineal germinoma, showing polygonal tumour cells and lymphocytes infiltrating brain.

Teratoma

While mature teratomas remain localised in the posterior third ventricle and slowly enlarge to produce pressure effects, the undifferentiated tumours in this group are highly malignant, infiltrate locally and disseminate by the CSF. They include embryonal carcinoma (analogous to that in the testis), choriocarcinoma (secreting human chorionic gonadotrophin) and yolk sac (endodermal sinus) tumour (secreting alphafetoprotein). Mixed tumours are again not infrequent and the presence of such elements, particularly of the sinister endodermal sinus tumour whose behaviour is very aggressive, limits the responsiveness to treatment of some germinomas of otherwise favourable prognosis.

Tumours Arising from the Pineal Parenchymal Cells

These tumours have classically been divided into two types: *pineocytoma* (a differentiated tumour resembling the normal gland), and the immature, undifferentiated *pineoblastoma*. However Rubinstein (1981) has pointed out that intermediate forms are frequent and that both cytologically and biologically the two are difficult to separate. Both are characterised by a malignant clinical behaviour which is associated with a liability to distant CSF metastasis. Such deposits, from either variant, invariably show the cytological features of pineoblastoma. Pineocytomas with neuronal, or mixed neuronal and astrocytic, differentiation (25% of cases) tended to remain localised, but in the demonstrable absence of this differentiation there was such a tendency to CSF spread as to have implications for treatment.

While pineal parenchymal tumours have in general no specific age or sex incidence there is one recently described and fascinating aetiological linkage: the association of pineoblastoma with retinoblastoma (Bader et al. 1980, Kingston et al. 1985). In the largest series Kingston et al. described 11 such cases, all occurring in families having the autosomal dominant retinoblastoma trait; the pineoblastoma occurred 14–70 months (median 47 months) after the retinoblastoma presentation and in all the pineoblastoma presented in the first 7 years of life. Those affected were predominantly females. These authors concluded that the incidence of familial pineoblastoma with retinoblastoma may be more frequent than suspected, since the incidence in this St Bartholomew's Hospital/Moorfields series was much higher in the CT scan era—the inference being that such children were previously diagnosed as having metastatic retinoblastoma. As with the sporadic variety of pineoblastoma, this familial form is highly malignant (Fig. 10.2a and b).

The concept of primitive neuroectodermal tumours arising at various intracranial sites in childhood and adolescence, showing varying degrees of differentiation and tending to disseminate by CSF pathways, has been discussed recently by Becker and Hinton (1983) of the Sick Children's Hospital in Toronto. They call attention to areas of neuroepithelial differentiation within brain teratomas, and we ourselves recently encountered areas of "medulloblastoma" within an otherwise classic teratoma of the fourth ventricle. Whilst some of these tumours may exhibit florid and highly typical features of a tumour arising in one particular location, much overlap occurs and frequently such neoplasms could be better classified as "primitive neuroepithelial tumours".

Fig. 10.2. **a** CT scan appearance of ectopic intracranial "retinoblastoma" (pineoblastoma) at the anterior end of the third ventricle in a child who had successfully received treatment for bilateral retinoblastoma. **b** CSF cytology of the same child demonstrating clumps of pineoblasts (retinoblasts).

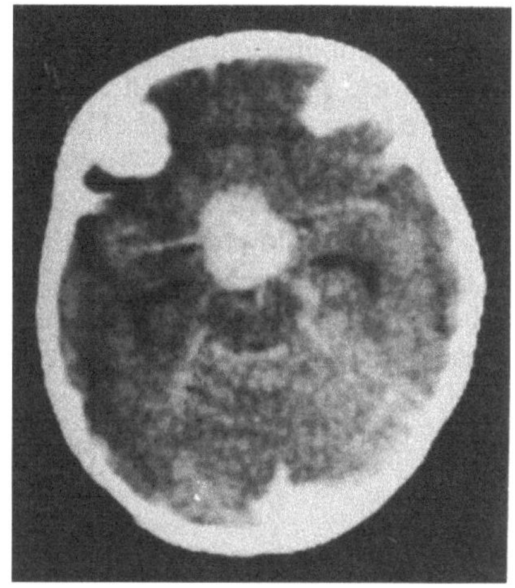

a

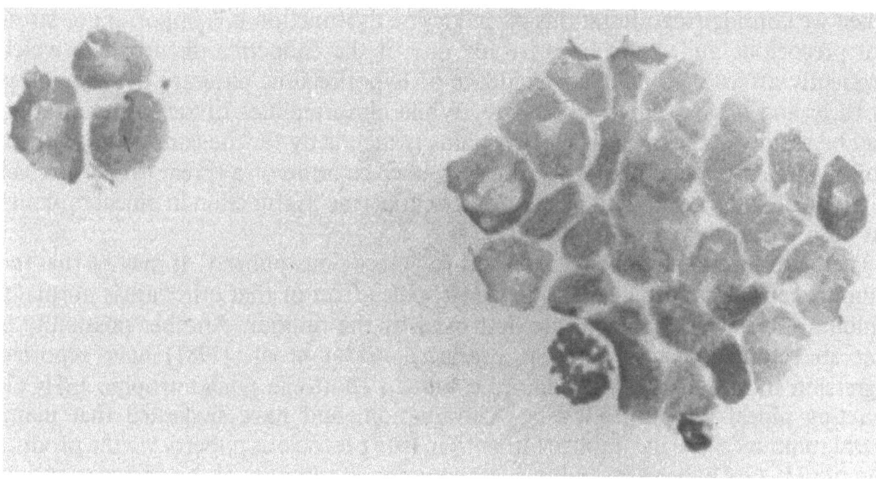

b

Clinical Diagnosis

General Aspects

Whatever the histological nature of a tumour of the posterior third ventricle the initial effects are those of CSF pathway obstruction, compression of the tectum of the mid-brain, and cerebellar dysfunction by interference with the superior cerebellar penduncles and dento-rubro-thalamic tracts. There is also disturbance of hypothalamic function from obstruction and growth in the floor of the third ventricle.

The duration of symptoms in our series varied from 2 weeks in children to as long as 4 years in adults. The clinical picture is of headache, vomiting and papilloedema or consecutive optic atrophy, often with restriction of eye movements known as Parinaud's syndrome (of which the main features are paralysis of upward gaze, dilated pupils fixed to light, and defective convergence). The supranuclear impairment of upward gaze is of course related to a lesion of the dorsal mid-brain and pretectal region involving pathways which traverse in or near the posterior commissure. Upward saccades (i.e. a flick of the eyes) rather than smooth pursuit movements are often the first to be affected. The neuro-ophthalmology of pineal tumours has been studied in detail by Wray at Boston (1977, 1983) and in 22 cases a mid-brain pupillary abnormality of light accommodation dissociation was in fact the leading sign. This was followed by paralysis of supranuclear upward gaze, with defects of saccadic eye movements ahead of those of pursuit. Paresis of convergence was the least frequent component of the triad. Nystagmus is common and there may be ataxia, central deafness, ptosis, internal strabismus and bilateral spasticity.

Endocrine Features

When we consider manifestations of endocrine dysfunction it is important to stress that precocious puberty in boys is only one of the endocrine disturbances which frequently affect such patients. Evidence of hypothalamic-pituitary dysfunction is an early and almost universal feature. While abnormalities of sexual maturation may be readily apparent, diabetes insipidus (which is by far the commonest abnormality) and anterior pituitary insufficiency may be more of a threat to the survival of a patient with germinoma. The range of endocrine dysfunction in pineal tumours has been well reviewed by Axelrod (1977).

There are several possible mechanisms for precocious puberty. It may be that the tumours cause loss of pineal antigonadotrophic effect or that other areas normally inhibiting sexual development are destroyed by the tumour. Another possibility is that an ectopic gonadotrophin is produced. Sklar et al. (1981) have reported regression of sexual precocity due to a human chorionic gonadotrophin (βHCG) secreting pineal tumour following X-irradiation, and have suggested that many pineal tumours cause incomplete rather than true precocious puberty via the production of βHCG. Diabetes insipidus is less common in tumours of the posterior end of the third ventricle than in those arising anteriorly, so that when it occurs it is usually due to anterior extension or metastasis of tumour rather than to simple ventricular obstruction.

Tumours affecting the anterior end of the third ventricle are more diverse in origin and type (Table 10.2). The characteristic initial presentation differs from that in posteriorly placed lesions with the triad of diabetes insipidus (often preceding other symptoms by months or years), visual disturbance from chiasmal compression and hypopituitarism dominating the picture. While these may be caused by any of the disorders listed in Table 10.2, Rubin and Kramer (1965) drew attention to ectopic pinealoma (germinoma) as a "radiocurable neuroendocrinological entity", and stressed that diabetes insipidus of unexplained aetiology should be carefully investigated during the first and second decades of life for associated visual disturbance and hypopituitarism. Twenty years later CT scanning would of course be the prime investigation. Craniopharyngioma, despite a greater frequency of raised pressure and hemianopia, less commonly causes diabetes insipidus unless it has been subjected to surgery. With growth and extension of the tumour hypothalamic involvement results in pyrexia, somnolence, hypernatraemia and profound muscle weakness.

Table 10.2. Third ventricular tumours: Anterior end

I Pituitary tumours	Prolactinoma Chromophobe Eosinophil Basophil
II Hypothalamic or stalk tumours	Craniopharyngioma Meningioma Optic chiasm glioma Germinoma Glioma Metastases Hamartoma
III Granulomas	Histiocytosis X Sarcoidosis Tuberculosis Syphilis
IV Miscellaneous	Including reticuloses

In a series of 10 cases of germinoma, of which 8 were suprasellar, one pineal and one in the caudate nucleus, Sklar et al. (1981) found pituitary deficits in all patients, with abnormal eye signs in 60%, short stature in 50% and abnormal pubertal development in 30%. The association of endocrine dysfunction with pineal and chiasmal tumours is important not only from the diagnostic viewpoint, as some other component of dysfunction may occur while the patient is under observation. Improvement in polyuria in a patient with diabetes insipidus may follow the development of anterior pituitary insufficiency, and this must always be considered when caring for these patients. The main investigations required initially are of course those for assessment of neurohypophyseal and adenohypophyseal reserve, and every effort should be made to assess quantitatively the reserve function of each component. It is unwise to start treatment on the basis of suggestive symptoms without careful assessment and laboratory confirmation.

Radiology

While the normal plain skull X-ray film will show pineal calcification in up to 60% of cases over the age of 20, this is rare below the age of 6. The abnormal skull X-ray film in pineal tumour may show premature irregular calcification and the pineal can be abnormally large and low in position due to hydrocephalus. The other signs of raised intracranial pressure may also be present (Grossman and Gonzalez 1977).

The advent of CT scanning in the 1970s revolutionised the further investigation of such tumours (Figs. 10.3 and 10.4). It has superseded the main contrast methods of ventriculography or pneumoencephalography which for half a century had been the mainstay of tumour delineation. Arteriography is now rarely used unless surgery is being considered. CT scanning can clearly define the majority of pineal tumours; it can recognise the adipose tissue of tectal lipomas, the fatty and osseous portions of teratomas, and the cystic and necrotic areas in a variety of tumours; it can indicate the presence of subarachnoid seeding; and it can assess the degree of ventricular enlargement.

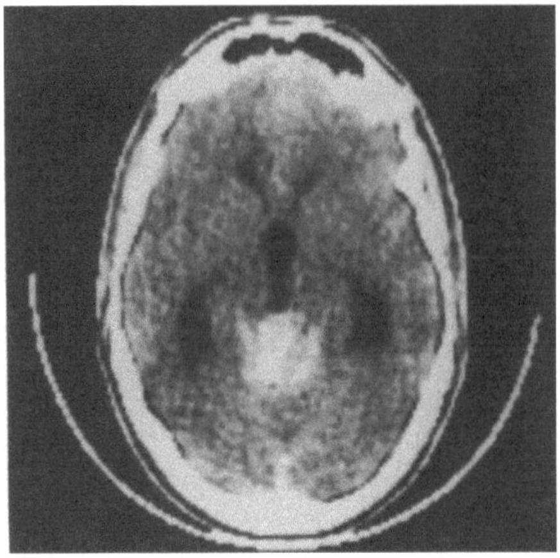

Fig. 10.3. CT scan (enhanced) demonstrating a pineocytoma.

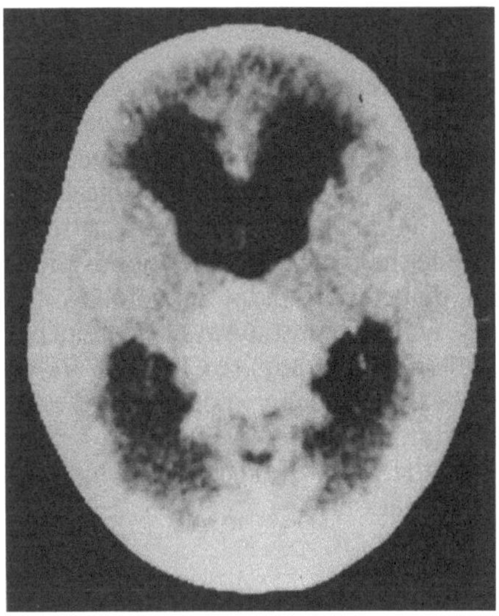

Fig. 10.4. CT scan (enhanced) demonstrating a pineoblastoma.

The question of the extent to which CT scanning can add further to the non-invasive assessment of tumour characteristics, particularly histology, has been considered in a number of reports in the last 5 years (Messina et al. 1976, Inoue et al. 1979, Zimmerman et al. 1980, Ueki and Tanaka 1980, Futrell et al. 1981, Wood et al. 1981, Jooma and Kendall 1983, Packer et al. 1984). For instance Zimmerman et al. (1980) found that abnormal calcification occurred most frequently in primary pineal tumours (pineocytoma and pineoblastoma). Early germinoma appeared as a well-defined mass of slightly greater than normal density, with uniform and marked contrast enhancement, but larger tumours were often poorly defined and infiltrated adjacent structures. There was a greater tendency to intratumoral calcification in the embryonal carcinomas than in the germinomas, and cystic changes were found in endodermal sinus carcinoma. These authors considered that the CT characteristics in conjunction with a patient's age and sex could often lead to histological prediction. Nevertheless this was imprecise and the same authors in another paper (Wood et al. 1981) in the context of treatment, considered that a tissue diagnosis was essential for management by surgery or irradiation.

While some have regarded periventricular contrast enhancement (Fig. 10.5) as virtually pathognomonic of germinoma (Dupont et al. 1977), diffuse ventricular spread or invasion of the mid-brain or basal ganglia can also occur with pineoblastoma or malignant teratoma (Jooma and Kendall 1983). A review of the relevant literature suggests, therefore, that accurate inferences as to histology cannot be made on the basis of CT scan appearances alone. This is underlined by a recent report (Whittle et al. 1983) of a tuberculoma mimicking a pineal tumour on CT scan.

We have therefore reviewed with Dr M. Charlesworth of the Department of Neuroradiology at St Bartholomew's Hospital the features of 22 cases in which the CT scans were available. The majority comprised germinoma or teratoma, and all showed contrast enhancement. However, there was no diagnostically useful pattern of boundary definition, or pre-contrast density, homogeneity or calcification. Seven cases of pineoblastoma from the "trilateral retinoblastoma" series (Kingston et al. 1985) usually showed well-defined boundaries with high density in the pre-contrast scan. They were usually homogenous throughout, but calcification was variable.

We can therefore conclude that, from the initial CT scan features alone, no firm conclusions regarding tumour type can be made. The information must be considered in the context of other investigations, and possible biopsy, before treatment. Nevertheless CT scanning can provide very accurate delineation of the lesion, particularly at the anterior end of the ventricle where actual involvement of the optic nerves by extension from a suprasellar mass may be seen (Fig. 10.6).

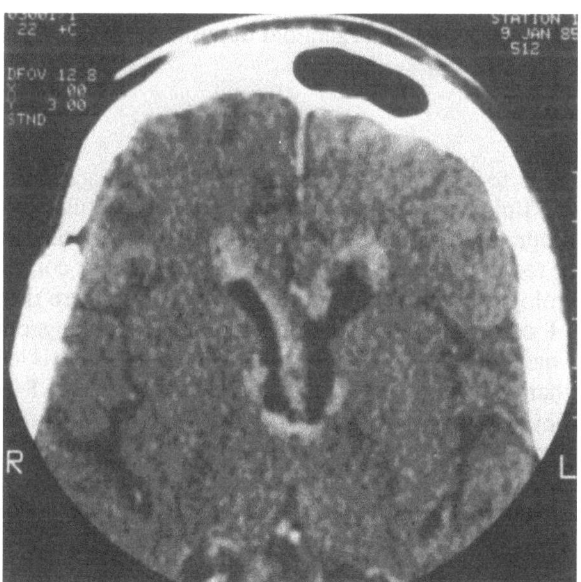

Fig. 10.5. CT scan (enhanced) demonstrating periventricular tumour infiltration by germinoma.

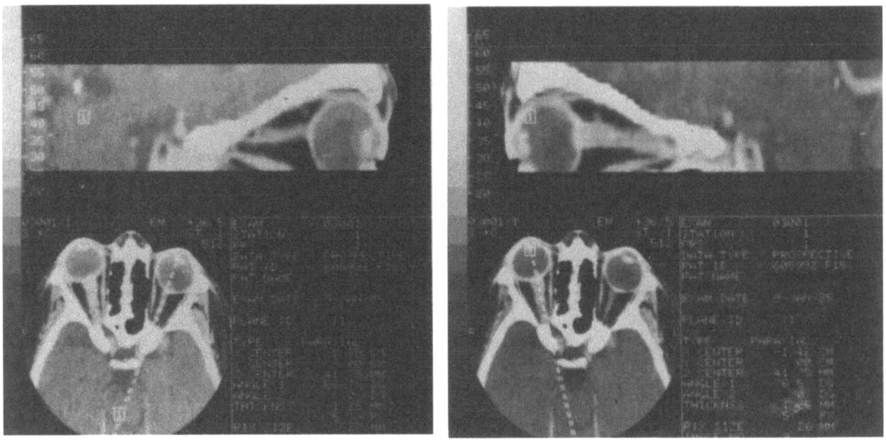

Fig. 10.6. CT scan demonstrating unilateral optic nerve infiltration by suprasellar germinoma.

Once treatment is undertaken CT scanning has an absolutely essential role in monitoring the effects of radiotherapy and chemotherapy. Germinoma and pineoblastoma are both extremely sensitive and it is now standard practice to plan to repeat the CT scan after a cumulative tumour dose of 15–20 Gy of fractionated irradiation as a so-called therapeutic test. The evidence of radiation response is then used to determine the policy of subsequent treatment, *qua* the need for craniospinal irradiation for tumours of high metastatic potential. Finally, of course, standard methods of neuroradiology may be required to recognise metastatic spread, particularly the use of myelography (Fig. 10.7) for subarachnoid deposits.

Cytology

The relationship of these tumours to the third ventricular CSF would suggest that cytological examination of the fluid for neoplastic cells could be useful in the diagnosis of the primary tumour, and of relapse and metastasis. However, the interpretation of CSF cytology requires great care. CSF has been found to contain malignant cells in cases of histologically proven germinoma as well as where there has been no histological proof of the primary tumour (Chapman and Linggood 1980, Pomerade et al. 1982, Amendola et al. 1984). In a large Japanese study Ueki and Tanaka (1980) suggested that epithelioid cells may be found in the CSF of 84% of patients with germinoma; they also suggested that ventricular fluid is more useful (17 out of 20 positive) than spinal fluid (11 out of 20 positive) for this examination. On the other hand Packer et al. (1984) found both ventricular and lumbar CSF to be free from malignant cells, on examination at diagnosis, in six cases of embryonal carcinoma. Chapman and Linggood (1980) obtained negative results from CSF cytology in patients where the histology showed a propensity for CSF spread; and Sung et al. (1978) reported 12 patients with spinal subarachnoid deposits in only three of whom the results of CSF cytology were positive.

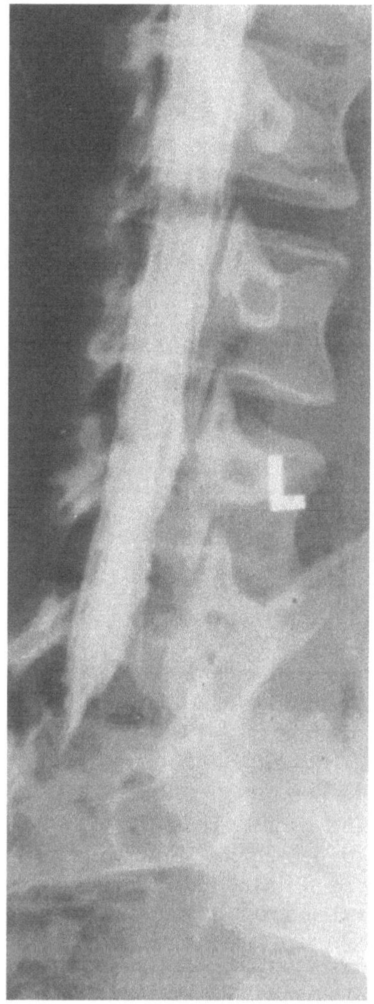

Fig. 10.7. Myelogram demonstrating "drop metastases" from pineocytoma.

The problems of CSF cytology are heightened by the diagnostic difficulties facing even the most experienced cytologist. They are demonstrated by the results from St Bartholomew's Hospital shown in Table 10.3. The CSF was examined at presentation in 11 cases, in six from lumbar fluid and in six from ventricular fluid. Of the lumbar fluid samples, two were reported as "suspicious" and one "possibly positive" (one germinoma, one ependymoma, and one case without histology); from ventricular fluid there was only one "probably positive" report and this from a patient with a negative therapeutic radiation test. Thus four cases out of 11 probably had detectable malignant cells in the CSF at presentation, but the type of cell could not be characterised in any. Whilst the same limitations apply when CSF is examined in relapsed patients (Table 10.3) a positive result can be unequivocal, as in a case of obviously malignant blasts from a relapsed patient with pineoblastoma (Fig. 10.2b).

Table 10.3. Diagnostic CSF cytology

Diagnosis	CSF cytology
Choriocarcinoma	– ve
Germinoma	Suspicious
Germinoma	– ve
+ ve therapeutic test (CSF βHCG = 60)	Probably – ve
– ve therapeutic test	– ve
– ve therapeutic test	Probably + ve
None	– ve
None	– ve
None	– ve
None	Suspicious
Ependymoma	Possibly + ve
Relapsed patients	
Pineocytoma	+ ve
Lymphoma	+ ve
Germinoma	– ve

Total 14 patients.

Tumour Markers

Examination of the CSF, blood and urine for biochemical markers has been found useful in the diagnosis of patients with histologically verified intracranial germ cell tumours (Nørgaard-Pedersen et al. 1978, Takeuchi et al. 1979, Allen et al. 1979, Pomerade et al. 1982, Wass et al. 1982, Packer et al. 1984).

The markers of interest in these tumours are comparable with those found in testicular tumours. Raised levels of alphafetoprotein (αFP) are associated with yolk sac elements. βHCG production is associated with choriocarcinoma and sometimes with germinoma. Embryonal cell carcinoma is associated with the production of both of these markers. The majority of studies on marker-secreting tumours show tumour product concentration gradients falling between the CSF and the blood (Nørgaard-Pedersen et al. 1978, Takeuchi et al. 1979, Allen et al. 1979, Wass et al. 1982, Packer et al. 1984), implying a high likelihood of contact by these tumours directly with the CSF. There are, however, exceptions where the gradient, as in one of our cases, may be reversed (Allen et al. 1979). It has also been suggested that the CSF to plasma gradient may be most apparent when lumbar rather than ventricular CSF is examined (Allen et al. 1979).

There are a number of reports documenting the use of markers to measure the response to treatment of intracranial germ cell tumours (Romshe and Sotos 1975, Nørgaard-Pedersen et al. 1978, Allen et al. 1979, Takeuchi et al. 1979, Kawakami et al. 1980, Wass et al. 1982) and in detecting recurrence, confirming the view that when tumours do produce markers they may be of great value in monitoring progress (Fig. 10.8). However, caution must be exercised. De Vere White et al. (1981) have questioned the accuracy of existing markers in testicular tumours, noting a false negative rate of 20%. Death may occur of patients with intracranial marker-producing tumours despite decreasing marker levels and with histological confirmation of tumour present at post-mortem (Takeuchi et al. 1979).

Our own experience with biochemical markers in these tumours is shown in Table 10.4. In 11 patients at diagnosis only three yielded positive markers. One patient with choriocarcinoma had a high CSF to plasma bHCG gradient. One with

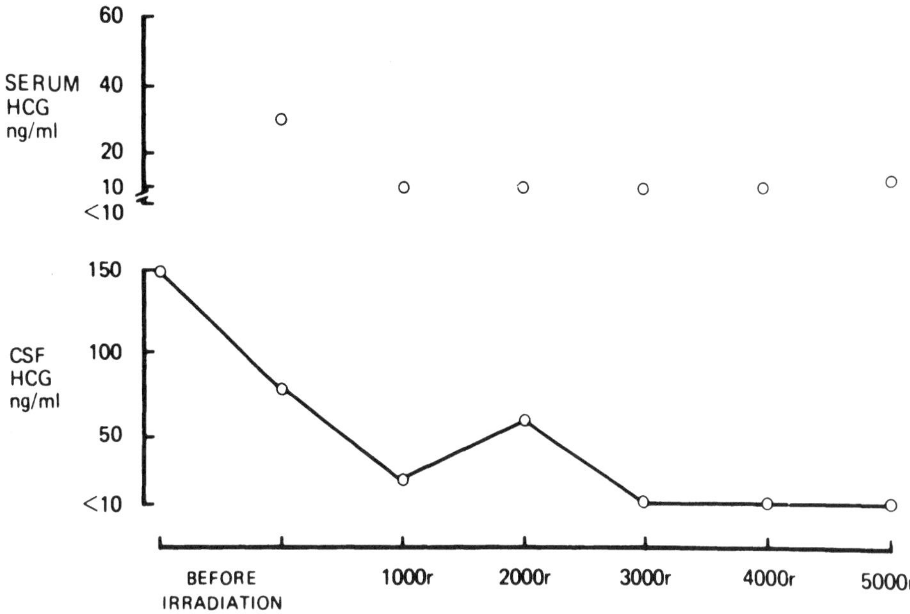

Fig. 10.8. Serial serum and CSF values of βHCG during cranial irradiation of pineal choriocarcinoma.

malignant teratoma also had a high CSF bHCG but unexpectedly the CSF to plasma gradient was reversed and no extracranial tumour was demonstrable. A third patient, with a positive therapeutic test, had a slightly elevated CSF bHCG level. In eight other patients no CSF markers could be demonstrated.

Other markers have been investigated in pineal tumours, but when new markers are being considered their specificity requires careful evaluation (Kaye and Bagshawe 1979). A tentative suggestion for melatonin as a pineal tumour marker was put forward (Wurtman and Moskawitz 1977, Barber et al. 1978) and the physiological basis for this has been reviewed by Wurtman and Moskawitz (1977). In fact

Table 10.4. Diagnostic marker studies in pineal tumours

Diagnosis	Blood		CSF	
	αFP (u/ml)	βHCG (iu/l)	αFP (u/ml)	βHCG (iu/l)
Germinoma	ND	– ve	ND	ND
Germinoma	– ve	– ve	ND	ND
Germinoma	– ve	– ve	ND	– ve
+ ve therapeutic test	ND	– ve	ND	– ve
+ ve therapeutic test	– ve	– ve	– ve	low + ve 60
Malignant teratoma	low + ve 61	+ ve 1029.0	– ve	+ ve 170.5
– ve therapeutic test	– ve	ND	ND	ND
– ve therapeutic test	– ve	– ve	ND	ND
Choriocarcinoma	– ve	+ ve up to 2587	– ve	+ ve up to 8800
Pineocytoma	ND	– ve	ND	ND
No tissue diagnosis	ND	– ve	ND	ND
Total no. of patients: 11	7	10	3	5

αFP, alphafetoprotein. ND, not determined.

Neuwelt and Lewy (1983) recorded the disappearance of plasma melatonin in one patient after removal of a neoplastic pineal gland. Currently studies are being done using placental alkaline phosphatase and immunoperoxidase-labelled antibodies in these tumours (T. Oliver pers. comm. 1985).

Tissue Diagnosis

Clearly with such a heterogeneous group of tumours a tissue diagnosis is desirable for planning management. For tumours at the anterior end of the third ventricle this has usually been available at craniotomy for decompression of the optic chiasm, but the situation at the posterior end of the ventricle has been very different. The mortality and morbidity of surgery in the pineal region was such that, in most historical series until the 1970s, initial histology was not available (Schmidek 1977). Even biopsy was hazardous because of the danger of damage to the veins and in any case 80% of the tumours would be malignant and dealt with by irradiation.

However, two major advances have occurred in the last decade to enable tissue diagnosis to be available in an increasing proportion of cases. In neurosurgery, brain retraction became much safer, particularly in children, as the result of developments in anaesthesia, corticosteroid control of oedema and the advent of microsurgery. Hoffman et al. (1983) showed that over a period of 30 years there was a reduction in the mortality from 66.7% to 4.3% at the Sick Children's Hospital in Toronto. The other important development has been in stereotactic biopsy based on CT scanning. While the main tumour types may be readily recognised, the problem of sampling error does occur (for instance teratoid elements may be missed) and more than one area may need to be sampled. From one or other of these methods a tissue diagnosis will increasingly be available in future, especially in young patients.

Management

Surgery

Since 70% of pineal and pineal-related tumours are radiosensitive surgical intervention was for decades reserved for those which had not responded to X-irradiation and a shunting procedure, as the surgical mortality was daunting. However, the recent advances in anaesthesia, and in the use of CSF diversion and glucocorticosteroids, together with the development of the operating microscope, have reduced the operative mortality associated with partial or total excision from 25%–70% to less than 5% (Schmidek 1977, Chapman and Linggood 1980, Wood et al. 1981, Sano 1983, Jooma and Kendall 1983, Packer et al. 1984, Rout et al. 1984). The value of stereotactic biopsy was stressed by Conway (1973) and by Schmidek (1977), who advocated irradiation or excision depending on the probable radiosensitivity of the tumour. Stereotactic biopsy is now being used with increasing frequency.

The swing in neurosurgical thought in certain major centres is reflected by two reports from the Massachusetts General Hospital (MGH) in Boston. In 1973 de Girolami and Schmidek, reviewing 53 patients treated there from 1920 to 1972, wrote "we believe that the risks of radiation damage to the brain are negligible compared with the hazards of subjecting all patients with posterior third ventricular tumour to immediate direct surgical intervention". However, Chapman and Linggood, who studied 22 cases treated from 1972 to 1977 at MGH (eight of whom had had direct operation), concluded in 1980 that neither radiation response nor CSF cytology were sufficient to determine optimal treatment. They found that direct operation, which was free from mortality or serious morbidity, was most useful in characterising these tumours for treatment.

There are several important questions relating to surgery for pineal tumours. These include the incidence of mortality and morbidity; the proportion of explored tumours found to be benign; the possibility that surgery may increase the dissemination of malignant tumours by the CSF; and the proportion of primarily irradiated tumours which prove to be radioresistant or which (like choriocarcinoma or mixed germinoma) may recur afterwards and require other measures.

Jooma and Kendall (1983) reported on 27 patients (mainly children and adolescents) from the National Hospital, Queen Square, and Hospital for Sick Children, Great Ormond Street, London, on whom surgery had been performed. There was no operative mortality, minimal morbidity, and no increase in subarachnoid seeding rate. The surgical results *qua* tumour cannot be assessed since most patients were referred for post-operative irradiation.

The question of the frequency with which tumours are revealed by operation is difficult to answer because of case selection. Lazar and Clark (1974) reported 50% (3/6); and the 2.4% incidence of Sano's series of 125 cases clearly reflects inversely the high incidence of germinoma in Japan. Rout et al. (1984) recently reviewed the evidence from collected series totalling 164 cases of surgical exploration and found the average incidence of benign lesions to be 15% (25/164). This incidence must, however, depend on the degree of investigation and the treatment policy of the individual centre.

The largest series of cases of pineal tumour verified histologically at surgery comes from Sano's clinic in Japan, where radiotherapy is the standard treatment for germinoma and surgical patients have post-operative irradiation. In the 42 cases there was no operative mortality. The 10-year survival was 74.9% for 32 pineal cases and 100% for 13 suprasellar cases, a difference which Sano himself relates to the greater operative reduction in tumour bulk in the suprasellar region before radiotherapy. From this experience the management policy which has been evolved in Japan hinges on tumour size. If less than 2 cm diameter, the tumour is irradiated to 20 Gy. If it disappears on CT scan, radiotherapy is continued; if not, direct surgery is performed. Larger tumours are surgically explored with a view to excision and post-operative irradiation.

The question of whether aggressive surgical techniques may result in higher spinal seeding rates has been raised on several occasions. In the US Children's Cancer Study Group (CCSG) series 14% (5/36) of the biopsy-proven germinomas had spinal metastases compared with 1.7% (1/59) of the unbiopsied group. While, *a priori*, piecemeal removal of these anaplastic and friable tumours would seem likely to promote metastasis, microsurgery may mitigate this risk, for in Sano's large series of 54 cases the incidence of metastasis was only 3.7% (2/54). It will certainly be difficult to prove this point now that patients with tumours of high metastasising potential are increasingly having whole neuraxis irradiation (see below).

Many neurosurgical centres at present do, however, adhere to the more conservative policy for posterior third ventricular tumours of relief of hydrocephalus by shunting together with radiotherapy as the mainstay of treatment. They only embark on direct surgical intervention if this is demanded by symptoms of persisting or recurrent disease. Torkildsen's operation (1939) of venticulocisternostomy has of course given way to ventriculo-atrial or ventriculo-peritoneal shunting, but it must be remembered that in this group of highly malignant tumours extracranial metastases have, if rarely, followed such procedures.

Disseminated haematogenous metastases have been described in germinoma (Howman-Giles et al. 1984). Three cases of abdominal metastasis of primary intracranial yolk sac tumour through a ventriculo-peritoneal shunt were reported by Wilson et al. (1979). This mode of spread occurred in one out of 15 cases documented by Salazar et al. (1979) and in one out of eight cases noted by Neuwelt et al. (1979), but in none of our six patients with ventriculo-peritoneal shunts has this been observed to date. Nevertheless, these results do argue the case for the need to use Millipore filters to minimise the risk of this bizarre mode of spread.

Radiotherapy

The high radiosensitivity of pineal and suprasellar germinomas is well known, as well as the more limited responsiveness of malignant teratoma. There is still difficulty, though, in establishing the normal parameters of radiotherapy because of both the rarity of the tumours and the lack of histological data in a considerable proportion of most series. The essential considerations are the level of radiation dosage required for a high probability of local cure, and the volume to be irradiated as determined by the propensity for spread in and around the ventricles and in the subarachnoid space.

Abay et al. (1981) at the Mayo Clinic analysed data from their 27 cases, treated with doses in the range of about 35–50 Gy, and found greater local control with increasing dose; there was 87.5% control after doses of 50 Gy or more. In the important study from the Columbia-Presbyterian Medical Centre in New York, Sung et al. (1978) reviewed 61 patients with midline pineal tumours and 16 with suprasellar tumours: of patients given 38–45 Gy to the primary site in 4–5 weeks 47% had local recurrence of tumour, while in only 10% of those given 50–55 Gy in 5–6 weeks did tumour recur. Although these doses were high, complications involving the hypothalamic-pituitary axis after 50–55 Gy were less of a threat than was treatment failure from inadequate dosage. The survival rate was 79% for midline pineal tumours and 77% for suprasellar germinomas, and there were no long-term complications. Obviously these dosages are much higher than those required to control the common extracranial germinoma (that is, seminoma) and the paradox is the greater when we consider the relatively small tumour mass in the pineal region. Almost certainly it is to be explained by the heterogeneity of tumour types which are radioresponsive and by the incidence of mixed forms of germinoma.

Estimates of the probable incidence of CSF dissemination, the main factor determining the volume to be irradiated, have varied greatly, ranging from less than 2% to as high as 33%. The evidence assembled from various collected series totalling 576 cases has been well set out by Bloom (1983), who found the overall incidence of spinal seeding to be 12%.

In the Columbia-Presbyterian series Sung et al. (1978) found that 10% of the midline pineal tumours and 37% of suprasellar germinomas had metastasised to the ventricular or spinal suparachnoid space within 6 months to 5 years. Consequently they advocated entire neuraxis irradiation for locally extensive tumours, for simultaneous pineal and hypothalamic lesions and for all biopsy-proven germinomas. A different view was taken in the report from the US CCSG (Wara et al. 1979) who reviewed 118 patients treated at CCSG institutions from 1960 to 1975. An incidence of spinal metastasis of 8% was found, which in their view did not warrant routine prophylactic irradiation in a growing child.

While most of the discussion has centred on germinoma it must be remembered that, of the true pineal tumours, it is not only pineoblastoma which behaves like medulloblastoma and is to be treated similarly. Pineocytoma also has a propensity for dissemination and unless very well differentiated (neuronal or astrocytic) needs to be considered with the germinoma group and pineoblastoma in planning treatment.

We consider that spinal irradiation as part of whole cerebrospinal axis treatment is usually indicated in all cases of biopsy-proven germinomas, pineocytoma/pineoblastoma or high-grade ependymoma; in those with a positive therapeutic radiation test; and in those with positive fluid markers for βHCG or alphafetoprotein. It should be remembered that in this latter group the irradiation may need to be phased with chemotherapy. While it would be ideal to be able to avoid irradiation of the spine in growing children, to postpone such irradiation until metastases become evident is a policy almost certainly doomed to failure for those unfortunate enough to develop late deposits.

Technique. The technique advocated by us for tumours of high metastatic potential is therefore whole-brain irradiation to a dosage (in adults) of 35 Gy in 20 fractions in 28 days, followed by local third ventricular irradiation using a three-field planned technique to an additional 15–20 Gy in 15 fractions in 21 days. The spinal axis is irradiated to 35 Gy in 23 fractions in 32 days, starting after 17 days of the whole-brain irradiation. A dose reduction is appropriate in young children. A high standard of precision is required, with plastic shell immobilisation in the prone position and great care in the apposition of junctions. Progress is monitored by repeat CT scans and examination of blood and CSF for tumour markers.

For tumours of indefinite nature we plan the irradiation by the reverse procedure. We treat an initial target volume which generously encompasses the third ventricle by a three-field technique and repeat the CT scan after a total dose of 20 Gy at the rate of 1.8 Gy per day. If by this therapeutic test the tumour is shown to be markedly responsive, the treatment is modified to become part of a full craniospinal regime (as above). If not, the local irradiation is continued to a dose of 50–55 Gy in a total of 42 days.

Chemotherapy

Drugs such as methotrexate, etoposide and cis-platinum which penetrate the blood–brain barrier, particularly when it has been disturbed, may be therapeutically useful. There have also been recent observations in patients with brain metastases from choriocarcinoma which suggest that chemotherapy can influence prognosis. Athanassiou et al. (1983) described 33 patients presenting with untreated choriocarcinoma and brain metastases who were managed by chemotherapy without cranial radiotherapy. These workers observed many responses to chemotherapy and had 16 survivors at 14–261 months (mean 111 months) from diagnosis. The chemotherapy regimes were not the same for all patients but high-dose systemic methotrexate (often alternating with intrathecal methotrexate) was common and etoposide and cis-platinum were included in the chemotherapy regimens latterly. A similar situation has been observed with regard to cerebral metastases from malignant germ cell tumours, notably those arising in the testis (E. S. Newlands 1985, pers. comm. 1985, T. Oliver pers. comm. 1985).

As the blood-brain barrier is regarded as deficient in the region of the pineal gland (the commonest site for CNS germ cell tumours) there is a good rationale for employing chemotherapy in assessable high-risk patients. Some authors have already concluded that it is effective (Siegal et al. 1983, Chan et al. 1984). It would be predicted that the immature germ cell lineage, including βHCG-secreting growths, would be most likely to respond.

In collaboration with Dr T. Oliver we have recently treated two patients with CNS recurrences after radiotherapy to primary brain germ cell tumours (one third ventricular germinoma, one fourth ventricular teratoma). Both have responded well to germ cell chemotherapy (bleomycin, VP-16, cis-platinum). We have also similarly treated a young male with a CNS recurrence after radiotherapy to a pineocytoma and not seen a worthwhile response. It may well be that chemotherapy, adjuvant to radiotherapy, has a role in brain germ cell tumours.

With regard to pineoblastomas, the morphological and surface marker homology with retinoblastoma and neuroblastoma have prompted us to pilot neuroblastoma chemotherapy. Although we have seen a partial response of a primary neuroectodermal brain tumour to such chemotherapy (cis-platinum, VP-16, cyclophosphamide and vincrisitine), we have not yet had the opportunity to pilot this regimen for pineoblastoma.

Results of Treatment

The surgical procedures employed in the 25 patients with third ventricular tumours referred to the Department of Radiotherapy at St Bartholomew's Hospital in the period 1962 to 1984 are shown in Table 10.5. The great majority had a shunt fashioned to relieve raised intracranial pressure, but three had biopsies and two had

Table 10.5. Surgical procedures in 25 patients with third ventricular tumours (pineal and ectopic) 1962–1984

	Initial surgery	Surgery at relapse/progression
Excisional surgery	2	3
Biopsy	3	1
Shunt	20	1

Table 10.6. Radiotherapy target volume in 25 patients 1962–1984; megavoltage X-ray therapy (4, 6, 8, 15, MV X-rays or ^{60}Co)

Local third ventricular target volume	15
Local third ventricular + whole brain	4
Local third ventricular + craniospinal	6

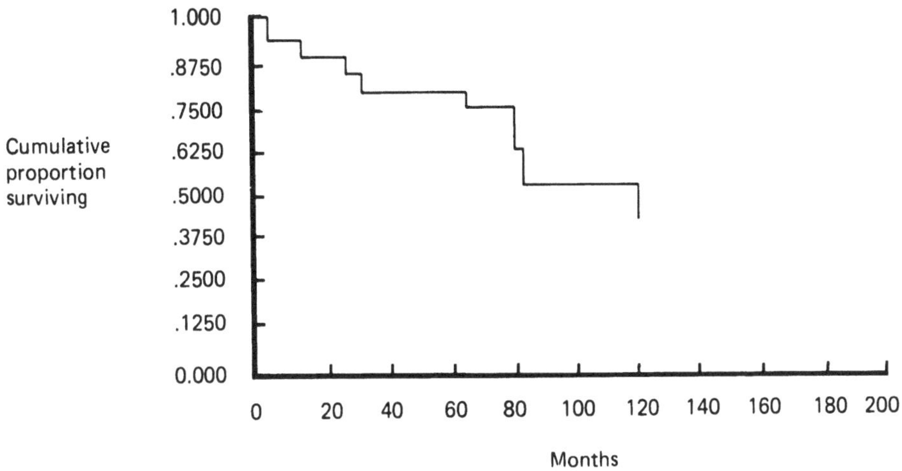

Fig. 10.9. Survival curve of 23 cases of pineal and third ventricular tumours presenting to the radiotherapy department of St Bartholomew's Hospital between 1962 and 1984.

excisional surgery as part of their initial management. Radiotherapy (Table 10.6) to the local third ventricular target volume was used in 15 patients, local third ventricular and whole-brain treatment was given to four, and whole-neuraxis irradiation to six patients. The results of these treatments in the 23 patients who have been followed up, indicate a median survival time of 120 months, with the 5-year survival being close to 80% (Fig. 10.9). These results are comparable to those reported in a large compilation of 478 patients with pineal region tumours and suprasellar germinomas, where the 5-year survival rate generally ranged between 50% and 75% (Bloom 1983).

Conclusions

For advance in the management of these rare tumours, the maximum of information is clearly desirable in each individual case. At the present time CT scanning, while excellent for delineation, is inadequate for tumour characterisation. Current biochemical markers when demonstrable in CSF or blood are most valuable in indicating a germinomatous lineage, but within this group they are insufficiently specific to separate completely the anaplastic teratomatous variants.

Most retrospective studies of pineal region tumours treated by by-pass and X-irradiation are to unknown degrees heterogeneous. With the increasing availablility of stereotactic biopsy, and its low morbidity in experienced hands, a definite tissue diagnosis should in future be the basis for management.

For the majority of such tumours radiotherapy which is based on adequate histological, imaging and marker studies remains the treatment of choice. Alone it is often inadequate in the anaplastic and teratomatous variants, where the role of pre- and post-irradiational surgery and the use of chemotherapy are currently being further explored.

It is a pleasure to express out thanks to our colleagues at St Bartholomew's Hospital for their collaboration, especially Dr M. Charlesworth (Department of Neurobiology), Dr G. Canti (Department of Cytology), Dr A. Stansfeld (Department of Histopathology), Professor T. Chard (Department of Reproductive Physiology), Dr T. Oliver (Department of Medical Oncology) and Professor G. M. Besser and Dr J. A. Wass (Department of Endrocrinology). We would also like to thank Miss Jenny Seems for her help in preparation of the manuscript.

References

Abay EO II, Laws ER, Grado GL, Bruckman JE, Forbes GS, Gomez MR, Scott M (1981) Pineal tumours in children and adolescents: Treatment by CSF shunting and radiotherapy. J Neurosurg 55: 889-895
Allen JC, Nisselbaum J, Epstein F, Rosen G, Schwartz MK (1979) Alphafetoprotein and human chorionic gonadotropin determination in cerebro-spinal fluid. J Neurosurg 51: 368-374
Amendola BE, McClatchey K, Amendola MA (1984) Pineal region tumours: Analysis of treatment results. Int J Radiat Oncol Biol Phys 10: 991-997
Athanassiou A, Begent RHJ, Newlands ES, Parker D, Rustin GJS, Bagshawe KD (1983) Central nervous system metastases of choriocarcinoma. Cancer 52: 1728-1735
Axelrod L (1977) Endocrine dysfunction in patients with tumours of the pineal region. In: Schmidek HH (ed) Pineal tumours. Masson Publishing USA, New York, ch 3
Bader JL, Miller RW, Meadows AT, Zimmerman LE, Champion LAA, Voute PA (1980) Trilateral retinoblastoma. Lancet II: 582-583
Barber SG, Smith JA, Cove DH, Smith SCH, London DR (1978) Marker for pineal tumours? Lancet II: 372-373
Becker LE, Hinton D (1983) Primitive neuroectodermal tumours of the central nervous system. Hum Pathol 14: 538-550
Bloom HJG (1983) Primary intracranial germ cell tumours. In: Bagshaw KD, Newlands ES, Begent RHJ (eds) Clinics in oncology: Germ cell tumours. WB Saunders, London, Philadelphia, Toronto, pp 233-257
Borit A (1981) History of tumours of the pineal region. Am J Surg Pathol 5: 613-620
Chan HSL, Humphreys RP, Hendrick EB, Chuang SH, Fitz CR, Becker LE (1984) Primary intracranial choriocarcinoma: A report of two cases and a review of the literature. Neurosurgery 15: 540-545
Chapman PH, Linggood RM (1980) The management of pineal area tumours: A recent reappraisal. Cancer 46: 1253-1257
Conway LW (1973) Stereotaxic diagnosis and treatment of intracranial tumours including an initial experience with cryosurgery for pinealomas. J Neurosurg 38: 453-460
Dupont MG, Gerard JM, Flament-Durand J, Baleriaux-Waha D, Mortelmans LL (1977) Pathognomic aspects of germinoma on CT scan. Neuroradiology 14: 209-211
Futrell NN, Osborn AG, Cheson BD (1981) Pineal region tumours: Computed tomographic-pathologic spectrum. Am J Radiol 137: 951-956
Girolami U De, Schmidek H (1973) Clinicopathological study of 53 tumours of the pineal region. J Neurosurg 39: 455-462
Grossman GB, Gonzalez CF (1977) Neuroradiology in the pineal region. In: Schmidek HH (ed) Pineal tumours. Masson Publishing USA, New York, pp 79-98
Hoffman HJ, Yoshida M, Becker LE, Hendrick EB, Humphreys RP (1983) In: Brihaye J et al. (eds) Abstract of 7th European Congress of Neurosurgery, Brussels, p 172
Howman-Giles R, Besser M, Johnston IH, Da Silva M (1984) Disseminated haematogenous metastases from a pineal germinoma in an infant. J Neurosurg 60: 835-837
Inoue Y, Takeuchi T, Tamaki M, Nin K, Hukuba A, Nishimura S (1979) Sequential CT observations of irradiated intracranial germinomas. Am J Radiol 132: 361-365
Jooma R, Kendall BE (1983) Diagnosis and management of pineal tumours. J Neurosurg 58: 654-665
Kawakami Y, Yamada O, Tabuchi K, Ohmoto T, Nishimoto A (1980) Primary intracranial choriocarcinoma. J Neurosurg 53: 369-374
Kaye SB, Bagshawe KD (1979) Clinical markers in spinal fluids for tumours of the central nervous system (CNS). In: Whitehouse JMA, Kay HEM (eds) CNS complications of malignant disease. Macmillan Press, New York, ch. 29
Kingston JE, Plowman PN, Hungerford JL, Bedford MA (1985) Management and prognosis of children

with ectopic intracranial retinoblastoma. Br J Ophthalmol (in press)
Lazar ML, Clark K (1974) Direct surgical management of masses in the region of the vein of Galen. Surg Neurol 2: 17-21
Messina AV, Potts G, Sigel RM, Liebeskind AL (1976) Computed tomography: Evaluation of the posterior third ventricle. Radiology 119: 581-592
Neuwelt EA, Lewy AJ (1983) Disappearance of plasma melatonin after removal of a neoplastic pineal gland. N Engl J Med 308: 1132-1135
Neuwelt EA, Glasberg M, Frenkel EP, Clark WK (1979) Malignant pineal region tumours: A clinico-pathological study. J Neurosurg 51: 597-607
Nørgaard-Pedersen B, Albrechtsen R, Arends J, Lindholm J, Sandberg E (1978) Two cases of primary intracranial germ cell tumours with elevated levels of alpha-fetoprotein and human chorionic gonadotrophin. Scand J Immunol 8: 1-4
Packer RJ, Sutton LN, Rorke LB, Rosenstock JG, Zimmerman RA, Littman P, Bilaniuk LT, Bruce DA, Schut L (1984) Intracranial embryonal cell carcinoma. Cancer 54: 520-524
Pomerade R, Czernichow P, Finidor J, Pfister A, Roger M, Kalifa C, Zucker JM, Pierre-Kahn A, Rappaport R (1982) Endocrine aspects and tumoral markers in intracranial germinoma: An attempt to delineate the diagnostic procedure in 14 patients. J Pediatr 101: 374-378
Romshe CA, Sotos JF (1975) Intracranial human chorionic gonadotropin secreting tumour with precocious puberty. J Pediatr 86: 250-252
Rout D, Sharma A, Radhakrishnan W, Rao VRK (1984) Exploration of the pineal region: Observations and results. Surg Neurol 21: 135-140
Rubin P, Kramer S (1965) Ectopic pinealoma: A radiocurable neuroendocrinologic entity. Radiology 85: 512-523
Rubinstein LJ (1981) Cytogenesis and differentiation of pineal neoplasms. Hum Pathol 12: 441-448
Salazar OM, Castro-Vita H, Bakos RS, Feldstein ML, Keller B, Rubin P (1979) Radiation therapy for tumours of the pineal region. Int J Radiat Oncol Biol Phys 5: 491-499
Sano K (1983) Pineal region tumours: Problems in pathology and treatment. Clin Neurosurg 30: 59-91
Schmidek HH (1977) Pineal tumours. Masson Publishing USA, New York
Siegal T, Pfeffer R, Catane R, Sulkes A, Gomori MJ, Fuks Z (1983) Successful chemotherapy of recurrent intracranial germinoma with spinal metastases. Neurology 33: 631-633
Sklar CA, Grumbach MM, Kaplan SL, Conte FA (1981) Hormonal and metabolic abnormalities associated with central nervous system germinoma in children and adolescents and the effect of therapy: Report of ten patients. J Clin Endocrinol Metab 52: 9-16
Sung D II, Harisiadis L, Chang CH (1978) Midline pineal tumours and suprasellar germinomas: Highly curable by irradiation. Radiology 128: 745-751
Takeuchi J, Handa H, Oda Y, Uchida Y (1979) Alpha-fetoprotein in intracranial malignant teratoma. Surg Neurol 12: 400-404
Torkildsen A (1939) A new palliative operation in cases of inoperable occlusion of Sylvian aqueduct. Acta Chir Scand 82: 117-123
Ueki K, Tanaka R (1980) Treatment and prognosis of pineal tumours: Experience of 110 cases. Neurol Med Chir (Tokyo) 20: 1-26
Wara WW, Jenkin DT, Evans A, Ertel I, Hittle R, Ortega J, Wilson CB, Hammond D (1979) Tumours of the pineal and suprasellar region: Children's cancer study group treatment results 1960-1975. Cancer 43: 698-701
Wass JAH, Jones AE, Rees LH, Besser GM (1982) hCGβ producing pineal choriocarcinoma. Clin Endocrinol 17: 423-431
White R de Vere, Karian S, Hong WK, Olsson CA (1981) Testis tumour markers: How accurate are they? J Urol 125: 661-663
Whittle IR, Allsop JL, Besser M (1983) Tuberculoma mimicking a pinealoma. J Neurosurg 59: 875-878
Wilson ER, Takei Y, Bikoff WT, O'Brien MS, Tindall GT, Boehm WM (1979) Abdominal metastases of primary intracranial yolk sac tumours through ventriculo-peritoneal shunts: Report of three cases. Neurosurg 5: 356-364
Wood JH, Zimmerman RA, Bruce DA, Bilaniuk LT, Norris DG, Schut L (1981) Assessment and management of pineal-region and related tumours. Neurology 16: 192-210
Wray SH (1977) The neuro-ophthalmic and neurologic manifestations of pinealomas. In: Schmidek HH (ed) Pineal tumours. Masson Publishing USA, New York, Ch 2
Wray SH (1983) Case records of the Massachusetts General Hospital. Weekly clinicopathological exercises. Cases 35-1983. N Engl J Med 309: 542-549
Wurtman RJ, Moskawitz MA (1977) The pineal organ. N Engl J Med 296: 1329-1333, 1383-1386
Zimmerman RA, Bilaniuk LT, Wood JH, Bruce DA, Schut L (1980) Computed tomography of pineal, parapineal and histologically related tumours. Radiology 137: 669-677

11 The Pharmacology of Brain Tumour Chemotherapy

P. Workman

Introduction: The Importance of Drug Delivery

Factors affecting the response of brain tumours to chemotherapy may be divided conveniently into two categories: those concerned with cellular sensitivity on the one hand and those concerned with drug delivery on the other. Relatively little work has been done on the cellular response of human brain tumours. Factors influencing response at this level will include the intrinsic sensitivity of the target site at the molecular level; repair; cell cycle status; the existence within the tumour of gradients of hypoxia, pH, nutrients, metabolites, etc.; the occurrence of cellular heterogeneity; and the acquisition of resistance. There seems to have been no enthusiasm to search for molecular peculiarities of brain tumours which might allow the design of highly specific and selective chemotherapeutic agents. The drugs used most commonly are among those employed in the treatment of solid tumours in other sites.

Numerous studies have been carried out on the response to chemotherapy of established rodent brain tumour cell lines, both in vitro (e.g. Wheeler et al. 1975) and in vivo (e.g. Shapiro 1973). For example in the case of rat glioma 9L cells treated in vitro with the widely used nitrosourea BCNU, a 1 log cell kill can be brought about by a nominal 1 hour exposure to a concentration of about 6 μg/ml (Wheeler et al. 1975). Studies with human brain tumour lines have been accumulating. Response is determined by increase in life span of the recipient or growth delay for tumours grown as xenografts in imunosuppressed mice (Shapiro et al. 1979, Houchens et al. 1983) or by isotope uptake or clonogenic assay in vitro (M. L. Rosenblum et al. 1981, Darling and Thomas 1983, Bogdahn 1983). From biopsies of 10 human malignant gliomas disaggregated and treated in vitro with BCNU for

2 hours, M. L. Rosenblum et al. (1981) have demonstrated a wide heterogeneity of response, with 10 μg/ml producing up to a 2 log cell kill in some cases and no effect in others. In this and other reports good correlations with clinical response have been observed (see chapter by Thomas in this book).

Overall it seems that we have no reason to think that the spectrum of response of human brain tumours will necessarily differ from that of other tumour types. However, two lines of evidence suggest that drug delivery to brain tumours may be a particular problem (Greig 1984). Firstly, there is the fact that human tumours metastatic to brain are often insensitive to agents to which the same tumours may respond in other sites. Secondly, these agents may likewise be effective against experimental rodent tumours and human xenografts grown extracranially but ineffective against these tumours growing in the brain.

Local factors influencing drug delivery from capillaries to cells within solid tumours are summarised in Table 11.1 (Levin et al. 1981). An adequate blood flow is required to deliver the drug to the tumour capillaries. The surface area of the tumour capillaries and their permeability to the drug together control the rate of passage from capillary lumen to the extracellular tissue space. Intracellular drug concentrations are dependent upon the permeability of the tumour cell membrane and the cellular/extracellular distribution ratio. The stability of the drug, both extracellularly (possibly dependent on chemical breakdown) and intracellularly (perhaps controlled by metabolism), is critical for its delivery to the target site within the cell. Finally, the drug may have to traverse several hundred micrometres, or even some millimetres, to reach the cells most distant from capillaries, and the drug diffusion coefficient may be a controlling factor.

Table 11.1. Local factors controlling drug delivery to solid tumours. Reproduced from Levin et al. (1981) with permission

1.	Blood flow
2.	Capillary surface area and permeability
3.	Cellular permeability
4.	Cellular/extracellular drug ratio
5.	Extracellular drug half-life
6.	Intracellular drug half-life

The Blood–Brain Barrier

As far as the entry of drugs is concerned the major difference between most areas of the brain and almost all other sites in the body is the presence of the blood–brain barrier (BBB). This has been reviewed in great detail by Rapaport (1976) and Bradbury (1979). Although somewhat controversial in the past, overwhelming functional and morphological evidence now implicates the cerebral capillary endothelial cells as the site of the barrier. Unlike most other capillaries these have tight intercellular junctions, devoid of fenestrae, which form continuous belts around the cells. This restricts passage of material between the endothelial cells. Since the capillary endothelial cells do not show pinocytosis and have no known transport capacity for anticancer agents, the uptake of these drugs into the brain extracellular space must occur by simple passive diffusion. The rate of uptake is proportional to the concentration gradient and it is dependent on the physicochemical properties of the drug molecule summarised in Table 11.2.

Table 11.2. Physicochemical properties of drugs affecting their uptake into the brain

1.	Partition coefficient (lipophilicity)
2.	Molecular weight (size)
3.	Fraction not-ionised (p*K*, pH)
4.	Plasma protein binding

Since the BBB is formed by the capillary endothelial cells with their tight junctions, its properties are those of a continuous cell membrane. To gain entry to the brain drugs must first dissolve in and then traverse the hydrophobic, lipid environment of the endothelial cell membrane. For most drugs of relatively low molecular weight ($\leqslant$400–500) the rate at which this process occurs is governed by the partition coefficient (*P*). This is usually measured between octanol as a model for the lipid compartment and water or buffer as a model for the aqueous compartment (Fig. 11.1).

A major factor responsible for partitioning behaviour is the ordered sheath of water molecules which surrounds lipophilic drugs in aqueous solution. This is removed on partitioning into a hydrophobic environment giving rise to a more disordered state which is favoured because of its lower energy. The lipophilicity of a molecule can be predicted by the number of hydrophilic and lipophilic substituents. Hydrophilic groups include hydroxyl, carboxyl, carbonyl, amine and amide groups. These undergo hydrophilic interactions, particularly hydrogen bond formation, and reduce the lipophilicity of the drug molecule. Lipophilic groups, e.g. alkyl groups and aromatic rings, participate in hydrophobic interactions and increase the lipophilicity of the drug molecule.

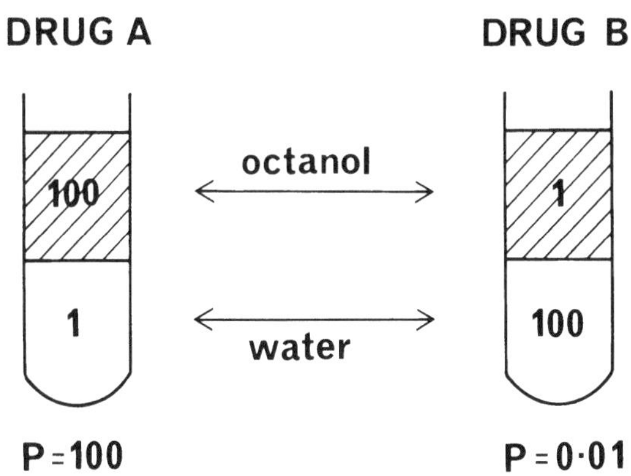

Fig. 11.1. Measurement of lipophilicity of a drug by the octanol/water partition coefficient (*P*), which is the ratio of its concentration in octanol to that in water or buffer. Drug A is very lipophilic with high affinity for lipid; drug B is hydrophilic with higher affinity for water. Reproduced from Workman (1982) with permission.

Molecular weight is also important for BBB penetration, with large, bulky molecules such as proteins being totally excluded. However, molecular weight also affects the rate of uptake of smaller molecules, with small drugs penetrating more rapidly than large ones.

The contribution of lipophilicity and molecular weight (MW) in determining drug permeability in the normal rat brain is illustrated very clearly by the data of Levin (1980) shown in Fig. 11.2. Details of the compounds studied are given in Table 11.3. With the exception of the circled values in the figure, there is an excellent relationship between capillary permeability and the expression $P(\mathrm{MW})^{-\frac{1}{2}}$. Let us consider first those agents of molecular weight $\leqslant 400$. Drugs with high permeability coefficients include BCNU (13), CCNU (15) and spirohydantoin mustard (21) and are all very lipophilic (Table 11.3). Those with intermediate permeability coefficients include procarbazine (14), the nitrosourea PCNU (17), 5-fluorouracil (6), dianhydrogalactitol (7), dibromodulcitol (20) and the radiosensitisers misonidazole (11) and metronidazole (8). These are of intermediate lipophilicity. The group with low permeability coefficients includes the methotrexate analogue Baker's antifol (23); such drugs are of low lipophilicity. Of the aberrant, circled compounds, water (1) exhibits such rapid uptake because of its very small size and, perhaps, the existence of small membrane "pores". Of more concern to us are the epipodophylotoxin VM 26 (25) and vincristine (26) which, despite their high lipophilicity, have very low permeability coefficients because of their large molecular weights (Table 11.3). Adriamycin (24) and bleomycin (27) have even lower permeability coefficients and are both large and hydrophilic. The latter four drugs are regarded as excluded from the normal brain.

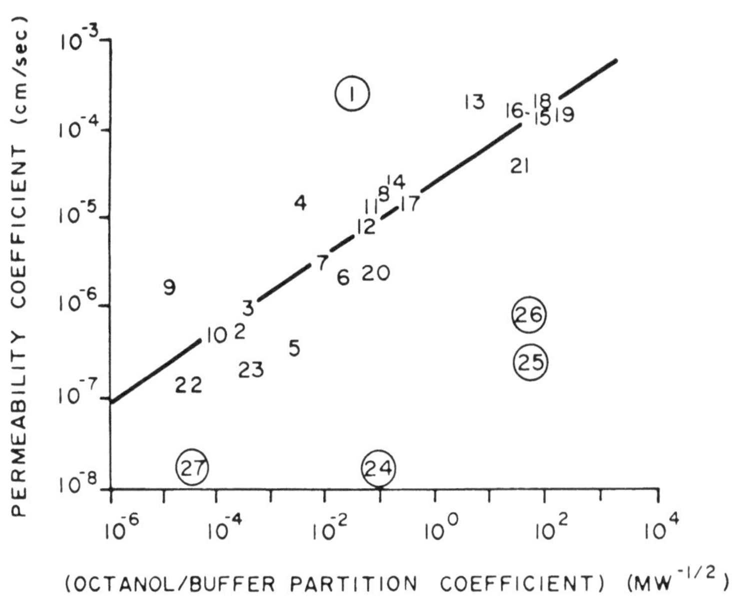

Fig. 11.2. Plot showing the effect of partition coefficient and molecular weight on the permeability of normal rat brain capillaries to various agents. Circled values were omitted from the best fit (continuous line). For identification of compounds see Table 11.3. Reproduced from Levin (1980) with permission.

Table 11.3. Molecular weight (MW), octanol/water partition coefficient (*P*) and rat brain capillary permeability coefficient (P_C). Reproduced with permission from Levin et al. (1980) with modification (V. A. Levin pers. comm.)

Number	Substance	MW	log *P*	*P*	($P_c \times 10^{-6}$(cm/s)
1	H_2O	18	−1.06	0.0871	200
2	Na^+	58	−3.40	0.000398	0.4
3	Urea	60	−1.66	0.0219	0.82
4	Glycerol	92	−1.75	0.0178	12
5	Creatinine	113	−1.77	0.0170	0.28
6	5-Fluorouracil	130	−0.95	0.112	1.7
7	Dianhydrogalactitol	146	−1.29	0.0513	2.5
8	Metronidazole	171	−0.16	0.691	14
9	Ascorbate	176	−4.04	0.0000912	1.3
10	Galactitol	182	−3.10	0.000794	0.39
11	Misonidazole	201	−0.37	0.427	10
12	Ftorafur	200	−0.48	0.331	6.4
13	BCNU	214	1.54	34.7	1.54
14	Procarbazine	221	0.06	1.15	19
15	CCNU	234	2.83	676	100
16	Pyrimethamine	249	2.69	490	120
17	PCNU	263	0.37	2.34	11
18	DDMP	269	2.82	661	150
19	DDEP	284	3.19	1549	110
20	Dibromodulcitol	308	−0.29	0.513	1.9
21	Spirohydantoin mustard	315	2.47	295	29
22	Sucrose	342	−3.01	0.000974	0.12
23	Baker's antifol	398	−2.46	0.00347	0.18
24	Adriamycin	543	−0.10	0.794	<0.014
25	Epipodophylotoxin	657	2.80	631	0.20
26	Vincristine	825	2.80	631	0.64
27	Bleomycin	1400	−3.3	0.000501	<0.014

Another way to compare capillary permeability is to use the extraction fraction, *E*, which is the fraction removed from the blood in one capillary passage through the brain. To give examples from the different permeability groups discussed above, *E* values are in the range 0.6–1.0 for BCNU and CCNU, and around 0.06 for procarbazine, 0.006 for 5-fluorouracil and 0.0006 for VM26 (see Groothuis et al. 1984).

Fig. 11.3 illustrates the penetration into normal mouse brain of a range of analogues of the radiosensitiser misonidazole that are similar in molecular weight but vary widely in lipophilicity. At *P* values >0.1 penetration is rapid, whereas at lower *P* values progressive exclusion from the brain is seen (e.g. SR 2508). With the exception of the most hydrophilic analogue, penetration into subcutaneous mammary tumour was independent of lipophilicity (Fig. 11.3).

Clinical data on penetration of anticancer drugs into normal brain are more difficult to obtain. Ames and Powis (1983) have summarised the limited data obtained with good analytical methodology on the uptake of nitrosoureas in the human central nervous system (CNS) (Table 11.4). For CSF a greater proportional uptake is seen with BCNU than with the more hydrophilic derivatives ACNU and MCNU. In our studies on tissue uptake of nitroimidazole radiosensitisers in a fairly large number of patients with brain tumours, we have found similar average uptake

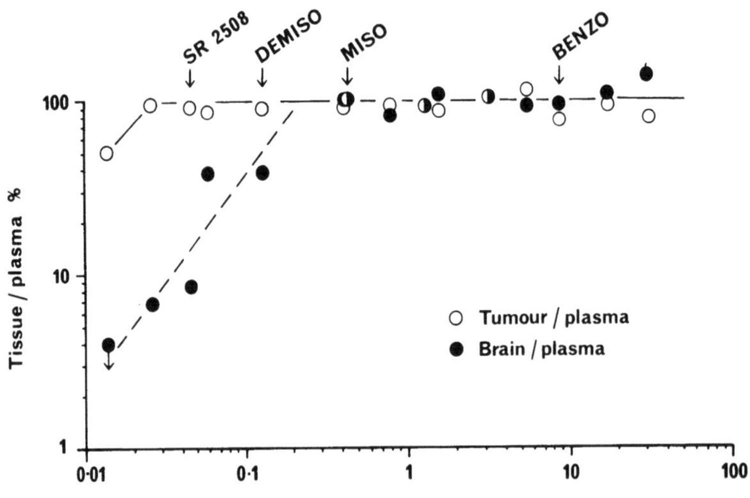

Fig. 11.3. Effect of lipophilicity on the penetration of misonidazole analogues into normal mouse brain and a subcutaneous mammary tumour in the mouse. Data from Brown and Workman (1980) and Workman (1982 and unpub.). Abbreviations: BENZO, benznidazole; DEMISO, desmethylmisonidazole; MISO, misonidazole.

Table 11.4. Uptake of unchanged nitrosoureas into human CNS. Reproduced with modification from Ames and Powis (1983) with permission

Drug	Tissue	Concentration (μg/g)	Tissue/blood %
BCNU	CSF	1	100
ACNU	CSF	0.6	30
	Glioma	>1	160
MCNU	CSF	0.4	30

for the three neutral compounds desmethylmisonidazole, misonidazole and benznidazole into "normal" brain (Table 11.5). All three have *P* values >0.1 but it is noteworthy that the least hydrophilic, desmethylmisonidazole, did exhibit lower tissue/plasma ratios at early time points (Bleehen et al. 1983). (Note also from Table 11.5 the large ranges observed and the fact that average tumour and "normal" brain uptake for these compounds was similar: we will return to both these points later.)

As well as lipophilicity and molecular weight, two additional factors affect brain capillary permeability towards anticancer drugs (Table 11.2). For agents which are ionised at physiological pH, only the uncharged form will be taken up to any appreciable extent. Thus penetration is determined by the fraction not ionised in the plasma, and this will be controlled by the p*K* of the drug and the plasma pH. The distribution coefficient *P** is often used in place of *P* for such drugs, and this is given by the product of *P* for the form not ionised and the fraction not ionised. We have studied the brain uptake of the nitroimidazole radiosensitiser Ro 03-8799. This is a weak base with a p*K* of 8.7 and the drug is therefore 95% ionised at plasma pH

Table 11.5. Penetration of radiosensitisers into human brain[a]

Sensitiser	Partition coefficient	Median tissue/plasma % (range)		n^{c}
		Tumour[b]	Normal	
Desmethylmisonidazole	0.13	66 (19–122)	78 (4–100)	11
Misonidazole	0.43	67 (27–100)	75 (0–114)	31
Benznidazole	8.5	83 (54–122)	69 (53–86)	11
Ro 03–8799	8.5 (0.40)[d]	329 (18–411)	381 (23–571)	9

[a] Data from Bleehen et al. (1983) and Roberts et al. (1984, 1985).
[b] Primary brain tumours.
[c] *n*, no. of patients.
[d] Distribution coefficient (P^*) in parentheses.

(7.4). Nevertheless Ro 03–8799 penetrates rapidly into the brain because of the high lipophilicity of the free base. Moreover, a three- to fourfold accumulation is seen (Table 11.5), and this is attributed to the protonation and consequent trapping of the ionised form in cells which are slightly more acidic than plasma. In contrast, fully ionised molecules such as quaternary amines are essentially excluded from the brain (Bradbury 1979).

The final factor to be considered is protein binding. Extensive and tight binding of anticancer agents to plasma proteins is likely to reduce the rate of uptake into the brain.

In summary then, in contrast to the situation in most other tissues, the BBB acts as a selective semipermeable membrane. Drugs which are very large or very hydrophilic are excluded. As a general rule for agents with molecular weights $\leqslant$400–500, those with P values >0.1 will penetrate the brain rapidly and their uptake will be limited by blood flow. For those with P values >0.1 (or molecular weights $>$400–500) uptake will be limited by BBB permeability. Uptake of drugs of intermediate lipophilicity will be dependent on both blood flow and capillary permeability. The fraction not ionised and non-protein-bound is also important.

In Table 11.6 we have listed some relevant antitumour drugs and divided them into those with high-intermediate capillary permeability and those with low capillary permeability in the normal brain. Those in the former group are of low molecular weight and of adequate lipophilicity. Hydroxyurea has been included in this category since, like urea (Table 11.3) which is also fairly hydrophilic, its low molecular weight is likely to facilitate uptake. Agents in the second category are of high molecular weight, or low lipophilicity, are highly ionised at plasma pH, or are extensively protein-bound. Nevertheless, several agents from this category are used in the treatment of brain tumours, e.g. vincristine, VP 16 and VM 26. The justification for using agents in the first category is clear, but why use those in the second?

Table 11.6. Brain capillary permeability of anticancer drugs

High–intermediate	Low
BCNU	Adriamycin
CCNU	Bleomycin
MeCCNU	Cyclophosphamide
PCNU	Chlorambucil
Procarbazine	Melphalan
5-Fluorouracil	Methotrexate
Pyrimethamine	Vincristine
Misonidazole	Vinblastine
Metronidazole	Chlorozotocin
Ro 03-8799	Cis-platinum
Dianhydrogalactitol	VP 16
Dibromodulcitol	VM 26
AZQ	Razoxane
Spirohydantoin mustard	SR 2508
Hydroxyurea	

The Blood–Brain Barrier in Tumours

To answer the question at the end of the last paragraph we need to consider the blood flow and capillary permeability characteristics of brain tumours. These parameters have been studied in great detail in experimental models, particularly by Blasberg and co-workers (e.g. Blasberg et al. 1981, Groothuis et al. 1984) using elegant quantitative autoradiographic techniques. The findings can be summarised under the following five points:

1. A characteristic of brain tumours is the enormous range of capillary permeability and blood flow, even within the same tumour.
2. Blood flow in tumours may increase, decrease or remain unchanged with respect to the uninvolved normal brain, but most commonly blood flow is found to decrease.
3. Capillary permeability may be unchanged but frequently increases.
4. Where they occur, these changes may become progressively more apparent with increasing tumour size, but do not always correlate with size or histology. Some very large, invasive tumours can exhibit normal capillary permeability.
5. Finally, in the normal brain immediately adjacent to the tumour (BAT) both blood flow and capillary permeability may be decreased.

Until quite recently it remained a matter of controversy as to whether the BBB existed at all in brain tumours (see Levin et al. 1975, Vick et al. 1977). There is now a clear consensus that the BBB may be intact and normal in some regions, whereas in others the microvasculature can be characterised by a fenestrated and discontinuous endothelium where the barrier function is markedly impaired. Similar conclusions are now being reached for human tumours using the rapidly advancing and highly elegant techniques of X-ray computerised axial tomography, positron emission tomography and magnetic resonance imaging (see chapters by Moseley, Bydder and Beaney in this book).

As far as drug delivery is concerned then, there are three distinct environments to be considered:

1. A region where the BBB is normal: Tumour cells located here would be expected to be reached by drugs previously categorised as having high-intermediate permeability coefficients with respect to normal brain, but not by those having low permeability coefficients.
2. A region where the barrier is leaky: Other things being equal, tumour cells located here would be expected to be reached equally well by drugs with high or low permeability coefficients calculated with respect to the normal brain.
3. The BAT, which probably contains the most actively proliferating cells: Because of reduced permeability and blood flow, concentrations of all drugs may be lower than in the normal brain.

Although these variations are often considered on a fairly gross scale, it seems likely that disparities in capillary permeability and blood flow will also operate at the level of individual capillaries.

As far as drug delivery is concerned then, it seems we can justify, in theory at least, the use of drugs from both categories in the treatment of brain tumours. There are likely to be some tumours, or regions of tumours, which will be reached better by smaller, more lipophilic drugs; other regions may be reached equally well by larger, more hydrophilic agents.

To what extent do we have data to confirm or refute the theoretical justification for using drugs which have low capillary permeability coefficients in the normal brain? In the studies described above capillary permeability was determined using model substances. As Groothuis et al. (1984) have pointed out, although increased brain tumour capillary permeability has been demonstrated for such a diverse range of compounds as γ-aminobutyric acid, urea, sucrose, insulin, Evans blue bound to serum albumin, and horseradish peroxidase, studies need to be carried out with individual chemotherapeutic agents in order to validate predictions based on model substances.

Penetration of Anticancer Drugs into Brain Tumours

No formal studies have been published in which brain tumour capillary permeabilities have been determined for individual anticancer drugs. Levin et al. (1976b) determined permeability coefficients for various drugs in normal brain and tumour in experimental animals. Although data were not shown, he commented that values were similar for lipophilic drugs, but about 1 log higher for tumour in the case of other drugs. His group have also shown in a mouse model (Levin et al. 1972) that methotrexate concentrations were only 3%–4% of plasma concentrations in normal brain compared with 13% at the brain-tumour interface, 32% in the main intracerebral tumour and 45% in the same tumour implanted subcutaneously. 5-Fluorouracil levels were higher in tumour than in normal mouse brain and intermediate in the BAT (Levin and Chadwick 1972), while dianhydrogalactitol also penetrated tumours more rapidly than rat brain (Levin et al. 1976a).

In addition, a series of studies have been carried out on the penetration of nitroimidazole radiosensitisers into normal brain and tumour in man (Table 11.5) and Stewart and co-workers have reported data for a a variety of other chemotherapeutic agents (Table 11.7). Samples were obtained at neurosurgery. Results are expressed as median tumour/plasma ratios and the ranges and number of patients are also given. Several of these investigations had reasonable numbers, whereas others were more anecdotal. Throughout these studies a consistent feature was the wide variation in tumour penetration (often ranging from undetectable to 100% or more), presumably reflecting differences in capillary permeability and blood flow.

Table 11.7. Penetration of various chemotherapeutic drugs into brain tumours in man [a,b]

Drug	Median tumour/plasma %	Range	*n*[c]
VM 26	23	0–313	13
Cis-platinum	128[d]		12
PALA	63	25–126	8
Pentamethylmelamine	0	0–1360	7
Methylglyoxal bis(guanylhydrazone)	547	58–705	6
AZQ	44	22–70	4
3-Deazauridine	75	18–176	1
Vinblastine	129		1

[a] Data from Stewart et al. (1979, 1980, 1982, 1983a, b, 1984), M.G. Rosenblum et al. (1981) and Savaraj et al. (1983).
[b] Primary and metastatic brain tumours.
[c] *n*, no. of patients.
[d] Plasma concentrations not reported; ratio estimated from plasma data reported by others.

All four nitroimidazoles studied in our laboratory were fairly lipophilic ($P>0.1$). Tumour penetration was generally similar to that in brain which was not directly involved, the ratios being 66%–83% for the neutral analogues and 329% for the weak base Ro 03-8799 (see earlier). It is interesting to note that misonidazole distributed rapidly and uniformly in normal brain and tumour in a rat model (Horowitz et al. 1983).

As predicted, AZQ shows good penetration into human cerebrospinal fluid (CSF) and BAT (Schilsky et al. 1982, Savaraj et al. 1983). Pentamethylmelamine was found in rather low levels in human CSF and BAT (Stewart et al. 1983a) but exhibited excellent penetration into normal mouse brain (C. J. Rutty pers. comm.), a finding more in keeping with its lipophilic character. The remaining compounds in Table 11.7 are essentially excluded from normal brain. It is significant, therefore, that such agents as VM 26 and cis-platinum clearly do penetrate into human brain tumours.

Broadly speaking, for the compounds in Tables 11.5 and 11.7 concentrations in intracerebral tumours were similar to those in extracerebral tumours or tissues such as muscle. Drug concentrations were sometimes lower in necrotic regions than in viable regions and cyst fluid levels were invariably low. CSF concentrations were likewise often poorly predictive of tumour levels. In some studies it was possible to show that concentrations decreased progressively in the BAT region; as well as being predictable from permeability considerations described earlier, a "sink effect" is also likely to apply, whereby drug entering the tumour periphery diffuses away down a concentration gradient into the surrounding brain. In addition, for pentamethylmelamine and VM 26 there was some evidence of lower penetration in glioblastoma compared with brain metastases, though this may have been due to chance. Nevertheless, these data do support the idea that drugs normally excluded from the brain are able to penetrate human brain tumours, at least on a fairly gross scale. There are, of course, likely to be differences at the microdistribution level. We have focussed on permeability considerations but other factors (Table 11.1) also play a role. Diffusion or bulk flow to distant sites such as CSF; poor penetration over large intracapillary distances; and rapid intratumour metabolism are factors which may be particularly important. Levin et al. (1980) have carried out heuristic modelling of drug delivery to brain tumours, illustrating the problems involved with drug diffusion from a well-vascularised 'leaky' region (*a*) outward to the BAT and normal brain where the BBB is intact and (*b*) inward to a central, poorly perfused core where intercapillary distances may be high. BCNU is one of the few drugs able to arrive at cells 200 μm away with less than a 50% decrease in concentration. Binding and/or metabolism produced much greater concentration gradients for 5-fluorouracil, vincristine and particularly adriamycin. Horowitz et al. (1983) obtained indirect evidence of heterogeneous nitroreductive metabolism of misonidazole in a rat brain tumour.

Circumventing the Blood–Brain Barrier

Because of the importance of drug delivery to brain tumours and the at least partially restrictive nature of the BBB, great efforts have been made to circumvent it. The strategies under experimental and clinical development are summarised in Table 11.8.

Prolonged infusions have the advantage of allowing greater time for equilibration between brain and plasma. For a drug with a fairly low extraction of 0.1, 15 and 30 minutes would be required for tumour concentrations to reach 50% and 90% of the plasma concentration respectively, even without tissue metabolism (Groothuis et al. 1984). Many anticancer drugs are cleared from plasma very rapidly. A disadvantage of prolonged infusion is that peak plasma concentrations are lower than with rapid injection. Administration of higher doses should increase brain concentrations at least proportionally, and possibly more if, for example, the drug exhibits saturable plasma protein binding. High-dose methotrexate with leucovorin rescue (Bleyer and Poplack 1978) and high-dose BCNU with marrow transplantation (Fingert and Hochberg 1984) are examples of this approach. Higher peak concentrations of circulating nitrosoureas can be produced in some patients by administering the radiosensitiser benznidazole prior to oral CCNU (Roberts et al. 1984). The mechanism

Table 11.8. Strategies for circumventing the blood–brain barrier

1.	Prolonged infusion
2.	High dose
3.	Intrathecal, intraventricular and intratumour administration
4.	Intra-arterial administration
5.	Reversible opening by physical or chemical means
6.	Chemical modification of drug

involves inhibition of drug-metabolising enzymes (Lee and Workman 1984) and has been shown to result in improved tumour response and therapeutic index in mice (Twentyman and Workman 1983).

Higher local exposures can be achieved without further risking, or even decreasing, systemic toxicity by direct administration into the CNS using intrathecal, intraventricular or intratumour injection (Blasberg et al. 1975, Bleyer and Poplack 1978, Collins 1983, Stewart 1984). Problems with administration into CSF include limited penetration because of rapid washout for drugs such as BCNU and thio-TEPA, and rapid metabolism of cytosine arabinoside in brain. Methotrexate appears more promising in terms of brain penetration (Ushio et al. 1974) but heterogeneity of distribution is still likely to be a problem. The intraventricular route produces higher CSF levels than the intrathecal route (Bleyer and Poplack 1978). It should be noted, however, that the latter study has also shown CSF methotrexate concentrations to be as high (10^{-7} to $5 \times 10^{-5} M$), more prolonged (48 hours), and more homogeneous with a high-dose infusion protocol. It is interesting that, compared with methotrexate, reduced folates penetrate the BBB very rapidly, apparently by transport in the form of $N_{(5)}$-methyltetrahydrofolate (Levitt et al. 1971, Spector and Lorenzo 1975). A rescue agent with reduced brain permeability may therefore be of interest, such as the enzyme carboxypeptidase G1 which degrades methotrexate directly (Bertino 1977).

Intratumour administration appears to result in rapid but uneven distribution of methotrexate (Tator and Wassenaar 1977) and this probably applies to other agents. Intra-arterial administration is another means of increasing target concentrations while potentially reducing systemic exposure (see Fenstermacher and Gazendam 1981, Stewart 1984). A two- to fourfold increase in drug concentration can be achieved for tumours in the field of perfusion. It has a particular advantage for an agent like BCNU where drug breakdown during the first pass may be high, or when poor blood flow is rate limiting. An advantage has also been seen for VM 26, though that with methotrexate is fairly small. Disadvantages include technical difficulties, problems with drug vehicles containing alcohol, incomplete mixing of drug with blood leading to uneven distribution, and the fact that the infused artery may supply only part of the tumour.

A further sophistication to intra-arterial administration is the immediate pre-administration, via the same artery, of hypertonic solutions of water-soluble solutes. This results in the so-called reversible osmotic opening of the BBB, apparently caused by shrinkage of the capillary endothelial cells (Neuwelt 1984). The effect is "all-or-none" and may last for up to 30 minutes. Hypertonic manitol (25%) is commonly used. For example, in dog brain methotrexate concentrations were improved up to 90-fold while adriamycin concentrations increased from undetectable to 4.5 μg/g (Neuwelt 1984). Neurotoxicity appears to be a problem with adriamycin as with bleomycin, mitomycin C, 5-fluorouracil and cis-platinum, while cyclophosphamide and methotrexate are more promising.

Other techniques for barrier opening can also be used experimentally (Rapaport 1976, Greig 1984) including Metrazole seizures, arterial hypertension and hypercapnia. Extremely high doses of X-rays (100 Gy) increase permeability within a few days, but clinical doses usually produce changes only months to years later. Doses of up to 2–25 Gy had little or no acute effect on brain uptake of methotrexate in mice (Griffin et al. 1977) or on uptake of bleomycin and VM 26 in rats (Levin et al. 1979). Microwaves have been reported to increase brain capillary permeability, but recent work suggests the effects were due to increased blood flow secondary to the hyperthermic effect (see Greig 1984). Likewise, in contrast to earlier findings, neither dimethylsulphoxide nor 5-fluorouracil has an effect on barrier permeability (see Greig 1984). Amphotericin B has been reported to increase permeability in some situations but not others (Levin et al. 1976b, Stewart et al. 1984). Glucocorticoids may in fact reduce brain capillary permeability (Levin et al. 1976b, Workman 1980).

Each of the above techniques is under clinical investigation, but the invasive nature of most of these technically difficult, potentially hazardous strategies makes them of limited general appeal. Of potentially wider application is the modification of drug structure to facilitate BBB penetration of a systemically administered agent. Some of the possibilities are as follows:

Optimisation of the Partition Coefficient

The importance of the partition coefficient was dealt with earlier. Several studies have been carried out to optimise *P* for nitrosoureas in experimental brain tumours. Hansch et al. (1972) found a parabolic dependence on log *P* for activity against the L1210 tumour implanted intracerebrally, with an optimum *P* of 0.25 (i.e. rather hydrophilic); Montgomery et al. (1974) saw a parabolic relationship with an optimum log *P* of 6.3 (more lipophilic) with the Lewis lung tumour outside the brain; and Levin and Kabra (1974) observed a linear relationship with the 9L tumour implanted intracerebrally, maximum activity being seen with PCNU for which *P* is 2.3 (quite lipophilic). None of the optimum compounds was as lipophilic as the more commonly used nitrosoureas. One of the difficulties with this type of analysis, especially with small numbers, is the variation of other properties such as alkylation and carbamoylation, which also govern activity. PCNU is undergoing clinical trial.

The aziridinyl benzoquinone AZQ is an agent for which the partition coefficient was optimised to allow CNS penetration and activity against experimental brain tumours while retaining sufficient aqueous solubility for intravenous administration (Khan and Driscoll 1976, Chou et al. 1976). Early clinical studies confirmed that CNS penetration is good (Schilsky et al. 1982) and trials are continuing.

A number of anthracyclines are becoming available with partition coefficients considerably higher than that of adriamycin: e.g. aclacinomycin and AD32. Molecular weights remain large, however, and this will impair uptake where the BBB is intact. It will also restrict diffusion over large distances, as will high affinity for DNA. Smaller molecules, some of which do not bind to DNA, are under development and these may have a role in CNS chemotherapy. Size may also be a problem with lipophilic derivatives of methotrexate.

Masking Polar Groups

This strategy involves masking lipophilic (e.g. -OH and -NH) residues with lipophilic substituents, which can then be removed by metabolism after uptake into the brain. The oldest example of this is the acetylation of morphine to yield the more lipophilic heroin, which is taken up more rapidly before being deacetylated to monoacetyl morphine and morphine itself (Bradbury 1979). This approach could be taken with many anticancer agents, and dialkyl esters of methotrexate have been synthesised (Johns et al. 1973). However, concentrations of γ-monobutyl ester were similar to those of methotrexate in Rhesus monkey CSF, apparently because of extensive protein binding (Rosowsky et al. 1982).

An exciting example of this prodrug approach is based on the work of Bodor and colleagues (Bodor and Brewster 1982). It involves the coupling of a drug to a dihydropyridine carrier which penetrates the brain rapidly; the redox potential in the brain favours rapid oxidation to the quaternary pyridinium ion which is then trapped in the brain. Dopamine, testosterone and an antidote to organophosphate poisoning can be delivered in this way, and the application of the technique to anticancer agents is under development.

Exploiting Accumulation/Transport Systems

Although many metabolic substrates are actively transported across the BBB (e.g. sugars, amino acids, folates, vitamins, peptides and proteins), it is thought that anticancer agents are not. Even melphalan, which is normally taken up by amino acid carriers, and methotrexate, normally accumulated via the folate carrier, do not appear to utilise these carriers at the capillary endothelium. There seems to be scope for further development here.

Accumulation of weak bases (in the way that the radiosensitiser Ro 03-8799 is accumulated) is also worthy of further study.

In an attempt to capitalise on the known accumulation of diphenylhydantoin in the brain and especially brain tumours (Rosenblum and Stein 1963) the nitrogen mustard derivative spirohydantoin mustard was synthesised specifically for CNS tumours (Peng et al. 1975). This is highly lipophilic, penetrates the normal rat brain rapidly (Table 11.3), enters CSF in dog (Plowman et al. 1977) and shows good activity against brain tumours (Peng et al. 1975). Clinical trials are in progress.

Antibody Targeting

In regions where the BBB is destroyed the possibility exists for using monoclonal antibodies to products expressed by brain tumours for targeting radionuclides or drugs (Bourdon et al. 1984). These are unlikely to be of value where the BBB is intact unless osmotic opening is used, and will share the problems of specificity and biodistribution that exist with other antibody-drug conjugates.

The Future

Despite considerable efforts the response of brain tumours to chemotherapy is very poor. The development of more selective drugs is surely an approach to be pursued, though very little has been done to define exploitable biochemical mechanisms in brain tumours. Brain tumour cells are clearly active metabolically (Rosenblum et al. 1984). The 9L rat brain tumour cell line has been shown to possess high levels of the reductive enzyme DT-diaphorase (Rosenblum et al. 1984) and preferential nitro-reduction of misonidazole appears to occur in RT-9 brain tumour cells compared with normal brain (Horowitz et al. 1983). Further study of agents activated by bioreductive enzymes (see Workman 1983), e.g. quinones and nitro compounds, is therefore warranted. More subtle dissection of the biochemical peculiarities and molecular biology of brain tumours may allow the rational design of drugs of even greater specificity.

Until such compounds are produced the aim must be to deliver existing drugs or their analogues in an optimal fashion. There is no doubt that even with the most widely accepted agents, BCNU and CCNU, drug concentrations are clearly sub-optimal for tumour cell-kill. Cellular dose-response curves for nitrosoureas frequently have large shoulders followed by a steep exponential region (e.g. Wheeler et al. 1975, M. L. Rosenblum et al. 1981) and concentrations to give even a 1 log cell kill for a nominal 1-2 hour exposure are in the range 3-30 μg/ml (see Lee et al. 1985). After maximum tolerated doses administered conventionally, peak plasma concentrations of BCNU after intravenous administration are 1-2 μg/ml (Levin et al. 1978) and CSF concentrations are similar (Table 11.4). After oral CCNU no parent compound is detected, but peak concentrations of the equally active hydroxylated metabolites are about 1 μg/ml (Lee et al. 1985). Thus for both nitrosoureas, average peak brain concentrations are unlikely to greatly exceed 1-2 μg/g, and some regions may see considerably less drug. In most cell lines these exposures would produce less than a 1 log cell kill. In view of these considerations and the fact that a small but significant response to BCNU and CCNU is seen in some clinical settings, there is clear justification for strategies to increase delivery of even the most lipophilic drugs. For those drugs which are often highly effective against tumours in other sites but which are excluded from certain regions of brain tumours, the need to overcome the BBB is perhaps even more pressing. Intra-arterial administration and osmotic opening appear particularly promising areas for research. The synthesis of novel prodrugs should also be encouraged.

Finally a comment may be made on the design of clinical trials of brain tumour chemotherapy. Whereas the importance of various other prognostic variables is now accepted, brain tumour permeability is not normally included. Now that regional permeability can be readily measured, particularly by positron emission tomography, it seems appropriate to build this variable into future studies. It should be possible to ask sensible questions about the relationship between BBB permeability and chemoresponsiveness for both lipophilic drugs and those excluded from more normal brain. A greater sophistication would be to use positron emission tomography together with antitumour agents labelled with appropriate positron-emitting radionuclides to ask more direct questions about barrier permeability, drug uptake and tumour response in individual patients.

References

Ames MM, Powis JS (1983) Pharmacokinetics of nitrosoureas. In: Ames MM, Powis G, Kovach JS (eds) Pharmacokinetics of anticancer agents in humans. Elsevier, Amsterdam, pp 113-134

Bertino JR (1977) Rescue techniques in cancer chemotherapy: Use of leucovorin and other rescue agents after methotrexate. Semin Oncol 4: 203-216

Blasberg RG, Patlack C, Fenstermacher D (1975) Intrathecal chemotherapy in brain tissue profiles after ventriculo-cisternal perfusion. J Pharmacol Exp Ther 195: 73-83

Blasberg RG, Kobayashi T, Patlack CS, Shinohara M, Miyoaka M, Rice JM, Shapiro WR (1981) Regional blood flow, capillary permeability, and glucose utilisation in two brain tumour models: Preliminary observations and pharmacokinetic implications. Cancer Treat Rep 65 [Suppl 2]: 3-12

Bleehen NM, Grant RM, Jones DH, Roberts JT, Workman P, Gleave JRW, Hardy DG, Holmes AE (1983) The penetration of misonidazole and desmethylmisonidazole into brain tumours and other central nervous system tumours in man. Br J Radiol 56: 859-863

Bleyer WA, Poplack DG (1978) Clinical studies in the central-nervous-system pharmacology of methotrexate. In: Pinedo HM (ed) Clinical pharmacology of antineoplastic drugs. Elsevier, Amsterdam, pp 115–131
Bodor N, Brewster M (1982) Problems of drug delivery to the brain. Pharmacol Ther 19: 337–386
Bogdahn U (1983) Chemosensitivity of malignant human brain tumours. J Neuro-Oncol 1: 149–166
Bourdon MA, Coleman RE, Bigner DD (1984) The potential of monoclonal antibodies as carriers of radiation and drugs for immunodetection and therapy of brain tumours. Prog Exp Tumor Res 28: 79–101
Bradbury M (1979) The concept of a blood-brain barrier. Wiley, Chichester
Brown JM, Workman P (1980) Partition coefficient as a guide to the development of radiosensitisers which are less toxic than misonidazole. Radiat Res 82: 171–190
Chou F, Khan AH, Driscoll JS (1976) Potential central nervous system antitumour agents. Aziridinylbenzoquinones II. J Med Chem 19: 1302–1308
Collins JM (1983) Pharmacokinetics of intraventricular administration. J Neuro-Oncol 1: 283–291
Darling JJ, Thomas DGT (1983) Results obtained using assays of intermediate duration and clinical correlations. In: Dendy PP, Hill BT (eds) Human tumour drug sensitivity testing in vitro. Academic Press, London, pp 269–280
Fenstermacher J, Gazendam J (1981) Intra-arterial infusions of drugs and hyperosmotic solutions as ways of enhancing CNS chemotherapy. Cancer Treat Rep 65: 27–37
Fingert HJ, Hochberg FH (1984) Megadose chemotherapy with bone marrow rescue. Prog Exp Tumor Res 28: 67–78
Greig NH (1984) Chemotherapy of brain metastases: Current status. Cancer Treat Rev 11: 157–186
Griffin TW, Rasey JS, Bleyer WA (1977) The effect of photon irradiation on blood-brain barrier permeability to methotrexate in mice. Cancer 40: 1109–1111
Groothuis DR, Molnar P, Blasberg RG (1984) Regional blood flow and blood-to-tissue transport in five brain tumour models. Prog Exp Tumor Res 27: 132–153
Hansch C, Smith N, Engle R, Wood H (1972) Quantitative structure-activity relationships of antineoplastic drugs: Nitrosoureas and triazenoimidazoles. Cancer Treat Rep 56: 443–456
Horowitz M, Blasberg R, Molnar P, Strong J, Kornblith P, Pleasants R, Fenstermacher J (1983) [^{14}C]misonidazole distribution in experimental RT-9 brain tumours. Cancer Res 43: 3800–3807
Houchens DP, Ovejera AA, Riblet SM, Slagel DE (1983) Human brain tumour xenografts in nude mice as a chemotherapy model. Eur J Cancer 19: 799–805
Johns D, Farquhar D, Wolpert M, Chabner B, Loo T (1973) Dialkylesters of methotrexate and 3,5-dichloromethotrexate. Synthesis and interaction with aldehyde oxidase and dihydrofolate reductase. Drug Metab Dispos 1: 580–589
Khan AH, Driscoll JS (1976) Potential nervous system antitumour agents. Aziridinylbenzoquinones I. J Med Chem 19: 313–317
Lee FYF, Workman P (1984) Inhibition of liver microsomal metabolism of CCNU by nitroimidazoles: Correlation with chemosensitization activity. Br J Cancer 50: 267 (abstr)
Lee FYF, Workman P, Roberts JT, Bleehen NM (1985) Clinical pharmacokinetics of oral CCNU (lomustine). Cancer Chemother Pharmac 14: 125–131
Levin VA (1980) Relationship of octanol/water partition coefficient and molecular weight to rat brain capillary permeability. J Med Chem 23: 682–684
Levin VA, Chadwick M (1972) Distribution of 5-fluorouracil-2-^{14}C and its metabolites in a murine glioma. J Natl Cancer Inst 49: 1577–1584
Levin VA, Kabra P (1974) Effectiveness of the nitrosoureas as a function of their lipid solubility in the chemotherapy of experimental rat brain tumours. Cancer Treat Rep 58: 787–792
Levin VA, Clancy TP, Ausman JI, Rall DP (1972) Uptake and distribution of ^{3}H-methotrexate by murine ependymoblastoma. J Natl Cancer Inst 48: 875–883
Levin VA, Freeman-Dove M, Landahl HD (1975) Permeability characteristics of brain adjacent to tumours. Arch Neurol 32: 785–791
Levin VA, Freeman-Dove MA, Maroten CE (1976a) Dianhydrogalactitol (NSC-132313): Pharmacokinetics in normal and tumour-bearing rat brain and antitumour activity against three intracerebral rodent tumours. J Natl Cancer Inst 56: 535
Levin VA, Kandahl HD, Freeman-Dove MA (1976b) The application of brain capillary permeability coefficient measurements to pathological condition and the selection of agents which cross the blood-brain barrier. J Pharmacokinet Biopharm 4: 499–519
Levin VA, Hoffman W, Weinkam RJ (1978) Pharmacokinetics of BCNU in man: A preliminary study of 20 patients. Cancer Treat Rep 62: 13505–1312
Levin VA, Edwards MS, Byrd A (1979) Quantitative observations of the acute effects of x-irradiation on brain capillary permeability: I. Int J Radiat Oncol Biol Phys 5: 1627–1631

Levin VA, Patlack CS, Landahl HD (1980) Heuristic modeling of drug delivery to malignant brain tumours. J Pharmacokinet Biopharm 8: 257–296

Levin VA, Landahl HD, Patlack CS (1981) Drug delivery to CNS tumours. Cancer Treat Rep 65 [Suppl 2]: 19–25

Levitt M, Nixon PF, Pincus JH, Bertino JR (1971) Transport characteristics of folates in cerebrospinal fluid, a study utilising doubly labelled 5-methytetrahydrofolate and 5-formyltetrahydrofolate. J Clin Invest 50: 1301–1308

Montgomery JA, Mayo JG, Hansch C (1974) Quantitative structure-activity relationships in anticancer drugs. Activity of selected nitrosoureas against a solid tumour, the Lewis lung carcinoma. J Med Chem 17: 477–480

Neuwelt EA (1984) Therapeutic potential for blood-brain barrier modification in malignant brain tumour. Prog Exp Tumor Res 28: 51–66

Peng G, Marquex V, Driscoll J (1975) Potential central nervous system antitumour agents: Hydantoin derivatives. J Med Chem 18: 846–849

Plowman J, Lakings D, Owens E, Adamson R (1977) Initial studies on the penetration of spirohydantoin into the cerebrospinal fluid of dogs. Pharmacology 15: 359–366

Rapaport SI (1976) Blood-brain barrier in physiology and medicine. Raven Press, New York

Roberts JT, Bleehen NM, Lee FYF, Workman P, Walton MI (1984) A phase 1 study of the combination of benznidazole and CCNU in man. Int J Radiat Oncol Biol Phys 10: 1745–1748

Roberts JT, Bleehen NM, Walton MI, Workman P (1985) A phase 1 toxicity study of Ro 03-8799: Plasma, urine, tumour and normal brain pharmacokinetics. Br J Radiol (in press)

Rosenblum MG, Stewart DJ, Yap BS, Leavens M, Benjamin RS, Loo TL (1981) Penetration of methylglyoxal bis(guanylhydrazone) into intracerebral tumours. Cancer Res 41: 459–462

Rosenblum ML, Dougherty DV, Deen DF, Wilson CB (1981) Potentials and limitations of a clonogenic assay for human brain tumours. Cancer Treat Rep 65 [Suppl 2]: 61–66

Rosenblum ML, Gerosa MA, Bodell WJ, Talcott RL (1984) Tumor cell resistance. Prog Exp Tumor Res 27: 191–214

Rosenblum T, Stein A (1963) Preferential distribution of diphenylhydantoin in primary brain tumours. Biochem Pharmac 12: 453–454

Rosowsky A, Abelson HT, Beardsley GP, Ensminger WD, Kufe DW, Steele G, Modest EJ (1982) Pharmacologic studies on the dibutyl and γ-monobutyl esters of methotrexate in the rhesus monkey. Cancer Chemother Pharmac 10: 55–61

Savaraj N, Lu K, Fenn LG, Leavens MEL, Stewart D, Burgess MA, Benjamin RS, Loo TL (1983) Intracerebral penetration and tissue distribution of 2,5-diaziridinyl 3,6-bis(carboethoxyamino)1,4-benzoquinone (AZQ NSC-182986), J Neuro-Oncol 1: 15–19

Schilsky RL, Kelly JA, Ihde DC, Howzer DM, Cordes RS, Young RC (1982) Phase 1 trial and pharmacokinetics of aziridinylbenzoquinone. Cancer Res 42: 1582–1586

Shapiro W (1973) Malignant brain tumour chemotherapy. I. Experimental studies. Clin Bull 23: 58–62

Shapiro WR, Basler GA, Chernik NL, Posner JB (1979) Human brain tumor transplantation into nude mice. J Natl Cancer Inst 62: 447–453

Spector R, Lorenzo AV (1975) Folate transport in the central nervous system. Am J Physiol 229: 777–782

Stewart DJ (1984) Novel modes of chemotherapy administration. Prog Exp Tumor Res 28: 32–50

Stewart DJ, Benvenuto JA, Leavens M, Hall SW, Benjamin RS, Plunkett W, McCredie KB, Burgess MA, Loo TL (1979) Penetration of 3-deazuridine into human brain, intracerebral tumour and cerebrospinal fluid. Cancer Res 39: 4119–4122

Stewart DJ, Leavens M, Friedman J, Benjamin RS, Moore EC, Bodey GP, Valdivieso M, Burgess MA, Wiseman C, Loo TL (1980) Penetration of *N*-(phosphonacetyl)-L-aspartate into human central nervous system and intracerebral tumour. Cancer Res 40: 3163–3166

Stewart DJ, Leavens M, Maor M, Fenn L, Luna M, Bonura J, Caprioli R, Loo TL, Benjamin RS (1982) Human central nervous system distribution of cis-diamminedichloroplatinum and its use as a radiosensitizer in malignant brain tumours. Cancer Res 42: 2474–2479

Stewart DJ, Benvenuto JA, Leavens M, Smith RG, Cabanillas F, Benjamin RS, Loo TL (1983a) Human central nervous system pharmacology of pentamethylmelamine and its metabolites. J Neuro-Oncol 1: 357–364

Stewart DJ, Lu K, Benjamin RS, Leavens ME, Luna M, Yap H-Y, Loo TL (1983b) Concentrations of vinblastine in human intracerebral tumour and other tissues. J Neuro-Oncol 1: 139–144

Stewart DJ, Richard MT, Hugenboltz H, Dennery J, Nundy D, Prior J, Montpetit V, Hopkins HS (1984) Penetration of teniposide (VM-26) into human intracerebral tumours. J Neuro-Oncol 2: 315–324

Tator CH, Wassenaar W (1977) Intraneoplastic injection of methotrexate for experimental brain-tumor chemotherapy. J Neurosurg 46: 165–174

Twentyman PR, Workman P (1983) Chemosensitization by lipophilic nitroimidazoles. Br J Cancer 48: 17–26
Ushio Y, Hayakawa T, Mogami H (1974) Uptake of tritiated methotrexate by mouse brain tumours after intravenous or intrathecal administration. J Neurosurg 40: 706–716
Vick NA, Khandekar JD, Bigner DD (1977) Chemotherapy of brain tumors: The 'blood–brain barrier' is not a factor. Arch Neurol 34: 523–526
Wheeler KT, Tel N, Williams ME, Sheppard S, Levin VA, Kabra PM (1975) Factors influencing the survival of rat brain tumour cells after in vitro treatment with 1,3-bis(2-chloroethyl)-1-nitrosourea. Cancer Res 35: 1464–1469
Workman P (1980) Drug interactions with misonidazole: Effects of dexamethasone and its derivatives on the pharmacokinetics and toxicity of misonidazole in mice. Biochem Pharmac 39: 2769–2776
Workman P (1982) Lipophilicity and the pharmacokinetics of nitroimidazoles. In: Breccia A, Rimondi C, Adams GE (eds) Advanced topics on radiosensitizers of hypoxic cells. Plenum Press, New York, pp 143–163
Workman P (1983) New drugs against hypoxic cells: II. Cancer Topics 4: 54–57

12 Chemotherapy of Brain Tumours

D. G. T. Thomas

Introduction

The invasive nature of cerebral glioma accounts for the failure of neurosurgical therapy in these tumours (Dandy 1928, 1933, Matsukado et al. 1961). Although the tumour may appear macroscopically limited at operation, nearly always microscopical examination reveals infiltrating neoplastic cells in surrounding brain. In one autopsy series of 28 cases 75% had interhemispheric spread across the corpus callosum (Maxwell 1946), while in a similar series of 100 cases 47% showed bilateral tumour extension (Matsukado et al. 1961). Thus, the long-term results of treatment of malignant glioma by surgery are very poor, with median survival in the region of 14–23 weeks (Frankel and German 1958, Walker and Gehan 1976). The 2-year survival is virtually zero (Grant 1956, Earle et al. 1957, Frankel and German 1958, German 1961). Grade 4 gliomas have a 1-year survival of 8%–9% when treated with surgery alone (Sheline 1977, Salcman 1980). However, surgery is a vital element in therapy of such tumours. The initial role is to establish a definite diagnosis. Secondly symptomatic relief of distressing symptoms by reduction of tumour bulk, and therefore of raised intracranial pressure, is valuable. It is also probable that such surgery may make more effective the adjuvant methods of radiotherapy and chemotherapy. Post-operative radiotherapy appears to increase survival in patients with glioma (Sheline 1977, Walker et al. 1978). The benefit to be derived from chemotherapy for these tumours is more controversial.

Selection of Drugs

Empirical treatment with many agents has been attempted (Shapiro and Ausman 1969, Thomas 1982, for reviews). Novel forms of drug delivery have also been tried, including intracarotid infusion as described first by Woodhall et al. (1959), and direct introduction into the cerebrospinal fluid (CSF) or tumour cavity (Rubin et al. 1966, Ommaya et al. 1965). The nitrosourea drugs are effective chemotherapeutic agents against brain tumours, and recently trials of BCNU, CCNU and methyl CCNU, including randomised prospective studies, have been carried out (Edwards et al. 1980). The most distinctive advantage shown has been a modest improvement in the proportion of long-term survivors, for example 19% 18-month survival in patients receiving adjuvant BCNU therapy compared with 4% in patients treated only with radiotherapy after surgery (Walker et al. 1978). The effect of procarbazine has been shown to be similar to BCNU in phase two (Kumar et al. 1974) and phase three trials (Green et al. 1983).

BCNU (Schabel et al. 1963) and CCNU (Carter et al. 1972) were developed as lipophilic chemotherapeutic agents. On theoretical grounds lipophilicity is desirable in delivery of treatment to an intracerebral tumour (see chapter by Workman in this book). It has been proposed that the chief beneficial activity of nitrosoureas is via alkylation, while carbamoylation may be responsible for their toxic effects (Wheeler et al. 1974). Studies with labelled BCNU have shown penetration into brain and CSF, with persisting levels at 12 hours in monkeys and 9 hours in man (de Vita et al. 1967). CCNU probably behaves in a similar manner. These agents are active against cerebral glioma (Edwards et al. 1980).

Procarbazine was synthesised as a monoamine oxidase inhibitor but was identified as an anticancer agent in animal tumour models (Bollag 1963). Its mode of action is unclear; however, it enters CSF well after oral ingestion (Oliverio et al. 1964).

Vincristine is a plant alkaloid which binds tubulin and has a phase-specific chemotherapeutic effect by blocking mitosis in tumour cells (Calabresi and Parks 1975). The vinca alkaloids are relatively poorly absorbed by CSF and brain (Stewart et al. 1983). However, vincristine has been incorporated into combination chemotherapeutic regimes for cerebral glioma (Levin et al. 1980).

Combination therapy has the theoretical advantage of adding the beneficial activities of agents with different modes of action without added toxicity when they have differing individual toxicities (de Vita and Schein 1973). Because the effects of useful single agents in cerebral glioma are modest there has been considerable clinical interest in combination therapy trials. Unfortunately, because so few even modestly effective single agents exist the variety of combinations is also limited. The combination of CCNU, procarbazine and vincristine appears effective in both adjuvant (Gutin et al. 1975) and primary chemotherapy (Shapiro and Young 1976).

One explanation of the finding of a responsive minority of cases in trials could be a heterogeneity of response of individual gliomas of similar histological grade to particular chemotherapeutic agents (Barranco et al. 1973, Kimball and Brattain 1980). There is evidence of histological heterogeneity in such tumours (Russell and Rubinstein 1977) and further, recent evidence of heterogeneity in other respects (Bradley et al. 1978, Shapiro et al. 1981, Bigner et al. 1981, Bullard et al. 1981a). Several experimental attempts have been made to display heterogeneity in chemosensitivity of human gliomas in vitro or in vivo (Easty and Wylie 1963, Gazsim and

Afra 1969, Mealey et al. 1974, Saez et al. 1977, Kornblith and Szypko 1978, Rosenblum et al. 1978, 1983, Shapiro et al. 1979, Bullard et al. 1981b). It is these attempts which have led to the use of surgical biopsy specimens from human glioma to perform in vitro tests of the chemosensitivity of individual tumours.

Methods for in vitro Chemosensitivity Assessment

The idealised in vitro chemosensitivity test would be applicable in all cases, give reproducible quantitative answers in a time frame suitable for control of clinical management, and would be cheap and not labour intensive. The human cerebral glioma can generally readily be cultured in vitro, and specific markers may be used to show that the resulting cultured cells are both glial in origin and tumorigenic (Freshney 1980).

One approach to in vitro chemosensitivity testing has been the colony-forming, or clonogenic, assay, as such tests are theoretically simple. Single-cell suspensions from tumours are treated with drugs and then cultured in soft agar or on surfaces of tissue culture dishes. Each viable cell is potentially capable of cell division to form a colony of cells which may be seen and counted. Comparison of control cultures with those treated can give quantitative results. In experimental animal tumours it seems probable that such surviving colonies come from tumour stem cells (Steel 1977 for review). Such cloning assays have been used to study effects of drugs on glioma cells in vitro (Guner et al. 1977, Rosenblum et al. 1983). In a study of the glucocorticoid steroid, dexamethasone, remarkably consistent effects on cloning and proliferation were found (Guner et al. 1977). Increasing doses of steroid enhanced colony formation and proliferation, and only very high doses caused inhibition of cloning and of proliferation. Such asssays are expensive in time and labour, and tend to give answers in a minority of cases (Rupniak and Hill 1980).

An alternative method of in vitro assay which has been applied to cerebral glioma is based on growth in soft agar of aggregated clusters of cells known as multicellular spheroids (Darling and Thomas 1983). Such spheroids are capable of progressive growth, the rate of which may be varied by exposure to chemotherapeutic agents. The diameter and volume of the spheroid may be measured optically and the growth delay effects caused by different agents assessed. This method, like the clonogenic assay, is biologically attractive but is also time-consuming and labour intensive.

A third approach to in vitro chemosensitivity assay has been the use of microtitration assays as indicators of metabolic activity such as nucleic acid or protein synthesis (Thomas et al. 1979). The results of this assay have been correlated with the clinical results obtained in a series of grade 3 and 4 cerebral gliomas treated with adjuvant chemotherapy (Thomas et al. 1985).

Results of in vitro Predictive Testing

A chemotherapy adjuvant regime of vincristine (1.4 mg/m^2 intravenously as a single dose), CCNU (80 mg/m^2 orally as a single dose) and procarbazine (100 mg/m^2 per day orally over 10 days) has been used at the National Hospitals for Nervous Diseases, London, and three associated centres in the treatment of grade 3 and 4 cerebral gliomas referred for surgery. One hundred and seventeen patients with histologically verified tumours were treated post-operatively with a combination of radiotherapy and the adjuvant chemotherapy described above (Thomas et al. 1985). Twelve cycles of adjuvant therapy were planned at intervals of 6 weeks over an 18-month period. Computerised tomographic (CT) scanning was performed at intervals of 3 months during chemotherapy and at intervals of 6 months thereafter. Disease progression was determined by clinical deterioration which correlated generally with worsening CT scan. The relapse-free interval was calculated from the time of surgery. The end-points in follow-up after neurosurgery which are useful in comparing results of different therapies are the relapse-free interval and survival. The latter end-point is generally accurately measured, but factors like hospitalisation in the terminal stage may greatly affect it (Hildebrand and Brihaye 1975). Relapse-free interval may be determined by clinical and radiological means (Levin et al. 1977, Edwards et al. 1980), and is not influenced by variable terminal care.

Surgical biopsy samples were sent to the tissue culture laboratory in 48 cases, in addition to those sent to the routine diagnostic biopsy for histopathological examination. Forty of the samples thus provided grew and were maintained until evaluable by in vitro chemosensitivity testing. Six (12.5%) failed to grow and two (4%) became contaminated. Primary cultures were set up of disaggregated cells and testing was performed on cells at passage numbers one or two (Thomas et al. 1979, 1985, Morgan et al. 1983). The tumour cells were exposed in vitro to 3 days of drug treatment with graded concentrations of CCNU, procarbazine and vincristine. At variable periods of recovery after drug removal, residual protein synthesis was estimated by amino acid uptake on autofluorography. The effect of each drug on protein synthesis was measured in this way. The dose of drug which caused 50% inhibition in the treated cells compared with control was termed the Inhibitory Dose 50 (ID_{50}). Previous studies have shown that at 3–5 days after drug exposure there is a good correlation between the apparent in vitro chemosensitivity of tumour measured by this microtitration assay and that measured by an alternative clonogenic assay (Morgan et al. 1983). A tumour was reported as sensitive if the ID_{50} values were below the median ID_{50} of a panel of 123 glioma cultures tested previously. Twenty-two of the tested gliomas were sensitive when judged this way, and 18 were insensitive. Of the sensitive gliomas a larger proportion were grade 3 (16/20 or 80%) than grade 4 (6/20 or 30%). However, in both types of tumour the apparent in vitro chemosensitivity was prognostic for the relapse-free interval on treatment (Thomas et al. 1985). Previously, Kornblith et al. (1981) have found that grade 3 tumours are more sensitive than grade 4 tumours to BCNU while Rosenblum et al. (1982) found an inverse correlation between apparent in vitro sensitivity to BCNU and the patient's age. However, in the series of Thomas et al. (1985) the in vitro chemosensitivity was found to be significantly independent of both tumour grade and age.

Conclusions

The next stage in the use of such assays of chemosensitivity, based on surgical biopsy, should be to proceed to prospective trials in which an individual patient's adjuvant chemotherapy is determined by chemosensitivity results. An additional field of application may be in screening of new agents suitable for treating gliomas.

The preclinical screening and assessment of cytotoxic drugs for use in cancer chemotherapy depends at present mainly on determining their activity in animal tumour models. In the United States National Cancer Institute, for example, about 15 000 new substances are tested annually (de Vita et al. 1979). Phase 1 clinical trials on a few of the most effective drugs from this screen follow, to determine toxicity and possible activity against human tumours in vivo. In this scheme it is generally only in phase 2 studies that the specific question of a drug's use against glioma is addressed. The use of in vitro chemosensitivity tests offers the possibility of testing such agents against a panel of brain tumours, specifically malignant glioma, and may possibly increase the detection rate of agents useful for these specific tumours.

References

Barranco SC, Drewinko B, Humphrey RM (1973) Differential response by human melanoma cells to 1,3-bis(2-chloroethyl)-1-nitrosourea and bleomycin. Mutat Res 19: 277–280

Bigner SH, Bullard DE, Pegram CN, Wikstrand CW, Bigner DD (1981) Relationship of in vitro morphologic and growth characteristics of established human glioma-derived cell lines to their tumorigenicity in athymic nude mice. J Neurpathol Exp Neurol 40: 390–409

Bollag W (1963) The tumour-inhibitory effects of the methylhydrazine derivative Ro 4-6467/1 (NSC-77213). Cancer Chemother Rep 33: 1–4

Bradley NJ, Bloom HJG, Davies AJS, Swift SM (1978) Growth of human gliomas in immune deficient mice: A possible model for preclinical studies. Br J Cancer 38: 263–271

Bullard DE, Bigner SH, Bigner DD (1981a) The morphologic response of cell lines derived from human gliomas to dibutyryl adenosine 3':5'-cyclic monophospate. J Neuropathol Exp Neurol 40: 231–246

Bullard DE, Schold SC, Bigner SH, Bigner DD (1981b) Growth and chemotherapeutic response in athymic mice of tumours arising from human glioma-derived cell lines. J Neuropathol Exp Neurol 40: 410

Calabresi P, Parks RE Jr (1975) Alkylating agents, antimetabolites, hormones and other antiproliferative agents. In: Goodman LS, Gilman A (eds) The pharmacological basis of therapeutics, 5th edn. Macmillan, London, pp 1254–1307

Carter SK, Schabel FM Jr, Broder LE, Johnstone TP (1972) 1,3-bis(2-chloroethyl)-1-nitrosourea (BCNU) and other nitrosoureas in cancer treatment: A review. Adv Cancer Res 16: 273–332

Dandy WE (1928) Removal of right cerebral hemisphere for certain tumours with hemiplegia. J Am Med Assoc 90: 823–825

Dandy WE (1933) Physiological studies following extirpation of the right cerebral hemisphere in man. Bull Johns Hopkins Hosp 53: 31–51

Darling JL, Thomas DGT (1983) Results obtained using assays of intermediate duration and clinical correlations. In: Dendy PP, Hill BJ (eds) Human tumour drug sensitivity testing in vitro: Techniques and clinical applications. Academic Press, London, pp 269–280

de Vita VT, Schein PS (1973) The use of drugs in combination for the treatment of cancer. Rationale and results. N Engl J Med 288: 998–1006

de Vita VT, Denham C, Davidson JD, Oliverio VT (1967) The physiological disposition of the carcinostatic 1,3-bis(2-chloroethyl)-1-nitrosourea (BCNU) in man and animals. Clin Pharmacol Ther 8: 566–577

de Vita VT, Oliverio VT, Muggia F (1979) The drug development and clinical trials program in the Division of Cancer Treatment, National Cancer Institute. Cancer Clin Trials 2: 195–216

Earle KM, Rentschler EH, Snodgrass SR (1957) Primary intracranial neoplasms: Prognosis and classification in 513 verified cases. J Neuropathol 16: 321–331

Easty DM, Wylie JAH (1963) Screening of 12 gliomata against chemotherapeutic agents in vitro. Br Med J i: 1589–1592

Edwards MS, Levin VA, Wilson CB (1980) Brain tumour chemotherapy: An evaluation of agents in current use for phase I and II trials. Cancer Treat Rep 64: 1179–1205

Frankel SA, German WJ (1958) Glioblastoma multiforme. Review of 219 cases with regard to natural history, pathology, diagnostic methods and treatment. J Neurosurg 15: 489–503

Freshney RI (1980) Tissue culture of glioma of the brain. In: Brain tumours: Scientific basis, clinical investigation and current therapy. Butterworths, London, pp 21–50

Gazsim LR, Afra D (1969) Study on the effect of actinomycins in tissue cultures from human brain tumours. Acta Neurochir (Wien) 21: 139-152
German WJ (1961) The gliomas: A follow-up study. Clin Neurosurg 7: 1-20
Grant FC (1956) A study of the results of surgical treatment in 2,326 consecutive patients with brain tumour. J Neurosurg 13: 479-488
Green SB, Byar DP, Walker MD and fifteen others (1983) Comparisons of carmustine, procarbazine and high-dose methyl prednisolone as additions to surgery and radiotherapy for the treatment of malignant glioma. Cancer Treat Rep 67: 121-132
Guner M, Freshney RI, Morgan D, Freshney MG, Thomas DGT, Graham DI (1977) Effects of dexamethasone on in vitro cultures from human astrocytoma. Br J Cancer 35: 439-447
Gutin PH, Wilson CB, Kumar ARV, Boldrey EB, Levin V, Powell M, Enot KJ (1975) Phase II study of procarbazine, CCNU and vincristine combination chemotherapy in the treatment of malignant brain tumours. Cancer 35: 1398-1404
Hildebrand J, Brihaye J (1975) Malignant gliomas: Prognostic factors and criteria of response. In: Staquet MJ (ed) Cancer therapy: Prognostic factors and criteria of response. Raven Press, New York, pp 307-318
Kimball PM, Brattain MG (1980) Isolation of a cellular subpopulation from a human colonic carcinoma cell line. Cancer Res 40: 1574
Kornblith PL, Szypko PE (1978) Variations in response of human brain tumours to BCNU in vitro. J Neurosurg 48: 580-586
Kornblith PL, Smith BH, Leonard LA (1981) Response of cultured human brain tumours to nitrosoureas: Correlation with clinical data. Cancer 47: 255-265
Kumar ARV, Renaudin J, Wilson CB, Boldrey EB, Enot KJ, Levin VA (1974) Procarbazine hydrochloride in the treatment of brain tumours. Phase 2 study. J Neurosurg 40: 365-371
Levin VA, Crafts DC, Norman DM, Hoffer PB, Spire JP, Wilson CB (1977) Criteria for evaluating patients undergoing chemotherapy for brain tumours. J Neurosurg 47: 329-335
Levin VA, Edwards MS, Wright DC, Seager ML, Schimberg TP, Townsend JJ, Wilson CB (1980) Modified procarbazine, CCNU and vincristine (PCV 3) combination chemotherapy in the treatment of malignant brain tumours. Cancer Treat Rep 64: 237-241
Matsukado Y, McCarthy CS, Kernohan JW (1961) The growth of glioblastoma multiforme (Astrocytomas, grades III and IV) in neurosurgical practice. J Neurosurg 18: 636-644
Maxwell HP (1946) The incidence of interhemispheric extension of glioblastoma multiforme through the corpus callosum. J Neurosurg 3: 54-57
Mealey J Jr, Chen TT, Shupe R (1974) Response of cultured human glioblastomas to radiation and BCNU chemotherapy. J Neurosurg 41: 339-349
Morgan D, Freshney RI, Darling JL, Thomas DGT, Celik F (1983) Assay of anticancer drugs in tissue culture: Cell cultures of biopsies from human astrocytoma. Br J Cancer 47: 205-214
Oliverio VT, Denham C, de Vita VT, Kelly MG (1964) Some pharmacologic properties of a new antitumour agent, *N*-isopropyl-γ-(2-methylhydrazine)-*p*-toluamide hydrochloride (NSC-77213). Cancer Chemother Rep 42: 1-7
Ommaya AK, Rubin RC, Henderson ES, Rall DP, Gieseke FC, Bering EA, Bagan M (1965) A new approach to the treatment of inoperable brain tumours. Med Ann DC 34: 455-458
Rosenblum ML, Vasquez DA, Hoshino T, Wilson CB (1978) Development of a clonogenic cell assay for human brain tumours. Cancer 41: 2305-2314
Rosenblum ML, Gerosa M, Dougherty DV, Reese C, Barger GR, Davis RL, Levin VA, Wilson CB (1982) Age-related chemosensitivity of stem cells from human malignant brain tumours. Lancet I: 885-887
Rosenblum ML, Gerosa MA, Wilson CB, Barger GR, Pertuiset BF, de Tribolet N, Dougherty DV (1983) Stem cell studies of human malignant brain tumours. I. Development of the stem cell assay and its potential. J Neurosurg 58: 170-176
Rubin RC, Ommaya AK, Henderson ES, Beriny EA, Rall DP (1966) Cerebrospinal fluid perfusion for central nervous system neoplasms. Neurology 16: 680-692
Rupniak HT, Hill BT (1980) The poor cloning ability in agar of human tumour cells from biopsies of primary tumours. Cell Biol Int Rep 4: 479-486
Russell DS, Rubinstein LJ (1977) Pathology of tumours of the nervous system, 4th edn. Edward Arnold, London
Saez RJ, Campbell RJ, Laws ER (1977) Chemotherapeutic trials on human malignant astrocytomas in organ cultures. J Neurosurg 46: 320-327
Salcman M (1980) Survival in glioblastoma: Historical perspective. Neurosurg 7: 435-439
Schabel FM Jr, Johnston TP, McCaleb GS, Montgomery JA, Laster WR, Skipper HE (1963) Experimental evaluation of potential anticancer agents. VIII. Effects of certain nitrosoureas on intracere-

bral L1210 leukaemia. Cancer Res 23: 725–733
Shapiro WR, Ausman JI (1969) The chemotherapy of brain tumours: A clinical and experimental review. In: Plum F (ed) Recent advances in neurology. Blackwell Scientific Publications, Oxford, pp 149–235
Shapiro WR, Young DF (1976) Chemotherapy of malignant glioma with CCNU alone and CCNU combined with vincristine sulfate and procarbazine hydrochloride. Trans Am Neurol Assoc 101: 217–219
Shapiro WR, Basler GA, Chernik NT, Posner JB (1979) Human brain tumour transplantation into nude mice. J Natl Cancer Inst 62: 447
Shapiro JR, Yung WKA, Shapiro WR (1981) Isolation, karyotype and clonal growth of heterogeneous subpopulation of human malignant gliomas. Cancer Res 41: 2349–2359
Sheline GE (1977) Radiation therapy of brain tumours. Cancer 39: 873–881
Steel GG (1977) Growth kinetics of tumours: Cell population kinetics in relation to the growth and treatment of cancer. Clarendon Press, Oxford
Stewart DJ, Lu K, Benjamin RS, Leavens ME, Luna M, Yap HY, Loo TL (1983) Concentrations of vinblastine in human intracerebral tumour and other tissues. J Neuro-Oncol 1: 139–144
Thomas DGT (1982) Chemotherapy of cerebral glioma: Current research and its application to clinical practice. In: Rice Edwards JM (ed) Topical reviews in neurosurgery. J Wright, Bristol, pp 93–121
Thomas DGT, Darling JL, Freshney RI, Morgan D (1979) In vitro chemosensitivity assay of human glioma by scintillation autofluorography. In: Paoletti P, Walker MD, Butti G, Knerich R (eds) Multidisciplinary aspects of brain tumour therapy. Elsevier/North-Holland Biomedical Press, Amsterdam, pp 19–35
Thomas DGT, Darling JL, Paul EA, Mott TJ, Godlee JN, Tobias JS, Capra LG, Collins CD, Mooney C, Bozek T, Finn GP, Arigbabu SO, Bullard DE, Shannon N, Freshney RI (1985) Assay of anti-cancer drugs in tissue culture: Relationship of relapse free interval (RFI) and in vitro chemosensitivity in patients with malignant cerebral glioma. Br J Cancer 51: 525–532
Walker MD, Gehan EA (1976) Clinical studies in malignant gliomas and their treatment with the nitrosoureas. Cancer Treat Rep 60: 713–716
Walker MD, Alexander E, Hunt WE and nine others (1978) Evaluation of BCNU and/or radiotherapy in the treatment of anaplastic gliomas. J Neurosurg 49: 333–343
Wheeler TK, Dendy PP, Dawson A (1974) Assessment of an in vitro screening test of cytotoxic agents in the treatment of advanced malignant disease. Oncology 30: 362–376
Woodhall B, Hall K, Mahaley S Jr, Jackson J (1959) Chemotherapy of brain cancer: Experimental and clinical studies in localised hypothermic cerebral perfusion. Ann Surg 150: 640–652

13 Combined Modality Treatments in Malignant Supratentorial Gliomas

J. Hildebrand

Introduction

This review addresses the most common type of malignant brain tumour of the adult: the supratentorial malignant gliomas (SMG). These include a variety of tumours such as glioblastomas multiforme, astrocytomas grades 3 and 4 (or malignant astrocytomas), oligodendroglioblastomas and ependymoblastomas. Although these various tumours are mixed in therapeutic trials, retrospective analyses have shown that they have different biological behaviours. Thus the survival of patients with glioblastoma multiforme is significantly shorter than that of patients with malignant astrocytoma. There are other prognostic factors which have emerged from retrospective analyses of large studies, the most important of which are age and performance status (Karnofsky index). The distribution of at least these three factors should be given in future studies, and we have selected for the present review trials which provide, at least partially, such data.

Four treatment modalities have been applied to the treatment of patients with SMG: radiotherapy, immunotherapy, corticosteroids and chemotherapy. As in other neoplasms these agents have been tested as adjuvant treatments (i.e. given immediately after the neurosurgical removal of the tumour) or at the time of recurrence. Combined modality therapy was tested mainly as adjuvant treatment. Radiotherapy is the only modality which has been shown to be unequivocably active as adjuvant treatment, and is therefore part of all the tested combination treatments. It usually consists of 55-60 Gy given in 6 weeks and prolongs the survival time of patients with SMG by 30%-100% (Walker and Gehan 1972, Trouillas 1973, Walker et al. 1978, Kristiansen et al. 1981). We are now left with the question as to whether other treatment modalities improve the efficacy of radiotherapy.

Combination of Radiotherapy with Radiosensitisers of Anoxic Cells

The encouraging results of Urtasun et al. (1976), who combined high doses of metronidazole with relatively low doses of radiotherapy, have not been confirmed in larger and more recent trials using misonidazole associated with either a conventional radiotherapy schedule (Bleehen et al. 1981) or a modified regimen aiming to give misonidazole during irradiation at a higher daily dose (3.5 Gy) (EORTC Brain Tumour Group 1983).

Combination of Radiotherapy with Immunotherapy

Two trials reporting conflicting results concerning the efficacy of the immunotherapy were published in 1973. Important differences in methodology may account for the fact that, when compared with radiotherapy used alone, immunotherapy was found effective by Trouillas (1973) but ineffective by Bloom et al. (1973). Thus Trouillas used four to ten injections of saline tumour extract also containing Freund's adjuvant, and the administration of corticosteroids was avoided in his study. Bloom et al., on the other hand, injected irradiated autologous tumour cells and allowed steroid therapy. The lack of information concerning the distribution of the main prognostic factors and the small number of patients included in each of the four arms of the Trouillas study makes comparison between the two trials even more difficult.

Combination of Radiotherapy with the Administration of Corticosteroids

Corticosteroids are probably the most effective treatment for symptomatic relief of signs due to brain tumours. This effect, which is rapid and unrelated to the pathological nature of the tumour, is attributed primarily to the reduction of the peritumoral oedema. However, the possibility that corticosteroids, especially in high doses, may act as cytotoxic agents is suggested by data from animal tumours and experiments using cultures of human glioma cells (Chen and Meakey 1973).

The effect of high intermittent monthly doses of methylprednisolone (400 mg/m^2 5 times a day) on the survival of patients with SMG was recently tested by the National Cancer Institute brain tumour group and shown to be ineffective. Thus the percentage of 24-month survivors among patients treated with prednisolone was lower than that in patients who received BCNU; and in the group of patients treated with BCNU the addition of prednisolone made no difference (Green et al. 1983).

Combination of Radiotherapy with Chemotherapy

Chemotherapy has been investigated more extensively than the three other treatment modalities. There is no doubt that single-agent chemotherapy using nitrosourea derivatives (BCNU, CCNU or MeCCNU) or procarbazine (Wilson et al. 1976, EORTC Brain Tumour Group 1976, 1981, Levin et al. 1984) is able to produce objective remissions in patients with recurring symptoms and signs caused by SMG. The percentage of such remissions varies considerably, from 15% to 60%, between studies. It is our feeling that the discrepancies are mainly due to differences in defining objective remission and the criteria used to distinguish the activity of chemotherapy from the effects of corticosteroids. On the other hand, there is no firm evidence that any combination of drugs is superior to single-agent chemotherapy in the treatment of SMG.

There is more debate concerning the effectiveness of chemotherapy when used as an adjuvant treatment. In studies aiming to answer this question, three parameters have been evaluated: (a) the length of the free interval (time to clinical recurrence), (b) the length of survival time from the operation, and (c) the percentage of long-term survivors. The first two parameters are fairly well correlated, whereas the third appears to be independent of the other two.

Two agents, bleomycin and 5-hydroxyurea, were tested as "radiosensitisers" and given during irradiation therapy. Bleomycin was ineffective (Kristiansen 1981) whereas 5-hydroxyurea was marginally active in the glioblastoma multiforme group but not in malignant astrocytomas (Levin et al. 1979).

BCNU was found able to prolong the median survival time in a study containing a relatively small number of patients (Armentrout et al. 1974). The National Cancer Institute brain tumour study group has tested BCNU in two much larger studies (Walker et al. 1978, 1980), where various prognostic factors were reported and were equally distributed between the trial arms. The total survival time measured in the two trials was 37.5 and 51 weeks respectively in patients treated with 55–60 Gy, and 40.5 and 41 weeks in those who received BCNU in addition to irradiation. The difference between these survival times was not statistically significant. However, the number of survivors at 18 months was statistically increased in the first study from 4% to 19% by the addition of BCNU, and the same trend was also observed in the second trial (15% to 27%).

In another large study, by Chang et al. (1983), the total survival time for all the age groups was similar in patients treated with radiotherapy alone (9.9 months) and in those who in addition received BCNU (10.0 months). But in the subgroup of those aged 40–60 years the addition of BCNU was beneficial. The trend towards an increase in the number of survivors at 18 months (19% to 29%) in the arm treated with radiotherapy plus BCNU was also seen in this study.

CCNU has also been shown to be active as an adjuvant chemotherapeutic agent, at least in terms of its effect on time to recurrence, in a trial with a relatively small number of patients (Band et al. 1974). But these favourable results could not be confirmed by the EORTC Brain Tumour Group, who failed to show any effect of CCNU on length of the tumour-free interval or survival time when used alone (EORTC Brain Tumour Group 1976) or in combination with VM 26 (EORTC Brain Tumour Group 1981).

The activity of the third currently used nitrosourea derivative, MeCCNU, appeared comparable or slightly inferior to that of BCNU (Walker et al. 1980).

Finally, dibromodulcitol has been reported to increase median survival time (Afra et al. 1983), but this single study awaits further confirmation.

Summary

1. Radiotherapy is the only unequivocably active adjuvant treatment in SMG of the adult.
2. Radiosensitisers such as misonidazole are not effective in SMG.
3. The administration of high intermittent doses of corticosteroids is not effective as an adjuvant treatment.
4. Immunotherapy has been tested in only a few trials using different methodologies, and results have been conflicting.
5. Various chemotherapeutic agents are able to produce objective remissions in patients with recurring symptoms and signs due to SMG. However, they do not prolong the mean (or median) survival time nor the time to recurrence. BCNU has been shown, in some studies, to increase the number of long-term survivors.

References

Afra D, Kocsis B, Dobay J, Eckhardt S (1983) Combined radiotherapy and chemotherapy with dibromodulcitol and CCNU in postoperative treatment of malignant gliomas. J Neurosurg 59: 106–110

Armentrout SA, Foltz E, Vermund H, Otis PT (1974) Comparison of postoperative irradiation alone and combination with BCNU (NSC-409962) in the management of malignant gliomas. Cancer Chemother Rep 58: 841–844

Band PR, Weir BKA, Urtasun RC, Blain G, McLean D, Wilson F, Mielke B, Grace M (1974) Radiotherapy and CCNU in grade III and IV astrocytoma. ASCO Abstr 15: 161

Bleehen NM, Wiltshire CR, Plowman PN et al. (1981) Randomised study of misonidazole and radiotherapy for grade III and IV cerebral astrocytoma. Br J Cancer 43: 436–442

Bloom HJG, Peckham MJ, Richardson AE, Alexander PA, Payne PH (1973) Glioblastoma multiforme: A controlled trial to assess the value of specific active immunotherapy in patients treated by radical surgery and radiotherapy. Br J Cancer 27: 253–267

Chang CH, Horton J, Schoenfeld D et al. (1983) Comparison of postoperative radiotherapy and combined postoperative radiotherapy and chemotherapy in the multidisciplinary management of malignant gliomas. Cancer 52: 997–1007

Chen TT, Meakey J Jr (1973) Effects of corticosteroids on protein and nucleic acid synthesis in human glial tumour cells. Cancer Res 33: 1721–1723

EORTC Brain Tumour Group (1976) Effect of CCNU on survival rate, objective remission and duration of free interval in patients with malignant brain glioma. First evaluation. Eur J Cancer 12: 41–45

EORTC Brain Tumour Group (1981) Evaluation of CCNU, VM-26 plus CCNU and procarbazine in supratentorial brain gliomas. J Neurosurg 55: 27–31

EORTC Brain Tumour Group (1983) Misonidazole in radiotherapy of supratentorial malignant gliomas in adult patients: A randomised double-blind study. Eur J Cancer Clin Oncol 19: 39–42

Green SB, Byar DP, Walker MD et al. (1983) Comparisons of Carmustine, procarbazine and high dose methylprednisolone as additions to surgery and radiotherapy for the treatment of malignant glioma. Cancer Treat Rep 67: 121–132

Kristiansen K, Hagen S, Kollevold T et al. (1981) Combined modality therapy of operated astrocytomas grade III and IV: Confirmation of the value of postoperative irradiation and lack of potentiation of bleomycin on survival time: a prospective multicenter trial of the Scandinavian Glioblastoma Study Group. Cancer 47: 649–652

Levin VA, Wilson CB, Davis R et al. (1979) A phase III comparison of BCNU, hydroxyurea and radiation therapy to BCNU and radiation therapy for treatment of primary malignant gliomas. J Neurosurg 51: 526–532

Levin VA, Resser KJ, McGrath L, Vestnys P, Nutik S, Wilson CB (1984) PCNU treatment for recurrent malignant gliomas. Cancer Treat Rep 68: 969–973

Trouillas P (1973) Immunologie et immunothérapie des tumeurs cérébrales. Etat actuel. Rev Neurol 128: 23–38

Urtasun R, Band P, Chapman JD, Feldstein ML, Mielke B, Fryer C (1976) Radiation and high-dose metronidazole in supratentorial glioblastomas. N Engl J Med 294: 1364–1367

Walker MD, Gehan EA (1972) An evaluation of 1-3-*bis*(2-chloroethyl)-1-nitrosourea (BCNU) and irradiation alone and in combination for the treatment of malignant glioma. In: Proceedings of the 63rd Meeting of the AACR. Proc Am Assoc Cancer Res 13: 67

Walker MD, Alexander E Jr, Hunt WE et al. (1978) Evaluation of BCNU and/or radiotherapy in the treatment of anaplastic gliomas. A cooperative clinical trial. J Neurosurg 49: 333–343

Walker MD, Green SB, Byar DP et al. (1980) Randomised comparisons of radiotherapy and nitrosoureas for the treatment of malignant glioma after surgery. N Engl J Med 303: 1323–1329

Wilson CB, Gutin P, Bolderey E, Crafts D, Levin V (1976) Single agent chemotherapy of brain tumors. Arch Neurol 33: 739–744

Subject Index

MIX
Papier aus verantwortungsvollen Quellen
Paper from responsible sources
FSC® C105338

If you have any concerns about our products,
you can contact us on
ProductSafety@springernature.com

In case Publisher is established outside the EU,
the EU authorized representative is:
Springer Nature Customer Service Center GmbH
Europaplatz 3, 69115 Heidelberg, Germany

Printed by Libri Plureos GmbH
in Hamburg, Germany